Revolutionary
Medicine

Revolutionary Medicine

The Founding Fathers and Mothers
in Sickness and in Health

JEANNE E. ABRAMS

NEW YORK UNIVERSITY PRESS

New York and London

NEW YORK UNIVERSITY PRESS
New York and London
www.nyupress.org

References to Internet websites (URLs) were accurate at the time of writing.
Neither the author nor New York University Press is responsible for URLs that
may have expired or changed since the manuscript was prepared.

LIBRARY OF CONGRESS CATALOGING-IN-PUBLICATION DATA
Abrams, Jeanne E., 1951-
Revolutionary medicine : the Founding Fathers and mothers in sickness and in health /
Jeanne E. Abrams.
p. cm.
Includes bibliographical references and index.
ISBN 978-0-8147-8919-3 (cl : alk. paper)
1. Founding Fathers of the United States. 2. Public health—Philosophy. 3. Public health—
United States—History—18th century. 4. Public health—United States—History—19th
century. 5. Medical care—United States—History—18th century. 6. Medical care—United
States—History—19th century. I. Title.
E302.5.A37 2013
973.2--dc23
2013010673

New York University Press books are printed on acid-free paper, and their binding materials
are chosen for strength and durability. We strive to use environmentally responsible
suppliers and materials to the greatest extent possible in publishing our books.

Book design by Marcelo Agudo

Manufactured in the United States of America
10 9 8 7 6 5 4 3 2 1

CONTENTS

ACKNOWLEDGMENTS

Many years ago, as an undergraduate freshman in an American history class, I was assigned a term paper on a topic relating to the colonial era. The project necessitated a visit to the New York Historical Society, which led to a lifetime love affair with primary source documents and a deep and abiding interest in the lives and writings of America's founders. The founders highlighted in this study, including George and Martha Washington, John and Abigail Adams, Thomas Jefferson, Benjamin Franklin, and James and Dolley Madison, were unusually prolific writers; Thomas Jefferson alone wrote nearly eighteen thousand letters and numerous essays and documents. I have attempted to be judicious in choosing to use excerpts from only those letters that illustrate the themes of this book, but some readers might want to look at an even larger sampling of their work. We are very fortunate that over the last few years, in addition to robust print volumes, much of the founders' correspondence and many of their papers are now available in wonderfully convenient, accessible, on-line editions. Especially noteworthy are the Rotunda electronic imprint of the University of Virginia Press; the Library of Congress American Memory Project; the Adams Family Papers and the Thomas Jefferson Papers at the Massachusetts Historical Society; and the Papers of Benjamin Franklin made available through the auspices of the American Philosophical Society and Yale University.

* * *

As always, I am indebted to numerous friends, colleagues, and "boosters" along the way. First, I'd like to express my sincere appreciation to my distinguished colleague Dr. Alan Kraut of American University. He graciously read early drafts of many chapters in this book and astutely offered valuable suggestions for how to make my arguments more effective. As author E. B. White once observed, "It is not often that someone comes along who is a true friend and good writer," and Alan has filled both those roles admirably! I'd also like to thank Dr. Rebecca Tannenbaum of Yale University, Dr. Elaine Breslaw at the University of

Tennessee, and Dr. Joyce Goodfriend of the University of Denver for their excellent critiques and valuable feedback, as well as for their sharing of helpful resources at various stages in my writing and research. Dr. John Stagg, editor-in-chief of the *Papers of James Madison*, also generously shared his expertise with me.

At the University of Denver, Provost Gregg Kvistad and Dean Nancy Allen of Penrose Library offered encouragement from the beginning of this project, and I am especially grateful for having been awarded a Fall 2012 sabbatical leave with an enhancement as well as a Faculty Research Fund grant, both of which assisted in the completion of this book. Thank you to my colleague Thyria Wilson for her assistance with preparing for publication many of the photographs that appear in this book and to the staff at the U.S. National Library of Medicine and the Library of Congress for their helpful advice in accessing their marvelous historical photograph collection. At New York University Press, I am grateful to Deborah Gershenowitz for her enthusiastic support of this project from the beginning and her skillful editing and to Emily Wright, copyeditor par excellence. When Deborah moved to another press near the end of my writing phase, editorial assistant Constance Grady provided outstanding and highly efficient service and served as my lifeline to the press. Clara Platter, the new American history and law editor at NYU Press, stepped in with admirable energy and expertise and has been a wonderful source of support as I entered the final stages of revising and editing. This book is dedicated to my loving family for as always, my husband Lewis and our children and grandchildren, as well as dear friends too numerous to mention, have been a constant encouragement.

Introduction

Health and Medicine in the Era of America's Founders

> Experience learns us to be always anxious about
> the health of those whom we love.
> —*Thomas Jefferson to Martha Jefferson, April 7, 1787*

> Above all worldly goods, I wish you health, for
> destitute of that great Blessing, few others can
> be enjoyed.
> —*Abigail Adams to Thomas Boylston Adams, June 2, 1799*

Introducing the Founders

The literature about America's early leaders continues to proliferate, but instead of placing the usual emphasis on the political roles of the nation's founders or their personal relationships, this book will focus a lens on their experiences with health, illness, and medical treatment. The lives of America's founding mothers and fathers demonstrate that today's preoccupation with good health and illness is not a new one. Abigail Adams fretted over her family's health and particularly that of her husband throughout the American Revolution as well as John's days as president, although ironically Abigail was by far the more fragile of the two. Thomas Jefferson often involved himself in the treatment of ailments that affected his family and slaves. He professed and practiced a surprisingly modern outlook and regimen for fostering good health, and he and his contemporaries Abigail and John Adams took the controversial step at the time of making sure that they and their family members were immunized against smallpox. After the Continental Army was devastated by smallpox in 1776, George Washington insisted that all his soldiers be inoculated. Benjamin Franklin was an early and staunch advocate of smallpox inoculation and a primary initiator of the first voluntary public hospital and medical school in America. His inventions included bifocal glasses and a flexible urinary catheter, and his keen interest in what today would be termed preventative medicine led to numerous medical experiments as well as often sound advice on healthful living.[1]

Despite differences in personality and political outlook, George Washington, Benjamin Franklin, John Adams, Thomas Jefferson, and James Madison shared the revolutionary desire to make fundamental changes in American social and political relationships, including the role of government in the lives of individuals and government's ability to promote general welfare. As historian Peter Gay has observed of the Enlightenment era, "The most tangible cause for confidence lay in medicine. . . . Medicine was the most highly visible and the most heartening index of general improvement."[2] The founders recognized early on that government had compelling reasons to shoulder some new responsibilities with respect to ensuring the health and well-being of its citizenry. For example, on July 16, 1798, Adams signed a bill "to provide for the relief and maintenance of disabled seamen," creating the United States Marine Hospital Service. It gave rise to a network of hospitals located at sea and river ports across the United States, and slowly over the next century it ultimately evolved into the national American Public Health Service. In the beginning, in a process administered by their employers, sailors paid a twenty-cent tax every month out of their wages as their share toward a form of insurance for hospital care, which provided for doctors, room and board, and medicine, and the government directed the use of those funds and underwrote most of the real remaining costs. The tax was turned over quarterly to the United States Treasury, and it was used in the district where it was collected.[3]

With the Seaman's Act, for the first time in American history, the federal government mandated and paid for the temporary medical treatment of individuals who could not afford their own private care, creating a safety net for thousands of mariners. The seaman's bill was signed into law following a severe outbreak of yellow fever as sailors often brought a variety of serious diseases with them to ports, including smallpox, cholera, and malaria, and quarantine was sometimes necessary. Although it took almost a century to take hold, in essence the legislation established a precedent for federal intervention in the health care arena.

Forward-thinking political men such as Adams understood that the failure to address the illnesses of sailors endangered the well-being of all citizens in American port cities. Adams as well as Washington, Jefferson, Franklin, and Madison clearly recognized that the health of the nation was inextricably tied up with the health of individuals; improving general health care and the state of medicine could have far-reaching positive economic and social consequences and was therefore beneficial for all Americans. The founders were witnesses to the fact that epidemics not only brought personal devastation to individuals, families, and communities; they also played havoc with commerce.[4] It is telling that in his State of the Union Address on November 4, 1812, when the United States was embroiled in the War of 1812, Madison opened his remarks with a reference to the health of the nation, observing, "On our present meeting it is my first duty to invite your attention to the providential favors which our country has experienced in the unusual degree of health dispensed to its inhabitants" and tying the nation's good health to its prosperity and implicitly to its democratic republican form of government.[5] Although during that era public health still remained primarily a local responsibility, the contemporary debate over the federal role in health care had its roots with America's founders, who modeled a foundation for its development.

As historian Joseph J. Ellis has observed, Abigail and John Adams and, by extension, the other founding mothers and fathers lived "through the most tumultuous and consequential chapter in America's birth as a nation," a period in which they all played highly active and pivotal political roles during both revolution and independence.[6] However, in addition to their complex and visible public work, their private lives involved numerous personal relationships with family and friends. Even though they were part of the colonial elite, none of the members of the founding generation was immune to sickness and disease, and concerns over health frequently shaped the trajectory of their daily lives. Indeed, before the advent of modern antibiotics, one's life could be abruptly shattered by contagion and death, and debility from infectious diseases was commonplace in every ethnic group and class. Surgery was especially risky in an era when there were essentially no reliable anesthetics or antiseptics.

Abigail and John Adams were predeceased by four of their six children, and Franklin lost a much-beloved four-year-old son to smallpox, one of the greatest scourges of the age. Even given the grim mortality statistics of the day, Jefferson suffered what seems to have been a disproportionate number of family tragedies. He grieved deeply over the loss of his young wife, Martha, and the death in infancy and early childhood of four of their six children, as well as the later loss of an adult daughter only in her midtwenties. Washington battled a number of serious life-threatening illnesses and was predeceased by his two stepchildren, a favored nephew, and all his brothers, most of whom died of tuberculosis. His wife, Martha Custis Washington, sadly rivaled Jefferson in regard to family loss. By the time Martha was in her midtwenties, her young husband and two of her small children had succumbed to fatal illness, her remaining daughter died as a teenager as a result of an epileptic seizure, and her last surviving child, a son, died in his late twenties, probably from "camp fever" (typhus) contracted in a Revolutionary War army camp. Martha Washington's and Jefferson's experiences serve as extreme but far from unique reflections of the high rate of mortality among children and young adults at the time and demonstrate how easily illness could devastate a family.

Although it has been suggested that colonial- and revolutionary-era parents were inured to the death of children as a protective reaction to the high infant mortality of the era—as many as a quarter of infants died during their first year—the pain and grief the founding mothers and fathers exhibited at the loss of their children graphically demonstrates that this was not the case.[7] They were, however, all acutely aware of how often during their era life ended tragically early. In 1785, Abigail Adams penned a letter to her sister about the impending demise of a favorite aunt at a relatively young age. "It will be another memento to us of the fragility of the whole, and that duration depends not upon age," Abigail observed sadly.[8] Nearly a decade later Martha Washington lamented, "It is the case with all parents that have many children—they lose them as soon as they raise them generally."[9] The words of John C. Jackson to his sister-in-law Dolley Madison serve as a poignant reminder that death and illness were an almost daily occurrence at the time. Arriving home in the fall of 1808 shortly after he had lost his wife to disease, he found his children "very ill with a billious fever. . . . When shall sickness & death cease to terrify & distract me?" Jackson wrote in despair.[10] How this group of American founders coped with illness and tragedy and mustered the fortitude to go on with their lives reveals much about their characters as well as early American medical history.

Revolutionary Medicine provides an in-depth look at the health, illnesses, and medical endeavors of the collective group of America's founders highlighted above. It is based on close readings of literally thousands of their letters, their prolific writings, and hundreds of secondary sources. Over the last decades, serious scholarly examination of the subject has been limited. A few publications have studied the involvement of several founding fathers, most notably Jefferson and Franklin, in the growth of science in the Age of Reason, a handful have addressed, but only briefly or tangentially, their health experiences, and one recent monograph has even provided an admirable book-length examination of Franklin's "medical career."[11] However, these works have been limited in scope and have focused primarily on only one individual.

In contrast, this book has three main goals. The first is to demonstrate the critical but mostly overlooked roles these founders played in the development of a foundation for the country's later public health care system as they strove to effect "general" improvement of American society. Secondly, it reveals the dramatic, compelling stories of the founders' own personal encounters with illness and wellness issues, which encouraged them to support many surprisingly modern notions about health regimens and treatment. Finally, *Revolutionary Medicine* illuminates colonial and early-republic medical treatment and practice and provides salutary lessons for our time.

Public health in America was in its infancy under British rule. It was generally reactionary—prompted by epidemics and limited to often ineffective quarantines aimed primarily at avoiding contagion from diseases such as smallpox and yellow fever brought to America through passengers on incoming ships from foreign ports and at establishing rudimentary sanitary measures to control open sewers, protect water, and promote cleanliness in public streets in growing towns.[12] However, several American founders, particularly Jefferson, Franklin, and Washington, anticipated modern medicine and were on the cutting edge of public health advancement, beginning with small steps to promote community action in regard to disease, prompted by a strong sense of social responsibility. They personally advocated contemporary sanitary measures that led to cleaner thoroughfares and water, but at the same time they realized that municipal government could play a key role in their successful adoption.

All the founders were profoundly influenced by Enlightenment thought, which venerated scientific progress and empirical knowledge. Franklin and Jefferson were both elected as early presidents of the American Philosophical Society. Despite the somewhat misleading name, the organization's focus was the study of "useful" knowledge, to be utilized primarily as a stepping stone to increased liberty, prosperity, and even happiness. The concept of personal happiness was a fundamental theme in Enlightenment philosophy. In the new American nation that ideal was famously voiced in the Declaration of Independence, authored by Jefferson with the input of Franklin and Adams, in the phrase that all men were entitled to "life, liberty, and the pursuit of happiness." The European *philosophes* repeatedly connected contentment with good health, so medicine became a central focus; Voltaire famously declared that "there is no true happiness for the man who is not well." John Locke, the philosopher who most influenced America's founders, began his career as a physician, and he, too, emphasized the connection among health, happiness, and progress toward a better world.

Since the practice of medicine in the eighteenth century was largely theoretical and most medical knowledge and even a medical degree could be acquired by apprenticeship or study that emphasized "reading,"[13] educated and highly literate laypersons like Adams, Franklin, Washington, Jefferson, and Madison were well acquainted with what they considered simply another branch of science, albeit a highly practical one. Influenced by Enlightenment aspirations for general progress, they anticipated that medical treatments would develop rapidly, although they would undoubtedly have been disappointed to find that it would take decades for nineteenth-century American medicine to advance in any measurable degree.

Due to their privileged status, this circle of founders was assured of access to contemporary medical knowledge, trained physicians, and the best medications available, although until the Civil War, most health care took place in the home. Popular health guides of the era offered practical advice and even encouraged self-dosing. As one early historian noted, "Men of education and genius in varying paths of life did not consider it strange or peculiar to think, discuss, or write about medical matters."[14] Franklin and Jefferson, in particular, were perhaps as well versed in medicine as any contemporary learned medical practitioner, and women such as Abigail Adams, Martha Washington, and Dolley Madison were expected to treat family illness at home with their store of medicinal herbs and traditional remedies.

These particular founders were chosen deliberately for a variety of compelling reasons. All of them experienced dramatic and often tragic personal encounters with disease and epidemics. Not only does the prolific correspondence they left for posterity vividly and articulately describe these health "events," but their experiences are illustrative of the host of health challenges almost all early Americans faced. Moreover, this group of founders displayed a remarkably impressive grasp of medicine for the time, but viewed the subject from somewhat different perspectives. For example, Franklin and Jefferson were leaders in promoting scientific medicine based on empirical evidence, while Washington represents the outlook of what might be dubbed a "warrior healer," and Abigail and John Adams reflect a pragmatic approach to medical treatment. These founders' often progressive outlooks about medicine influenced their efforts to improve American medical practice and disease control. The high level of political power that Washington, Franklin, Adams, Jefferson, and Madison possessed enabled them at times to translate their concerns about public health into practical action.

This introduction will set the stage for an examination of the founders highlighted in this book against the backdrop of eighteenth-century medicine, including descriptions of the many illnesses and diseases they confronted and the remedies available at the time. The next chapters will focus on their individual medical/health stories, beginning with the Washingtons, moving on to Franklin and John and Abigail Adams, and ending with Jefferson. Space constraints did not allow for a full chapter devoted exclusively to Dolley and James Madison. However, the highlights of their often-harrowing encounters with disease and Madison's involvement with health care have been interwoven into several chapters in the book, most prominently in this introduction, the two chapters focusing on Thomas Jefferson, and the epilogue. Conversely, Jefferson's exceptional personal experiences with sickness and early death, his scientifically based, sophisticated understanding of medicine, and his prominent work in the battle to reduce smallpox in America during the early republic through the introduction of widespread vaccination resulted in two chapters focusing on his role.

Each chapter is biographical in nature but focuses on the book's three central themes: each founder's personal health, his or her individual experiences with illness and disease in terms of family and friends, and, for those who held political positions, his or her pursuit of public health policies. Not only did this elite cadre share a commitment to liberty and republicanism, but their lives frequently intersected in discussions about improving community health and concerns about sickness. Indeed, they all believed that a democratic republic was the most conducive environment for good health. They often shared their medical knowledge with their family members, neighbors, and the larger community and comforted one another in times of physical crisis and grief. In a variety of ways, each of them demonstrated early and active involvement in public health issues.

Illness and Disease in Early America

Because illness was so prevalent and often catastrophic in the colonial and revolutionary eras, disease was a constant fear embedded in the early American psyche—and with good reason, as such afflictions as tuberculosis, smallpox, malaria (intermittent fever or ague), yellow fever, typhoid, whooping cough, diphtheria (quinsy), cholera, measles, and dysentery (bloody flux) often reached epidemic and deadly proportions, and a "minor" infection such as bronchitis or strep throat, relatively simple to treat today with antibiotics, was serious enough to cause death. For example, complications from streptococcal or some form of throat infection (compounded by excessive bloodletting, which resulted in shock) is thought to have been the cause of the demise of George Washington.[15]

Before 1800, life expectancy at birth was startlingly low by modern standards, and there is evidence to suggest that the overall mortality rate in America actually increased in the nineteenth century before the Civil

War. Men in the eighteenth century on average lived into their late forties or early to middle fifties; women, who were at heightened risk due
to frequent pregnancies (fertile women could expect to give birth on an
average of every eighteen months to two years) and complications of
childbirth, could often expect to live only into their forties.[16] It is noteworthy that by contemporary standards all the American founders in
this study exceeded those expectations remarkably, perhaps aided, in
part, by their elite status, which gave them access to the best medical
care available at the time, good nutrition, and a high standard of living.[17]

As pioneer medical historian Richard Shryock put it over half a century ago, "In reviewing the circumstances of health in early America
one almost wonders that so many people survived and that the country
grew and prospered."[18] Historically, smallpox killed over 25 percent of
those infected with the disease and scarred for life most of those who
survived. In one New Hampshire town in 1735 nearly 20 percent of
the population succumbed to diphtheria, and the victims were almost
exclusively children. Due to the especially virulent disease environment, in southern colonies the child mortality rate was, tragically,
even higher. Over 85 percent of the babies in early South Carolina died
before they reached the age of two; more than a third of the babies in
one of the colony's parishes died before the age of five, many during the
peak malarial season through the summer and early fall.[19]

Cholera was another common and frightful disease, caused by a
micro-organism arising from contaminated water. Doctors and family members could do little but stand by as victims were wracked by
such severe diarrhea, stomach cramps, and vomiting that they became
so dehydrated that their lips turned blue and their faces often turned
purple. Most patients died within days. In 1793, by the time the yellow
fever epidemic in Philadelphia ended with the advent of cooler weather,
well over four thousand people, nearly 10 percent of the population,
died, and another nearly twenty thousand people fled, including many
government officials.[20] While many realized that a number of diseases
were contagious, the origins of the maladies and nature of the mecha-
nisms of transmission were not understood, and leading physicians and
sanitarians disagreed over both the cause and cure of most illnesses.

It is interesting to note that the lives of several of America's founders,
including Adams, Washington, Jefferson, and Dolley Todd Madison,

intersected during the epidemic, and the story of that infamous event is particularly instructive. Their experience of living in Philadelphia, at that time the nation's capital and largest city, during arguably the greatest single public health crisis of the century undoubtedly helped shape their thinking about community health issues and what level of responsibility government should have in what had normally been regarded as a private issue. Social, economic, and political life was disrupted over the summer and fall of 1793 as those who had the means to escape did so, leaving many who were poor or infirm behind to cope with the limited assistance of a core group of selfless city officials, physicians, and volunteer private citizens.[21] President Washington fled to Mount Vernon and Vice President Adams traveled to Massachusetts to avoid the terrifying path of illness and death, which sometimes killed as many as half of those who had contracted the disease. Jefferson, then the workaholic secretary of state, decried the panic and observed the epidemic from his airy rented country home on Philadelphia's outskirts with a scientific eye, noting its symptoms and duration. But as danger mounted he, too, made plans to leave for Monticello.

Jefferson remained in the area longer than most government officials and escaped illness, but Dolley Todd, at that time the wife of rising young lawyer John Todd Jr., was not so lucky. Tragically, the terrible epidemic claimed the lives of her beloved husband, her sickly six-week-old son William Temple, and her in-laws in one fell swoop, leaving her ill and weak from complications following childbirth and with her sick two-year-old remaining son John Payne to care for.[22] Dolley's correspondence and the details of her harrowing days in the midst of the epidemic provide graphic insight into the anguish experienced by the victims and family members affected by the yellow fever.

When the epidemic spread, Dolley's husband sent her and the children away to what was considered a safer area in the countryside at a farm near Gray's Ferry. However, John Todd remained in Philadelphia to care for his parents and conduct his law practice, and he visited his wife and children when he could. As the sad events unfolded, Dolley poured out her heart to her brother-in-law: "A revered Father in the Jaws of Death, & a Love'd Husband in perpetual danger. . . . I am almost destracted with distress & apprehension—it is too late for their removal . . . I wish much to see you, but my Child is sick & I have no way of getting to you."[23]

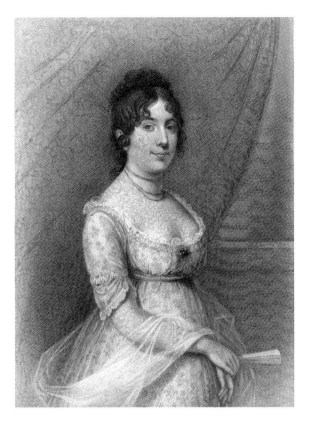

Engraving of Dolley Payne (Todd) Madison from a painting by Gilbert Stuart. (Courtesy Library of Congress)

Fortunately, the 26-year-old Dolley, as well as her mother, three brothers, and three sisters, survived the yellow fever epidemic, and Dolley remained especially close to them for the rest of their lives. An attractive widow, Dolley would marry future president James Madison in less than a year after Todd's death, but her tragic experience left her always especially anxious about the health of family members, particularly Madison and her remaining child. As she wrote to a friend in 1808 after the death of her youngest sister,

Oh God! We must bow our heads to thy decrees however awful—we cannot change or avert them . . . when I trace the sad events that have occurred to me, I feel as if I should die two [sic]. . . . My Husband is nearly well & I have exerted all my fortitude, all my religion, in order to live for him & my son. . . . I used to think I could not survive the loss of my Mother & my sisters yet am I still here & in all the bitterness of mourning striving to reconcile my heart to the great misfortune![24]

Those like Dolley who survived yellow fever acquired lifelong immunity, and pregnant women who encountered the illness could even pass on some level of protection to their newborn children for at least the first months of life. Over the next decade, yellow fever affected people in varying but serious degrees in most bustling port cities up and down the coast, most notably in Philadelphia, New York City, and Boston, and served as an impetus for heightened government involvement in public health and sanitation and the stricter inspection of incoming ships. The virus required an initial pool of infected humans, most often travelers on incoming ships from tropical ports, but was carried and spread through the sting of infected *Aedes aegypti* mosquitoes. The insects bred in stagnant fresh water containers, including holes dug for runoff from gutters and cisterns and puddles that collected rain water in crowded urban centers, particularly in warm regions. Jefferson appears to have had a better understanding of the disease's origins than most physicians of the time. In 1804 he wrote a friend that "on the question whether the yellow fever is infectious, or endemic, the medical faculty is divided into parties." By the next year, on the basis of his own studies Jefferson concluded that it was indeed "an endemic, and not a contagious disease" that could be communicated from one person to another by contact, and he would emphasize the importance of sanitation and the efficacy of fresh water and air, particularly in urban centers.[25]

Although yellow fever epidemics were deadly and frightening, the incidence of the disease in America, with its characteristic jaundice, high temperature, chills, purple bruises on the skin, and internal hemorrhaging that produced black vomit, was relatively infrequent. Infectious diseases generally rose and fell with the seasons; yellow fever and malaria thrived in the heat and humidity of hot summers, which encouraged the proliferation of breeding mosquitoes, while other diseases, like smallpox, tended to peak in winter, particularly in urban centers where it spread more easily as people congregated indoors. In reality, on a regular basis, respiratory infections and consumption (tuberculosis), enteric intestinal illnesses such as dysentery, and malaria caused more sickness and took more lives than outbreaks of the infamous smallpox, cholera, and yellow fever, but the latter illnesses appeared more dramatic and hence aroused more apprehension and spurred more robust community action.[26]

Infant mortality at the time was very common, with a grim rate estimated to have been as high as 40 percent during the revolutionary age, and if one survived childhood, young adulthood posed another host of health challenges, especially tuberculosis and other respiratory illnesses.[27] In Philadelphia, it is estimated that in the 1780s, half of all deaths occurred in those under the age of ten.[28] Illness and disease were a given in the lives of most people of the era, an unavoidable fact reflecting the fragility of life, and as Martha Washington stated so succinctly from personal experience, "sickness is to be expected."[29] But what was the state of American medicine during the colonial, revolutionary, and early national eras, when doctors had little understanding of the causes of illness or specifically how one differed from another? How did the country's early founders cope with a host of illnesses in the light of limited medical knowledge and practice and lack of effective medications?

Early Medical Theory and Treatment

As we will see, many of the founders not only educated themselves about health and new as well as traditional treatments but also advocated government-sponsored public health measures and sometimes became informal medical practitioners themselves. During the era, sickness and health were part of a communal agenda, and particularly during times of crises, families and communities often combined their medical knowledge and resources to aid one another.[30] Early Americans often resorted to a wide range of proposed cures. While some of those medical treatments, such as bleeding for virtually every ill, appear ludicrous to us today, we should be mindful that medical science has always been a moving target, characterized by trial and much error. Medical progress has never been uniform, but fragmented and sometimes contradictory. Even today there are frequent news stories concerning medications or treatments that were considered safe and effective, only to be recalled or denounced a few years later.[31]

Medical theory in colonial America had not developed far from that espoused by the Greek physician Galen in the second century, and many doctors continued to emphasize that good health was a result of the balance of four bodily humors, which included yellow and black bile, blood, and phlegm. Conversely, illness was seen as a result of an imbalance of those factors. The goal of "cure" was frequently the alleviation of outward signs, as the connection between symptoms and underlying illness and disease was poorly understood: in other words, symptoms were seen as the disease. Moreover, specific diseases with attendant particular causes and treatments were concepts to be developed in future modern medicine.

Galen espoused bloodletting (venesection) as a means of ridding the body of bad humors. Bleeding, for example, might be used to relieve a patient of excess blood that contained diseased morbid matter that was thought to have caused fever. Raising skin blisters using caustics such as cantharides derived from the crushed body of the Spanish fly was thought to counteract overactive blood or tissue. Many radical practices were thought to remove "poisons" from the system and restore proper balance and equilibrium through their stimulating or sedating powers. Challenges to accepted theory began to appear in England in the late seventeenth century. A handful of physicians began to advocate more direct patient intervention based on a doctor's own experience rather than theory alone, and some emphasized the healing power of nature through the use of drug remedies compounded from either plant extracts or chemicals. Mercury to treat syphilis is a prime example, although it often brought a host of dangerous side effects.[32] Franklin and Jefferson were among the first American leaders to argue for medical treatment based on scientific empirical evidence, and Jefferson frequently decried invasive measures such as bloodletting.

Despite modest advances, confusion characterized eighteenth-century medicine and even persisted into at least the first half of the nineteenth century. Although prevailing medical theory of the time emphasized imbalances of the humors, another popular strain of medical thought attributed all illness to "solidism," the alternating states of tensions and relaxation in the nervous and vascular systems. If blood vessels became "too excited," for instance, the situation might produce fever, which required "calming" by removing excess blood. Both systems relied on bleeding and purging to bring the body into better alignment.[33]

No one at the time understood the role of microbes and that diseases were frequently spread not only through direct physical contact but also through droplets in the air resulting from coughing and sneezing—although Franklin certainly entertained a nascent theory on contagion. The subject of contaminated food and drinking water, which contributed to gastrointestinal illnesses like dysentery and diseases such as typhoid and cholera, was a mystery as well, and ideas about the efficacy of good sanitation to prevent some of these types of sicknesses was just emerging. In the absence of knowledge about bacteria and viruses and their relationship to infection, a number of radical therapies and theories thrived during the colonial, revolutionary, and early national periods.

Contemporary medicine in the eighteenth century often pointed to miasmas, "morbid," noxious air and vapors rising from stagnant water, or decomposing filth and rotting garbage as the cause of virtually all common diseases such as malaria, yellow fever, and typhus, which we understand today as being viral in origin, with microbes transmitted either from person to person, through contaminated food and water, or by infected insects that multiplied in filthy, standing water. In the case of malaria, for example, hordes of *anopheles* mosquitoes hatched in stagnant pools became frequent hosts of malarial parasites, spreading the illness among hapless human victims by feeding on their blood through their infectious bites and in the process destroying red corpuscles in the human bloodstream. When the disease was treated by the common therapy of bleeding, it often made matters worse by producing severe anemia in the victim.[34]

Malaria, which affected a large number of early Americans, could result in death, but more often the victim experienced chronic or intermittent fever and chills, an enlarged spleen, which produced pain in the abdomen, headache, fatigue, and general malaise. Two early visitors to South Carolina, for example, reported, "Fevers prevail all the year, from which those who are attacked seldom recover; and if some escape their complexion becomes tawny [jaundiced]."[35] Washington and Madison, both Virginians, probably suffered from malaria and recurrent flare-ups throughout their adult lives.

Because the concept of bacterial or viral infection was unknown at the time, the highly regarded Dr. Benjamin Rush of Philadelphia insisted that when Benjamin Franklin died in 1790, the pleurisy that led to his death "was caught by lying with his windows open."[36] In Charlestown, South Carolina, an early statute maintained, "The air is greatly infected and many maladies and other intolerable diseases daily happen."[37] John Tennent's popular book titled *Every Man His Own Doctor*, authored in 1725 and reprinted several times by Benjamin Franklin, attributed "fevers, coughs, quinsies, pleurisies, and consumption" to "Fogs and Exhalations" in the air arising from marshes, swamps, and bodies of water.[38] Miasmas were considered most dangerous in warm climates, particularly during the "unhealthy months," but even people in northern states experienced their share of illnesses, including malaria. During the Revolutionary War, a high percentage of soldiers in some regiments were infected with parasites, which they introduced after returning home to New England.[39] Several serious malaria epidemics descended on the region in the late eighteenth century, encouraged in part by marshy areas created by milldams, which served as a breeding ground for the mosquitoes that spread the disease.

In late-seventeenth-century England, Dr. Thomas Sydenham was on the leading edge of early Enlightenment-inspired physicians who began to emphasize empirical clinical medicine based on observation and data, and his ideas later gained popularity in America. But even Sydenham began the treatment of virtually every disease by opening a vein with a lancet. In America, purging, blistering to raise pus-filled lesions from which to expel "harmful matter," sweating through the use of heat and steam, and especially bleeding—the ineffective but often detrimental taking of a pint or more of "bad" blood from the afflicted— also became the common medical therapies for almost all ills and were considered "best practices."[40]

Forward-thinking about health care in many other ways, Washington, Abigail Adams, and Franklin frequently recommended purging, bleeding, and blistering for their own families and friends and claimed to have personally experienced the benefits of the procedures, undoubtedly the result of a powerful psychological placebo effect.[41] Indeed, common medical wisdom recommended bleeding at least until 1835, when the French physician Pierre-Jean-George Cabanis demonstrated it to be worthless by using medical statistics to prove his case, although most American doctors still ignored his findings.[42] Many American doctors continued bleeding as well as purging with mercury taken in the pill form of calomel through the infamous cholera epidemics that took place between the 1830s and the 1850s.[43] Acrimonious debates about the efficacy of bloodletting and a variety of heroic drug therapies raged up to the Civil War,[44] before the procedures gradually faded into disuse.[45]

The use of these extreme "cures" was often worse than the illness itself, and many in an already weakened state died as a result of violent bleeding or purging. Today we know that mercury is poisonous, and many patients who were treated with calomel undoubtedly experienced deleterious effects. One revolutionary-era Boston physician distanced himself from the majority of doctors and violently criticized contemporary medical practice in early New England, which "was very uniform, bleeding, vomiting, blistering, purging, anodyne, etc. if the illness continued, there was *repetendi,* and finally *murderandi.*"[46]

Jefferson, who generally only turned to medical men as a last resort, took contemporary physicians to task in a similarly caustic manner and declared, "the inexperienced & presumptuous band of medical tyros let loose upon the world, destroys more of human life in one year, than all the Robinhoods, Cartouches & Macheaths do in a century."[47] In fact, he was not far off the mark. It is noteworthy that advanced medical ideas often stemmed from educated laymen like Jefferson and the other American founders included in this study rather than physicians, who often had little to offer seriously ill patients. Jefferson would undoubtedly have looked with approval on the early-nineteenth-century "revolt" against the excesses of heroic medicine and the heated rivalry between regular physicians and "irregular," unconventional natural homeopathic healers such as herbalist Samuel Thomson that flourished in the decades after Jefferson's death.[48]

Most early doctors, apothecaries, and lay healers compounded their own medicines, largely from combinations of chemicals, herbs, and plants. A number of "patent" medicines made use of plant-derived ingredients such as opium from poppies. After 1785, digitalis derived from the foxglove plant was used successfully for heart patients to treat "dropsy" or congestion. Homemade remedies mixed by laypeople often worked well for minor illnesses and spared them the expense of purchasing a patent medication, which was not inconsiderable. For example, doses of the popular laxative jalap in mid-eighteenth-century Virginia cost about the same as two pairs of shoes.[49] Indeed, we know that nature was the first source of medicine used to treat human illnesses, and even in modern times they remain an important avenue of healing.

Today's ubiquitous and remarkably effective medication aspirin was derived from willow bark, which was often used by early Americans to treat headaches, and penicillin famously evolved from a fungus that featured a substance that killed bacteria.

Many of the American founders were familiar with medicinal herbs and their reputed curative powers. They often espoused their own home remedies or "simples" recorded in family "receipt" books, or followed manuals explaining the specifics of mixing and administering herbal remedies. As we will see in later chapters, heads of households, including women like Abigail Adams, Martha Washington, and Dolley Madison and their contemporaries, often grew medicinal plants in their household gardens, learned how to brew their own potions, dress burns and wounds, staunch bleeding, reduce swelling, and treat common illnesses such as colic, measles, and whooping cough. As domestic healers, they often relied on a basic understanding of the humors to make a "diagnosis."[50] As one historian has noted, most women in the colonial era practiced some form of medicine, "whether they were housewives making herbal infusions for children or midwives delivering babies for their neighbors."[51]

In fact, home remedies often competed successfully with the many dubious patent medicines. Jefferson especially favored the healing power of nature and used thyme and lavender from his own garden at Monticello for stomach ailments and headaches. In 1759, Washington ordered drugs from London, including the ubiquitous cathartic calomel (mercurous chloride) and the emetic ipecac, but also purchased herbal tonics such as spirits of lavender and cinnamon water.[52]

In the absence of a reliable medication to relieve her painful symptoms of rheumatism, Abigail Adams recommended the application of cabbage leaves for those who suffered from the aches and pains of the ailment, which she characterized as "our family infirmity."[53] "Rheumatism" was the broad and general name then given to a variety of aches and pains, which most probably included arthritis, muscular inflammations, and strains. In addition to home remedies, for some people at the time, religion rather than medicine provided solace and the ability to cope with life's many vicissitudes.

Herbal remedies brought relief to some patients, and opiates were sometimes administered in a haphazard way to address pain. Opium in the liquid form of laudanum was introduced in England in the sixteenth century and often recommended for discomfort as well as insomnia and diarrhea. It was made from the concentrated juice of the poppy mixed with alcohol; the opium extract was often mixed into brandy. The name "laudanum" was derived from the Latin "*laudere*," meaning "to praise," and the popular remedy was used freely by most early Americans, including some founders. Jefferson, Franklin, and Abigail Adams relied on laudanum in their last years to help them sleep and mitigate severe physical discomfort. Dr. Sydenham maintained that "[m]edicine would be a cripple without it."[54]

In addition to laudanum, quinine derived from the bark of the cinchona tree (Jesuit's or Peruvian Bark) was another of the few therapeutically effective available drugs at the time, when it was used to treat malaria. Jesuit missionaries in South America introduced the bark to Europe in the 1630s, and it became the source for the later alkaloid quinine. Although quinine cannot prevent infection, it has the effect of poisoning the malarial parasite and preventing the outbreak of illness or minimizing its effects. Even though proposed cures for malaria have been documented back to the Romans, full understanding of the etiology of the disease did not emerge until 1897, when the British army surgeon Ronald Ross helped discover that the disease was transmitted by mosquitoes. Formerly, it had been thought that a malignant atmosphere produced the illness, and the name "malaria" literally means "bad air," "*mal aria*." Malaria is an insect-born disease, but the mosquito must be infected by a human host, and it was probably imported to the Americas through Europeans.[55] Still, even the use of the bark was only partially effective as an exact dosage was hard to determine, and quinine was not effectively isolated from cinchona until 1822. The diagnosis of malaria was elusive as its most prominent symptom, intermittent fever, was often confused with other illnesses, especially yellow fever. In many cases quinine was regarded as an efficacious tonic and ended up being used inappropriately for a hodgepodge of diseases.

Jefferson, Franklin, George and Martha Washington, John and Abigail Adams, and James and Dolley Madison certainly had access to popular medical guides, such as Dr. William Buchan's book *Domestic Medicine*, published in London in 1769, which appeared in Philadelphia by 1771. The manual offered practical advice and instructions for the treatment of a variety of diseases and their symptoms written in a clear, commonsense style intended for the general public.[56] It was so popular that it was reprinted numerous times in America.

Early Medical Practitioners

Buchan was a learned Scottish physician who had received his training at the famed University of Edinburgh. He hoped his publication would be of assistance primarily in the area of preventative medicine and the treatment of mild illnesses, but Buchan strongly recommended calling in a doctor promptly when more serious disease was suspected. Even regular physicians in America at the time encouraged reprinting of the book in the United States, reflecting contemporary appreciation for the role of domestic involvement in successfully treating illnesses.[57] By 1784, Abigail Adams was studying the volume on her sea voyage to join her husband John in Europe, and she concluded that "[h]e [Buchan] appears a sensible, judicious and rational writer."[58] The book's emphasis on prevention and the benefits of exercise, fresh air, clean water, cleanliness, and good nutrition must have been very appealing to Jefferson and Franklin, in particular, but Buchan still considered bleeding an effective treatment tool.

Although doctors like Buchan commanded respect, the formation of medicine was a laborious process, and not until the beginning of the twentieth century would American physicians fully consolidate their respected professional status and authority.[59] Popular feeling is encapsulated in the remarks of an early American observer in the 1750s who opined that "[q]uacks abound [here] like locusts in Egypt."[60] Understandably, colonial medicine mirrored contemporary practice in England. Physicians, surgeons, and apothecaries jockeyed for predominance in both locations, although the lines between the various health practitioners were often blurred, and many doctors were clearly rank amateurs. During the era, three spheres of medical "practice" held relatively equal sway: domestic household medicine, medicine practiced by doctors, who had undergone "formal" education or apprenticeship, and medicine practiced by experienced lay healers, including midwives and herbalists. To enhance their position, learned colonial doctors often referred disparagingly to medical competitors whom they viewed as having lesser qualifications or who did not follow the practices of orthodox medicine as mere "empirics" or "quacks," although the latter term was most often applied to dishonest charlatans who aggressively advertised outlandish treatments for financial gain.[61]

On the eve of the Revolution, there were about thirty-five hundred medical practitioners in America, but only about 10 percent actually held medical degrees.[62] However, by the mid-eighteenth century an academic degree became increasingly desirable, although it did not necessarily guarantee competence. University-trained physicians learned much about prevailing medical theories but often had limited contact with actual patients. Doctors with a university education could command twice the fee of those who had merely apprenticed, a cost that generally only the rich could afford. Scotland housed several respected medical schools, although England and the Continent also provided education for many aspiring colonial physicians.[63] English-born Dr. Robley Dunglison studied medicine in London, Paris, Edinburgh, and Bavaria, and later became a professor at the new University of Virginia in 1824 as well as Jefferson's personal physician in the former president's last years.[64]

Washington's personal physician for most of his adult life was the Scottish-born Dr. James Craik, who had also studied medicine at the University of Edinburgh. Dr. Benjamin Waterhouse, who with the active assistance of Thomas Jefferson introduced the effective and safer Jenner method of smallpox vaccination in America, was born in colonial Rhode Island in 1754. Following the typical pattern for aspiring early American physicians, Waterhouse attended medical school in Edinburgh in 1775, studied with a noted doctor in London in 1776, and received his diploma from Leyden in 1780, before returning to the United States. Waterhouse was revolutionary not only in his public health endeavors but also in his politics. It is said that his enrollment signature in the Leyden medical school was followed by the statement, "A citizen of the free and United States of America."[65]

The story of Dr. Benjamin Rush of Philadelphia (1745-1813) illuminates the state of medical training and practice in early America and attendant disagreements over therapies. The handsome, garrulous, and energetic Rush was perhaps the foremost American physician of the colonial and early national eras. Rush apprenticed with Dr. John

Redman in Philadelphia and was allowed to follow Redman in his rounds at the local hospital. His duties in Redmond's "shop," as he termed the doctor's medical practice, included "preparing and compounding medicines, visiting the sick and performing many little offices of a nurse to them . . . and exclusive charge of his books and accounts."[66]

Rush later trained under the famous Scottish physician and professor of medicine Dr. William Cullen, received his medical degree at the University of Edinburgh in 1768, and spent nearly two years in London and Paris gaining experience. Though Rush received strong academic instruction in addition to practical experience, most American physicians in the revolutionary era learned their craft through the apprenticeship system alone, and the medical profession in the United States was not regulated and did not become firmly established until the first half of the nineteenth century.[67] Pragmatic Americans tended to respect not only doctors who had acquired formal theoretical training in a university setting but also those who built reputations as experienced physicians, such as Rush, who had regular daily contact with patients. Those lacking even rudimentary knowledge competed with the more competent at the time, which resulted in a motley and surprisingly large assortment of medical practitioners, for "[t]hough many physicians were ill-trained, even-untrained, there were a good many of them."[68]

The first medical school founded in America opened in Philadelphia in 1765, with Benjamin Franklin's central involvement and encouragement, and was followed by a second academy, the King's College Medical School in New York, the following year. Both institutions were aimed at professionalizing and upgrading the state of medicine. Franklin served as a mentor to Rush and a number of prominent emerging Philadelphia doctors, who revered the older leader. On his return from Europe to Philadelphia in 1769, Rush launched his successful American practice and became a member of the College of Philadelphia medical school faculty as a professor of chemistry. As a measure of his elevated status, twenty years later Rush was elected professor of theory and practice of medicine at the college, and when the school became the University of Pennsylvania, he was named professor of the Institutes of Medicine.

Rush was the first to diagnose what he termed "billious remitting yellow fever" in August 1793, at the beginning of the notorious Philadelphia epidemic. Although he had at first been acclaimed as a popular hero,

Rush was later strongly criticized for his increasingly aggressive medical response by some physicians, particularly those who followed the French school of medicine, which emphasized moderation, the use of bark and a variety of herbal remedies, and the superiority of nature over heroic measures. In the wake of the negative publicity, an embittered Rush later resigned from the College of Physicians, America's most prestigious medical society at the time and one that he had helped found, and his medical practice declined precipitously by the late 1790s.[69]

During the duration of the epidemic, Rush exhausted himself working tirelessly to treat the yellow fever victims, often seeing as many as one hundred patients a day. His devotion to his patients during the crisis was exemplary, although ultimately as ineffective as the variety of treatments offered by all local physicians. In fact, Rush's radical depletion therapies, including violent purging with calomel combined with jalap and extreme bleeding, which at times ran to his calculation of four-fifths of the patient's circulating blood, probably hurried many of the sick to their deaths. His treatments sometimes caused gastrointestinal bleeding and certainly added some level of mercury poisoning and debilitating weakness to their conditions. Rush's view of the treatment of yellow fever is particularly instructive about the state of medicine during the age. Philadelphia at the time was the center of American medicine; at least eighty doctors worked in the city, and Rush, dubbed the "American Sydenham," was its most respected practitioner. Rush traced all disease to underlying excess stimulation in the blood vessels. As late as 1796, Rush still believed that "there was but one fever in the world . . . and one disease," the "morbid excitement induced by capillary tension" that responded best to the remedy of bloodletting and purging.[70]

As one historian observed, Rush and his fellow physicians "stood between medieval and modern medicine."[71] The era's greatest minds in American medicine were divided on the causes and treatment of yellow fever, some asserting that it was "imported" through foreigners arriving on ships from the West Indies and others blaming domestic conditions such as local climate and miasmas. Rush believed incorrectly that the disease stemmed from local "sensible and insensible qualities of the air." One solution put forward by members of the local legislature to rid Philadelphia of the fever was to set off cannons to clear the air, and at one point Rush pointed to exhalations from spoiled coffee on the local wharves as the culprit for the start of the epidemic! Rush noted the great infestation of mosquitoes that fateful summer, but made no connection between the insects and the spread of the disease.[72]

Walter Reed's discovery in the early 1900s that yellow fever was transmitted by biting mosquitoes and not by personal contact with people who had been infected by "noxious" air was still over a century away. Therefore, the illness could not be effectively prevented or treated by simply turning away foreigners, quarantine, fumigation, the large doses of bark and wine advocated by some doctors, or radical bleeding and purging.[73] Rush himself became ill but survived. As the epidemic continued to rage, he advised Philadelphia residents to flee the city if possible to escape contagion. The numbers of deaths only increased in September until the yellow fever slowly tapered out with the coming of colder weather, heralding the end of mosquito season, and finally ended in late November, when many Philadelphians who had left the city returned home.

Although Rush was tragically wrong about the yellow fever epidemic, he had many other positive attributes to commend him as both a physician and a patriot, one of the many early American physicians who became involved in politics. Rush, an American founding father in his own right, was active in the Continental Congress and signed the Declaration of Independence. As a surgeon general in the Continental Army from 1777 to 1778, he authored a tract about preventative health instructions for soldiers. A firmly committed republican, like most of the founders examined in this book, he believed that educated American citizens could take a direct role in managing their own health and once declared "the people rule here in medicine as well as government."[74]

In that view, Rush was reflecting republican thought that emphasized a connection between ably and sensibly managing one's own health and regulating and promoting the well-being of the nation as a whole. This philosophy was surely a driving force in Jefferson's efforts in his twilight years to introduce a medical curriculum at the University of Virginia, which he helped found. Jefferson's goal was not only to help provide high-level scientific training in medicine for future physicians but also to educate general students so that the "common" man would acquire basic knowledge about illness and treatment, which could be applied practically to help guide the health of their families and communities. Moreover, for America's founders, the "health" of the nation referred to far more than simply the physical state of its inhabitants and was inextricably linked to the country's political, economic, social, and cultural vitality.

A close friend of Franklin, Jefferson, and Abigail and John Adams, Rush played a pivotal role in the reconciliation of Adams and Jefferson in their later years after Jefferson defeated Adams for the presidency and their political differences had driven a wedge between the two American leaders. Because of his medical reputation and close relationship with the Adamses, Rush was consulted when their daughter Nabby was diagnosed with breast cancer when she was in her midforties. He was the physician who made the recommendation that Nabby Adams Smith undergo a mastectomy as her best chance for cure. Unfortunately, despite the operation, it was too late for Nabby, whose cancer had already spread. In old age, Jefferson turned to Rush for medical advice about a severe attack of rheumatism. Sensitive to the fact that Jefferson abhorred most drugs, Rush conservatively recommended botanical medications, including doses of sassafras tea and spirits of turpentine, and sent the former American president castile soap, opium, and camphor among other remedies to relieve the discomfort. Another time, Rush advised Jefferson that his feet be kept warm for they were "the avenues of half the paroxysms of all chronic diseases when cold."[75]

As an eminent and captivating teacher and a graceful medical writer, Rush was also fundamentally a champion of humanitarian social reform. He was a strong advocate for high-level academic medical education, the education of women, the abolition of slavery, alcohol temperance, and humane care for the mentally ill and the impoverished, many of whom he treated free of charge. He is often regarded as the father of modern American psychiatry. In his autobiography Rush recalled, "My shop [practice] was crowded with the poor in the morning and at meal time. . . . I often remained [in the houses of the poor] to administer my prescriptions, particularly bleeding and glisters, with my own hands."[76]

Although a caring man devoted to the cause of social welfare, and a physician who helped make Philadelphia a leader in American medicine, he was also, as we have seen, a proponent of radical heroic medical practices, particularly in times of serious epidemics—treatments that certainly caused much harm.[77] Yet it is important to note that Rush, like most trained physicians at the time, was just as certain as doctors today that his therapeutics were effective and an improvement over the past and reflected legitimate treatment based on empirical evidence. Rush sincerely believed he acted in an enlightened and scientific manner and that he followed the most advanced medical practices of his time.[78] Furthermore, once Rush administered what he viewed as the initial required therapies of bleeding, purging, and puking (vomiting), he generally followed a philosophy of letting nature take its course through the rest of the healing process.[79] Rush neither introduced heroic medical measures to America (where they had been popular for nearly two centuries), nor was he unusually extreme in his stand on bloodletting. His position as perhaps the leading physician in America at the time may have simply made him the most visible proponent of venesection.[80]

Rush's contemporary, Thomas Jefferson, had long displayed a keen interest in medicine. Probably influenced by his stay in France and admiration of French medicine, he understood before most American doctors the harmful effects of commonly practiced heroic measures employed in medicine at the time, such as the frequent use of the poisonous chemical mercury (calomel). While Jefferson staunchly opposed bleeding, even after the yellow fever epidemic, Rush still continued to believe strongly in its efficacy; when one of his "beloved" pupils later died, he maintained in his diary that "[h]is fever became fatal from the neglect of bleeding in one paroxysm of his fever."[81] Jefferson enjoyed a long friendship with Rush, but he sharply criticized the doctor's penchant for drastic measures. In 1814, Jefferson recalled that "in his theory of bleeding . . . I was ever opposed to my friend Rush, whom I greatly loved; but who has done much harm, in the sincerest persuasion that he was preserving life."[82] Yet, triumphantly reviewing "The Improvements, Progress and State of Medicine" in the eighteenth century, as late as 1800 the eminent American physician and politician Dr. David Ramsay praised Rush as the "pride and boast of his country."[83]

Although Jefferson valued the potential of the prestigious Philadelphia College to advance the state of medicine, that did not prevent him from scoffing at the doctors the school produced: "Our country is overrun with young lads from the Philadelphia school who, with their mercury and lancet in hand, are vying with the word of Bonaparte which shall shed the most human blood."[84] Despite his criticism of many of Rush's therapies, when Rush died in 1813, Thomas Jefferson wrote to Adams, "Another of our friends of 76 is gone. . . . And a better man than Rush, could not have left us, more benevolent, more learned, of a finer genius, or more honest."[85] Similarly, John Adams concluded, "I know of no Character living or dead, who has done more real good in America [than Rush]."[86]

Rush and most physicians in the colonies seemed to be somewhat more willing than English physicians to incorporate both traditional and emerging ideas, and doctors in both areas were often called in to treat a variety of illnesses, from treating infections to setting bones and pulling teeth. Surgery was generally limited to relatively minor procedures such as lancing boils and abscesses and bloodletting, and for the more daring and experienced, amputation, removing urinary tract stones, and aspirating fluids. At the same time, responsibility for medical care often fell to family members, who nursed the ill, often garnering their rudimentary expertise from books, newspapers, almanacs, or local experts such as midwives, apothecaries, and doctors.[87] Abigail Adams's sister reported tending to her dying nephew through many anxious days and nights, relieved at times by her young daughter and a paid "watcher."[88] Founding father Benjamin Franklin, always receptive to new ideas, played a pivotal role in American medicine during the colonial and revolutionary periods through his own experimentation and inventions and dissemination of medical information through his *Poor Richard's Almanac* and newspaper. His medical expertise earned him the respect of many physicians both in America and in Europe, where he received many honorary degrees and mentored many of America's rising young physicians studying on the Continent.

Launching the Battle against Smallpox

The introduction of variolation, popularly known as inoculation, against smallpox was probably the most significant advance in colonial medicine and occurred simultaneously with its early use in England.[89] As one historian put it succinctly, "Probably nothing in the field of early American medicine was more revolutionary."[90] Variolation could be traced back to ancient times in China, India, and Africa, but the first documented instance in England took place in 1718. Boston's erudite minister-physician Cotton Mather, who lost his wife and three of his children in 1713 in one episode of the many severe waves of the disease, was one of the first Americans to successfully advocate for the introduction of inoculation in the colonies. As John Adams's grandson, historian Charles Francis Adams, observed, the clergy were especially revered in early Massachusetts and they "not infrequently became the family physician," but many clergy opposed inoculation because they believed it went against the will of God.[91]

Mather had a genuine desire to improve social welfare through medical advances. He followed contemporary scientific developments closely and seems to have adhered to an early protean concept of "animalcular" or "germ theory" in his belief in the existence of tiny "animal" material causing disease.[92] Mather was also a strong voice for moderation in medical treatment, particularly decrying the excessive bloodletting of the day: "Before we go any farther, let this Advice for the Sick, be principally attended to: *Don't kill 'em!* That is to say, With mischievous Kindness." [93]

Mather was assisted in his pioneering preventative smallpox campaign of 1721 by Dr. Zabdiel Boylston, the great-uncle of John Adams. Boylston inoculated himself and his only son Thomas, who was six years old at the time, as well as Mather's younger children to demonstrate the efficacy and safety of the procedure. By the end of the outbreak, a total of 247 people underwent variolation, which involved inserting a small amount of live smallpox matter into the skin of a healthy person. Many contemporary doctors in Massachusetts, such as the university-trained William Douglass, initially opposed the procedure as both dangerous and medically unproven. Inoculation was so controversial at the time that Boylston was threatened with hanging and Mather's house was bombed (unsuccessfully) by an irate critic. Many colonies passed laws to prohibit inoculation, which over time gave way to regulation as its benefits became more appreciated.[94] Benjamin Franklin later observed that "the practice of Inoculation always divided the people into parties, some contending warmly for it, and the others against it."[95]

Still, inoculation was both risky and expensive at the time. The death rate for the procedure ranged from one to five in a hundred. To compound matters, the vulnerable poor sometimes found themselves infected by those who could afford inoculation and moved about in public while still contagious. Smallpox had an incubation period between ten and fourteen days before symptoms became noticeable. Dangers such as these prompted many conservative doctors to decry the inoculation process altogether because of the potential to spread smallpox if quarantines were not strictly enforced.

Then, as now, only those who could afford the cost received the best medical care, but most of America's founders were comfortably off if not actually affluent. Adams underwent the still-controversial procedure in 1764 in Boston when he was in his late twenties, and two years later, in 1766, Jefferson traveled from Virginia to Philadelphia at the age of twenty-three to be inoculated, signaling their forward outlook on disease prevention. Smallpox was one of the most serious threats to the health of early Americans. The widespread smallpox epidemic that ravaged the country from 1775 to 1782 killed more than a hundred thousand people and snuffed out many more lives than the British Army during the Revolutionary War, a phenomenon that prompted Washington to formulate his own public health policy of requiring inoculation among his troops and stressing overall good sanitation and other preventative measures for his soldiers. New recruits from more isolated country areas who had not developed immunity to diseases like typhoid and smallpox were especially vulnerable given the crowded and often unsanitary army conditions.[96]

Even for civilians, the war disrupted normal life across the colonies and promoted the spread of a variety of infectious illnesses. Despite its drawbacks and potential for spreading contagion, overall, inoculation played a significant role in reducing future outbreaks of smallpox. But a decade later, smallpox still disrupted American life. In 1794 Madison complained to Jefferson that a wave of smallpox in Virginia had not only caused fatalities but also delayed the mail.[97] Later, with the memory of war devastation in his mind and propelled by his keen interest in infectious diseases and public health, in the beginning of the nineteenth century Jefferson would play a pivotal role in the American introduction of the Jenner cowpox-based method of vaccination, first introduced in England in 1798. Influenced by the successful work of Boston's Dr. Waterhouse, Jefferson used his political power as president to make the government a major player in encouraging better preventative health care through providing smallpox vaccination around the country.

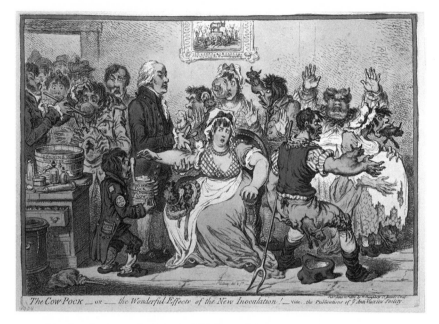

The Cow-Pock—or the Wonderful Effects of the New Inoculation, 1802.
This cartoon caricature of a Jenner vaccination scene in England by artist
James Gillray reveals that in 1802 the new smallpox preventative method
was still controversial. (Courtesy Library of Congress)

Madison followed in his mentor Jefferson's footsteps in addressing
the threat of smallpox. During Madison's presidency, on the eve of
the War of 1812, smallpox vaccination of soldiers was ordered by the
War Department. More significantly, in 1813 Madison went one step
beyond Jefferson when he signed into law a statute to encourage wider
smallpox vaccination, one of the nation's earliest public health bills.
The legislation was aimed at regulating the Jenner vaccine to protect
American citizens from unscrupulous purveyors who offered adulter-
ated versions. The Vaccine Act of 1813 was the first federal law to oversee drug purity with an eye toward consumer protection. It also gave
the president the power to "appoint an agent to preserve the genuine
vaccine matter, and to furnish the same to any citizen of the United
States." The medical officer was instructed to send packages of vaccine
weighing under a half an ounce free of charge through the U.S. mail to
all interested parties. The act was repealed in 1822, when the authority

to regulate vaccine was transferred to the states, but it established an important precedent.[98]

From the beginning, America's founders were willing to consider the benefits of health innovations. The spirit of the Age of Reason encouraged medical and scientific experiments, but they were not conducted in sterile laboratories with test tubes in the manner we are accustomed to today. Rather, as we have seen, humans served to verify procedures, and many medical innovators used themselves and their families as the test cases. Smallpox inoculation with human matter could be a dangerous business, but the willingness of Jefferson, Abigail and John Adams, and Franklin, among other American founders, to undergo the procedure is a testament to both their faith in scientific progress and their personal courage. American medicine was in transition during the late-eighteenth and early-nineteenth centuries, beginning slowly, as the first decades of the nineteenth century passed, to move away from age-old practices of heroic therapeutics. Considering that there was no real comprehension and acceptance of germ theory until the late nineteenth century, and no agreement that it was specific pathogens that caused particular illnesses, medical science was just beginning to emerge from the darkness. America's founders were among the small group of medical visionaries, although unfortunately many of their advanced ideas were lost over the next several decades.

The stories of America's founding fathers and mothers as they developed over the backdrop of eighteenth-century medicine reminds us that evolving science is not only complex but even today always subject to uncertainties, and medical progress continues to be challenged. Despite the advances of modern medicine in producing parasite-killing antimalarial drugs to combat the illness and in eliminating the deadly mosquitoes through chemical warfare in the form of DDT, or avoidance of insect bites, malaria is still a serious threat, primarily in the world's poorest countries, particularly in Southeast Asia, parts of South America, and sub-Saharan Africa.[99] Mosquitoes have gradually grown resistant to DDT, and some species of the wily malarial parasites have become more lethal. Others have adapted and become resistant to the most popular modern drugs that were thought to be superior to quinine, such as atebrin. Recent success in reducing mortality from malaria in Africa has resulted from an infusion of funds to pay for mosquito nets to prevent bites during sleep and the distribution of free antiviral drugs. Today, malaria-carrying mosquitoes infect between 250 million and 500 million people yearly, killing close to one million victims.[100] It is noteworthy that even in the era of modern medicine smallpox is the only major disease that has been eradicated.

America's founders not only helped navigate the road to independence, but in a variety of ways began to lay a framework for improvements in medicine and the development of a national public health program. As noted previously, in their minds republican ideals fostered a reciprocal connection between individual and national health. The founders' regular encounters with personal illness and the specter of epidemics and plagues that could and did devastate entire communities made men and women like George and Martha Washington, Benjamin Franklin, Thomas Jefferson, John and Abigail Adams, and James and Dolley Madison acutely sensitive to health issues. The state of medicine and public health today is still a work in progress, but these founders played a significant role in the conversation that helped shaped the contours of its development. Certainly the ongoing debate over American health care is hardly a new discussion.

1

George and Martha Washington

Health, Illness, and the First Family

The General has nothing more at heart, than the
Health of the Troops.
—*General Orders Issued by George Washington, August 5, 1776*

In passing down the vale of time, and in journey-
ing through such a mutable world as that in which
we are placed, we must expect to meet with a great
and continual mixture of afflictions and blessings.
—*Martha Washington to Mercy Otis Warren, June 12, 1790*

Against the effect of time, and age, no remedy has
yet been discovered; and like the rest of my fellow
mortals, I must (if life is prolonged) submit.
—*George Washington to Landon Carter, October 5, 1798*

In his many portraits, America's first president and "Foundingest
Father,"[1] George Washington, is depicted as a tall, commanding figure,
with an elegantly slim but strong, muscular physique. Indeed, at a little
over six feet, Washington towered above most of his contemporaries,
and by all accounts was a revered and imposing man who commanded
great respect. However, noticeably absent from the paintings are the
lightly pockmarked skin, which remained with him through adulthood as a result of smallpox contracted in his teens, the sunken cheeks
that resulted from the eventual loss of all of his teeth due to decay,

which was only partially relieved by ill-fitting dentures, and increasing debility as he aged due to numerous often vague but serious illnesses, including several severe bouts with malaria, pleurisy, influenza, and intestinal dysentery.

It was undoubtedly Washington's many personal illnesses and close friendships with many of the leading physicians of the day, coupled with his responsibilities as a plantation owner and commander of troops, that made him especially interested in medical matters. A largely self-educated man, Washington reflected the republican vision that American citizens could and should take a direct role in managing their own health and that of their communities and that individual health and the health of the nation were intertwined. Like so many of America's colonial leaders who had been influenced by Enlightenment philosophy, Washington looked forward to the development of a progressive medicine in a benevolent republic that would benefit all Americans.

Washington became quite familiar with symptoms and contemporary treatment of many diseases, and one early medical historian maintained that Washington's influence "in the prevention of smallpox in America was probably as great as that of Cotton Mather, Benjamin Franklin, or Thomas Jefferson."[2] Certainly in his military and political roles, Washington perceived the compelling need for government to take a role in health intervention, demonstrated most visibly in his insistence that his troops be inoculated against smallpox during the Revolutionary War. And it was as "warrior healer" that Washington made his most important medical contribution to America.

Personal health issues sometimes left Washington predisposed to intermittent depression and preoccupation with illness, although he was fearless on the battlefield. Considering his paternal genetic inheritance, which left the males in his family especially prone to tuberculosis, and the rather primitive state of contemporary medical treatment, it is a testament to Washington's underlying good health, his stoicism, and his determination that he lived to the age of sixty-seven, as his father died at age forty-eight, and his many siblings all predeceased him. Before Washington was three years old, he lost his older half-sister, Jane, and his baby sister, Mildred, passed away as an infant when George was still a young boy. Washington himself would later observe that "though I was blessed with a good constitution, I was of a short lived family."[3] The average life expectancy in Virginia when Washington was born was only about twenty-eight to thirty-five years of age.[4]

Washington's Early Health

George Washington was born in Wakefield, Virginia, on February 22, 1732, to the English-born Augustine Washington, a modestly successful planter, and his second wife, Mary Ball Washington, a strong-willed woman and often demanding mother. Augustine and his first wife had three sons and a daughter before he became a widower in 1729 at the age of twenty-nine. He soon remarried, and Augustine and Mary became the parents of six children. While there is scarce documentation, it is likely that the young George Washington contracted and survived the common and often life-threatening childhood illnesses of the time, including mumps and measles, because when he was exposed to those diseases as an adult he did not succumb to infection. Washington did not develop measles when his wife, Martha, contracted the illness during their marriage, and he was said to have been stricken with diphtheria, also known as "black canker," as a boy.[5]

As a young man, Washington developed an affinity for the outdoors and particularly enjoyed fox hunting and horseback riding, which probably helped to keep him fit and athletic. He was the first-born of his father's second marriage, and he felt a keen lifelong responsibility to all his siblings, but he developed an especially close relationship with his half-brothers. His father, Augustine, died of a respiratory ailment, possibly the result of underlying tuberculosis, contracted after a ride in stormy weather when George Washington was eleven. His half-brother Lawrence became a surrogate father to George, but Mary Washington was left to manage the family slaves and estate at Ferry Farm and to keep daily watch over her other five children. The death of his father put an end to formal studies for young Washington, who received only what we would consider an elementary school education. However, he read widely, including works of the Enlightenment philosophers, eventually acquired a library of some nine hundred books, and enjoyed cultural pursuits. At the age of sixteen, Washington trained for a practical occupation as a surveyor and acquired a license from the College of William and Mary, which launched him on his ambitious path to becoming a successful landowner.[6]

The young Washington's first experience with surveying, a respectable occupation at the time, began with his association with the aristocratic Fairfax family of Virginia, which was made possible by his half-brother Lawrence's marriage to Ann Fairfax, daughter of a wealthy aristocratic family. As a young man, Washington was successful both at surveying and at acquiring his own increasing parcels of land. Lawrence's sons all died as infants, and when he succumbed to tuberculosis at the age of thirty-four, he left to his two-year-old daughter his estate at Mount Vernon, which ultimately passed to the disciplined and capable George.

In 1749, in the course of his work as a surveyor in Virginia, the seventeen-year-old Washington first became exposed to what was termed "ague" at the time, which we know today as malaria. As he wrote to his sister-in-law, "I am deprived of the pleasure of waiting on you . . . by ague and fever which I have had to extremity."[7] "Ague" was also a contemporary catch-all term used to describe a variety of both fevers and chills. At the time Washington was growing up a number of diseases were rampant in America, including tuberculosis, typhoid, smallpox, influenza, and malaria. Seasonal outbreaks of amoebic dysentery and typhoid fever as a result of pollution of tidewater water sources especially contributed to the high mortality rate in the southern colonies and encouraged many residents to move farther inland to higher, healthier locations.[8] Early Virginia swamplands were particularly hospitable breeding grounds for malaria-carrying mosquitoes. However, in colonial America most sicknesses, such as malaria, were still attributed to "malignant" or "bad air" and humors gone awry, and there was little understanding of the true origin of the etymology of the disease.

During his lifetime, Washington would suffer numerous reoccurrences of malarial fever, which was characterized by a cycle of painful chills, high fever, and weakness. The disease taxed the blood system, and active episodes often occurred over several days and weeks. Malaria parasites often lay dormant in their victims, only to flare up in the summer and fall. It was still some time after Washington's first encounter with malaria as a young man before quinine derived from Peruvian Cinchona Bark, or the "Bark" as it was referred to at the time, would be used consistently and widely to treat the illness. However, we do know it would become one of Washington's favored medications, and the drug was used successfully for soldiers during the Revolutionary War.[9]

Throughout his lifetime, Washington exhibited a deep faith in the efficacy of bark. Many years later, in 1798, Washington would advise his secretary, Colonel Tobias Lear, that in regard to the treatment of ague and various fevers, "Bark is necessary to prevent a relapse."[10] By the time Washington's neighbor and personal physician, Dr. James Craik, began treating Washington's flareups of malaria, it was common for the doctor to first prescribe a cleansing cathartic followed by eight doses of bark. As he aged, the symptoms of malaria took a greater toll on Washington's health, and in his later years he is said to have lost twenty pounds while experiencing one attack in 1797.[11]

Following his first encounter with malaria, Washington's next experience with serious disease occurred in 1751 at the age of nineteen after he accompanied his sick brother Lawrence on a rough, 37-day voyage to Barbados in the futile hope of seeking a cure for the latter's tuberculosis in the warm West Indies climate. As early as 1749, Washington had alluded to Lawrence's illness when he wrote, "Dear Brother, I hope your cough is much mended since I saw you last."[12] Neither Lawrence's health-seeking trip to England nor an excursion to "take the healthful waters" at Warm Springs, Virginia, accompanied by George, succeeded in improving Lawrence's condition. In the eighteenth and nineteenth centuries, immersing in healing springs was thought not only to be curative for the sick but also invigorating for people in good health. Philadelphia's early leading physician, Dr. Benjamin Rush, for example, was a great proponent of taking mineral water internally, for both its healing and its tonic properties.[13]

A trip to the West Indies was Lawrence's last attempt to recover his health. After receiving an encouraging diagnosis from a local doctor after they docked in Barbados, both brothers were hopeful that the temperate climate and lush surroundings would cure Lawrence. Shortly after they found lodgings near Bridgetown, the two brothers accepted a dinner invitation from Gedney Clarke, a prominent local planter. It would prove an unwise decision, for as Washington remarked in his diary, "We went,—myself with some reluctance, as the smallpox was in his family." Even though he did not know the exact mechanism of transference, clearly George understood that smallpox was a dangerous and contagious disease. Two weeks later, on November 16th, he recorded in his diary that he had been "strongly attacked with the small Pox" and treated and nursed back to health by a local physician, Dr. John Lanahan.[14]

We cannot be sure of the exact trajectory of Washington's encounter with the smallpox virus, but it probably spread to his respiratory tract either through direct droplet contact with an infected Clarke family member or, less likely, through particles left in the air or on clothing or furniture, as the *Variola* virus can remain active for weeks outside the human body. A sneeze or a cough can be enough to transmit the infection. Smallpox is spread only from person to person, and unlike other diseases such as malaria or bubonic plague, it involves no animal vector. Washington's case was serious but relatively mild compared to those experienced by others in his day. The incubation period for the virus was normally ten to fourteen days. Typically the course of smallpox lasted three to four weeks from the initial fever to the separation of the telltale scabs.

According to his diary, Washington was confined to bed for three weeks, during which time he probably experienced the common symptoms of smallpox, including raging fever, unquenchable thirst, excruciating headache, and backache. This would have been followed by the infamous red sores and often spectacular rash, which in turn would evolve into pustules and scabs, leaving him at least lightly scarred for life. The most a doctor could do for a patient was to provide cold compresses, administer laudanum to dull the pain, and apply generally ineffective ointments for the rash. On the positive side, exposure to the disease also provided Washington with the lifetime immunity to withstand future smallpox epidemics when they ravaged the American colonies.[15]

Washington left Barbados in mid-December of 1751, but Lawrence remained. Unfortunately, the prolonged stay did little to improve Lawrence's health, and he died within the year. Clearly, the contagious nature of tuberculosis was not understood at the time. In nursing his brother, George Washington may have acquired a relatively mild case of pulmonary tuberculosis, which flared up when he returned to Mount Vernon and resulted in uncertain health for years. In May of 1752, at the age of twenty, Washington wrote to the father of a friend, "I was taken with a Violent Pleurisie which has reduced me very low."[16] The use of the word "pleurisy" at the time referred to a wide variety of respiratory ailments, so we cannot determine the exact nature of his illness, but incipient tuberculosis is possible.

Health and Illness on the Battlefield

Washington began his military career in earnest after Lawrence's death, first being appointed an adjutant general of the southern district of Virginia and then being promoted to the rank of major of the Virginia militia with a respectable salary at the age of twenty-one. By 1754, he had become a lieutenant-colonel, fighting on behalf of the British to repel increased French incursions in the area. Unsanitary, crowded conditions made military camps fertile breeding grounds for sickness and disease, and Washington contracted many common illnesses that often passed among the troops. For some time Washington's military fortunes during the French and Indian War waxed and waned, and during this period he suffered several episodes of bloody flux, or dysentery, an intestinal inflammation that produces severe diarrhea. It was often treated with some success by "Dr. James's Powders," a popular concoction of phosphate of lime, antimony, and the by now ubiquitous bark (quinine) introduced by an English physician in 1746 to combat fevers.

That first major bout with debilitating dysentery began in the summer of 1755 and left Washington extremely weak and in so much pain as a result of spasms and hemorrhoids that he could not ride his horse. Due to the illness, under his commander's orders and doctor's advice, Washington was at first left behind in the army camp. Subsequently, the 23-year-old Washington had to be carried by covered wagon to a battle near Fort Duquesne, where he was fortunate to be one of the few survivors of the bloody skirmish commanded by General Edward Braddock that left the French and Indians victorious and the British forces decimated. Washington had two horses shot out from under him and four bullets ripped through his jacket. Because so many of the officers were either wounded or died, Washington was forced to take charge despite his illness. By early July, he wrote optimistically to a friend (prematurely it turned out) that "I have been excessively ill, but am now recovering from violent Fevers & Pains, of wch my disorder consisted."[17]

After the battle Washington recovered at Fort Cumberland, Maryland, and on July 18th he reported the details of the battle and the state of his health to his mother, Mary: "I was not half recovered from a violent illness that had confin'd me to my Bed, and a Waggon, for above 10 Days; I am still in a weak and Feeble condn which induced me to halt here 2 or 3 Days in hopes of recovg a little Strength." Still, his sense of humor remained intact, for on the same day he wrote his brother John Augustine that "[a]s I have heard since my arrivl at this place, a circumstantial acct of my death and dying Speech, I take this early opportunity of contradicting the first, and of assuring you that I have not, as yet, composed the latter."[18]

The effects of Washington's illness lasted for over a month. From the battlefields he returned to Mount Vernon, where he spent nearly a month recuperating. As he reported to a friend in mid-August, "I am happily recover'd from the low ebb to w'ch I was reduced by a sickness of near 5 Weeks continuance."[19] Because of his bravery in battle, Washington developed a reputation as a military hero in the Virginia colony, and as a result, he was appointed commander of the combined Virginia military companies in the summer of 1755. Just two years later, in 1757, he again developed health problems and contracted yet another round of fever and violent dysentery, followed by pleurisy. An army comrade observed that Washington was "seized with stitches and violent pleuritic pains" and that "his strength and vigour diminished so fast."[20]

By November Washington was so weak he could hardly walk, and rumors of his death began to circulate once more. Washington was far from death, but his illness required a long period of recuperation that lasted over four months and prolonged treatment by his personal physician and friend, the Scottish-born and University of Edinburgh trained Dr. James Craik. Craik advised him that "your disorder hath been of long standing and hath corrupted the whole mass of blood,"[21] and in response bled him frequently. Washington had met Craik when the doctor served in a medical capacity in the British-Virginia Army in Pennsylvania, and he persuaded Craik to settle in Alexandria, Virginia, not far from Mount Vernon.[22]

But during the late fall and winter of 1757, Washington's health grew progressively worse, and Craik called in a local irregular medical practitioner, Reverend Charles Green, who prescribed dietary supplements, which included daily "doses" of wine and soft foods. When this regimen brought no relief, Craik, who by then feared for Washington's life, insisted on complete bed rest, but Washington displayed increasingly alarming symptoms, which included a high fever, chest pains, and a severe cough. By that time Washington was worried that he had developed tuberculosis and, unsurprisingly, became somewhat melancholic, or depressed as we would term it today. Given his bravery on the battlefield, it is ironic that anxiety over illness could frighten him so severely.

From a young age, Washington displayed two of his most enduring characteristics, self-control and ambition.[23] Although he possessed a "colossal" temper, for the most part he kept it tamped down, particularly after he assumed the presidency. A recent biographer has even characterized Washington as "a man of granite self-control."[24] These personality traits undoubtedly fueled his political ambitions, but they probably took a toll on his health and perhaps made him more susceptible to sickness.[25] Finally, in 1758 the health tide turned after Washington traveled to Williamsburg to consult Dr. John Amson, whose encouragement perhaps gave him the positive psychological tools with which to fight his combined illnesses. Two years later another bout with dysentery would send Washington home from military duty and back to Mount Vernon for recuperation. His superior at the time, a Colonel Stewart, reported that "[f]or upwards of three months past, Colonel Washington has labored under a bloody flux . . . with bad fevers," for which he was bled,[26] demonstrating once again how often bleeding was used, even in instances where the procedure appears to us today as clearly counterintuitive.

Martha Custis Enters Washington's Life

Although Washington had traveled to Williamsburg for advice about his precarious health, he felt well enough to soon return to his army duties during the French and Indian War. More importantly, while on leave in March he also began courting the charming 27-year-old Martha Dandridge Custis, perhaps the wealthiest widow in Virginia, whom he later married on January 6, 1759. Following his engagement to Martha and back on active military duty, Washington suffered from continued respiratory problems, perhaps a flareup of tuberculosis, and what was clearly a recurrence of dysentery. Washington became so anxious about his intestinal problems that Dr. Craik urged him to leave the army. Ill health and perhaps his perception of a limited future in the British military forced Washington to resign his military commission at the end of 1758, after five years of service, in order to return to full-time plantation life as a country gentleman at Mount Vernon. Soon Washington began to focus on the purchase of land in the West and on developing his farms.

In 1749, at the age of eighteen, the vivacious, petite Martha Dandridge, the daughter of a modestly successful Virginia planter, married the son of a socially prominent and rich landowner, Daniel Parke Custis. Martha's first husband was twenty years her senior, and when he died suddenly in 1757, after eight years of marriage and the birth of their four children, Martha inherited a substantial fortune, which included several large estates. Martha and Daniel's first child was born a year after their marriage. As was the custom during the era, Martha's children were delivered with the assistance of a midwife and female family members. Maternal and infant mortality was high at the time, but the fertile Martha was fortunate in delivering a robust baby boy, Daniel Parke Custis, in 1751, followed by a healthy baby girl named Frances Parke Custis (Fanny) in 1753, another son, John Parke Custis (Jacky) in 1754, and a second daughter in 1756, Martha Parke Custis (Patsy), who would turn out to be her last child. Tragically, the young Daniel died at the age of two of an undetermined fever. His death was a tragic blow for the affectionate young mother and reminds us of the fragility of childhood in colonial America, particularly in the South. One of Martha's recent biographers has observed that the toddler's death turned Martha into an overprotective mother.[27]

Martha's acute anxiety about the health of her children and later her grandchildren was palpable in her correspondence. In 1762, after she left her young son Jacky behind at Mount Vernon during a visit to relatives, she confided to her favorite sister, Nancy (Anna Maria) Bassett, that "I often fancied that he was sick or some accident happened to him."[28] Martha would experience yet another loss when Nancy later died suddenly in 1777 during the Revolutionary War at the age of thirty-eight after several years of ill health. The famous American artist Charles Willson Peale recalled that when he visited the Washingtons in the early 1770s, Patsy Curtis, who was epileptic, "Was subject to fits &

Mrs. Washington never suffered her to be a minute out of her sight."[29] Many years later, when her grandchildren were under her care, Martha wrote her niece Fanny that when her grandson had complained of a minor stomach ache, "I cannot say but it makes me miserable if ever he complains let the cause be ever to trifeling—I hope the almighty will spare him to me."[30]

Over time the ubiquitous presence of disease in eighteenth-century Virginia would prove that Martha had every reason to be concerned about the health of her family: in addition to the death of her eldest child, her older daughter, Frances, died in 1757, shortly before her fourth birthday, the younger daughter, Patsy, as a teenager, and Jacky as a young man in his twenties. Although only a limited number of Martha's letters have survived, those that remain are filled with frequent references to health and sickness, following the same pattern that characterizes the correspondence of Abigail Adams and Dolley Madison. For example, a year after her marriage to Washington, Martha wrote one of her sisters that "I am very sorry to hear my mammas complaints of ill health and I feel the same uneasiness on the account that you doe but hope . . . prescriptions will have the desired effect."[31] The following year, Martha begged off from a visit to her sister because "[t]he hooping coughs has put an end to all hopes for some time. I have had it so bad that I could not go out of the house for this four weeks past, the children are getting well but . . . I considered your little girl had not had it."[32] The letters of the founding mothers reveal the frequency of a variety of illnesses that could turn serious in moments and the pervasive fear of sickness and early death that hovered over all of America's founders and indeed their entire generation. While some of their families were more fortunate than others in regard to health and longevity, none of them escaped tragedies as a result of commonplace diseases.

The summer after Frances's demise, Martha's husband, Daniel, and their small son, Jacky, contracted an illness that probably contributed to Daniel's death at the age of forty-six. When the two ran a fever that did not respond to the usual treatments, she called in Dr. James Carter of Williamsburg. As the mistress of a large plantation Martha assumed the traditional female role of home nursing and was undoubtedly familiar with the herbal and patent medicine remedies she would often be called upon to administer. Indeed, preparing medicines at home was similar to cooking and preparing food.[33] A bill for drugs purchased from Carter's apothecary shop found in Daniel Custis's estate papers and dated November 28, 1757, lists many common medications of the time, including a variety of tonic cordials, rhubarb, often used as a purging laxative, the opium-based laudanum, and the popular emetic ipecac.[34]

Dr. Carter treated the patients conservatively with a honey-based compound rather than bleeding and purging. As was the norm during the colonial era, Martha provided personalized medical care by "watching" over her ill family members, sitting beside them, offering support and comfort, and administering food, drink, and medications.[35] It appears that both father and son suffered from severe throat infections, a condition that could easily be fatal at the time. Jacky survived but Daniel most likely literally suffocated to death as his swollen throat prevented air getting to his lungs. Despite her grief over the loss of a beloved husband, Martha was immediately forced to turn to taking over the responsibilities of the extensive family estates.[36] In a matter-of-fact manner, she wrote an agent of an English firm her husband had utilized that she was taking the "[o]pportunity to inform you of the great misfortune I have met with the loss of my late Husband Mr Custis," and simply proceeded with the business at hand.[37]

Washington's marriage to Martha brought the ambitious Washington the social position he had long craved, but he was also genuinely fond of the lively, attractive widow. Martha and George Washington seem to have been well suited and content in their marriage. While they do not appear to have had the same political and intellectual partnership and deep passion for one another that John and Abigail Adams experienced (Washington is said to have carried a lifelong torch for a young woman he had met earlier, Sally Cary Fairfax), by all accounts George and Martha respected one another and exhibited a loving relationship. Certainly Martha regarded her role as her husband's helpmate and the state of her husband's health as paramount to her happiness. Washington was known to have often extolled the marriage state on the basis of his own happy experience.

Wealthy southern planters often utilized traditional home cures, calling in physicians only for more serious ailments.[38] Like all capable wives at the time, Martha was experienced with treating a wide variety of everyday illnesses with popular contemporary medications, including the bark (quinine) so favored by her husband for fevers and mercury in the form of calomel as a laxative, and she certainly doctored the maladies of Washington's slaves. Medicinal compounds were often supplemented by herbal remedies handed down from generation to generation such as her "famous" cure for pinworms (especially common in the South), which included whiskey, wormseed, rhubarb, and garlic as ingredients.[39] In one of Martha's many letters to her niece Fanny, then the wife of Washington's secretary, Tobias Lear, she offered the opinion that her young great-niece's undiagnosed stomach ailment was caused by intestinal worms. This was a common but fallacious medical belief at the time, and Martha also criticized Fanny for "stuffing" her children with too much food. There is "nothing so pernicious as over charging the stomach of a child—with every kind of food that they will take," she scolded.[40]

The Washington Family

In addition to bringing home cures to her marriage, Martha Custis brought land, money, social status, and the two surviving children of the four she had borne, John Parke (Jacky) and Martha (Patsy) Custis. Washington never fathered any children; perhaps he was sterile as a result of one of his early illnesses. However, he was apparently very fond of children and was certainly disappointed at the lack of offspring from his marriage. Washington treated Martha's children as his own and dutifully oversaw their estates as their legal guardian. He was genuinely heartbroken when Patsy died at the age of sixteen after years of a combination of "fits" or seizures from what was presumably epilepsy, which may also have been compounded by early-stage tuberculosis. The first allusion to Patsy's illness is perhaps a letter Martha wrote to a friend in the fall of 1760 in which she optimistically reported that her "dear little girl is much better she has lost her fits & fevours both and seems to be getting well very fast."[41]

Washington's wide circle of friends had always included physicians, and at least sixty-seven doctors are mentioned in his diaries, including many of the leading medical lights of colonial America, including Dr. Benjamin Rush, Dr. John Morgan, Dr. William Shippen, and his personal physician, Craik. Washington's diary records visits by Dr. William Rumney, who attempted to treat Patsy Custis with a common botanical remedy, valerian, thought to control seizures. Dr. Hugh Mercer, who had received his medical education in Scotland, was also brought in to consult about Patsy's case. Mercer relied heavily on the popular contemporary therapies of bloodletting and purging in an effort to expel the supposed dangerous "blockages" and foreign bodies from Patsy's body that he thought caused the seizures. After the two doctors met, Rumney administered mercury in the form of calomel and a purge. In addition, a local blacksmith was called in to place iron rings on Patsy's fingers in an effort to stop her seizures through what appears to have been an alternative folk remedy, all to no avail.[42]

The following year, in 1769, Washington paid for medical treatment for Patsy from Dr. John de Sequeyra, a prominent Jewish physician of Sephardic descent, and Dr. William Pasteur, who ran an apothecary shop in Williamsburg. Also in 1769 Washington recorded in his diary that "Patcy being taken with a fit on the road by the mill, we turned back."[43] Patsy's condition continued to worsen, and Washington noted over the summer of 1770 that she had frequent seizures, sometimes as often as twice a day. In July 1770, Patsy's epileptic condition was compounded by a severe case of chills and fever that she contracted on a visit to Mary Washington's farm. Dr. Mercer arrived in haste to bleed Patsy and administer medications, and he visited his patient daily for over a week.[44]

A letter from Dr. John Johnson of Maryland to Martha in the spring of 1772 indicated that the physician sent a number of herbal remedies for Patsy's condition, including barley water and a phial of drops "to prevent faintness." Although Johnson's remedies were mild compared to the radical bleeding measures, they too proved ineffective. Still Johnson optimistically observed that "I have the greatest Hopes her Happiness will be much promoted by regular moderate Exercise, temperate living which she may think Abstemiousness and her being attentive to keep her Body cool."[45]

Although Washington showered Martha's daughter with presents to cheer her and spared no expense to seek a cure for Patsy, sadly she died on June 20, 1773. Both Washington and his wife were devastated. Martha wore black mourning for an entire year, and Washington did his best to ease her sorrow. The day following Patsy's death Washington confided to a friend that

[i]t is an easier matter to conceive, than to describe the distress of this Family . . . yesterday removed the Sweet Innocent Girl Entered into a more happy and peaceful abode than any she has met with in the afflicted Path she hitherto has trod. She rose from Dinner about four o'clock in better health and spirits than she appeared to have been in for some time; soon after which she was seized with one of her usual Fits, and expired in it, in less than two minutes without uttering a word, a groan, or a sigh.[46]

Patsy was buried in the family vault in haste because of the sweltering Virginia heat. Her death and the grief her mother and stepfather experienced underscore how helpless parents were at the time when a host of childhood diseases could carry their offspring away without warning. This would be the third of Martha Custis Washington's children who would die in childhood. Patsy's primary illness, probably some form of epilepsy, was poorly understood at the time and carried a stigma, and there was no medication available to control symptoms. Certainly the common treatments of bleeding and purging would have been totally ineffective.

Martha's remaining child, John Parke Custis, nicknamed Jacky, appears to have been a rather feckless young man, but Washington treated him generously. Washington attempted to provide Jacky with a good education and many other advantages when the boy was a child, teenager, and young adult. As Washington wrote Jacky's early tutor, the Reverend Jonathan Boucher, "nothing shall be wanted on my part to aid and assist him." Although Washington had little schooling, he certainly appreciated the benefits of knowledge and reading. Washington informed Boucher that "I conceive a knowledge of books is the basis upon which other knowledge is built,"[47] and indeed much of Washington's expertise about medicine was acquired by studying practical manuals. Although Washington and his wife became very fond of Eleanor (Nelly) Calvert, the daughter of a distinguished family, who became Jacky's fiancée, they initially opposed the marriage of the very young couple; Jacky was only nineteen and his bride sixteen. When they realized Jacky could not be persuaded to delay a wedding, the Washingtons gave in, but Martha, who was still in mourning for her daughter Patsy when Jacky and Nelly were married on February, 3, 1774, did not attend the ceremony.

The marriage helped to steady Jacky, and he was a devoted husband and father to the four children who arrived in quick succession. Washington urged Jacky to bring his young wife and family to Mount Vernon to be company for his wife while he was carrying out military duties. Later, Washington appointed his stepson as an aide de camp during his tenure as commander of the Continental Army in an effort to help Jacky make something of himself. Unfortunately, as the long war at last came to a victorious end for the American and French forces at Yorktown, during the celebrations Martha's son caught one of the many illnesses, probably "camp fever" (typhus), circulating through the crowded army barracks. Washington sent his stepson to Martha's sister and brother-in-law, the Bassetts, to be nursed through what he hoped would be a speedy recovery. However, the young man soon died, leaving a distraught wife, four young children, and a broken-hearted mother.

Martha and Nelly Custis had been at Mount Vernon when they heard that Jacky was seriously ill and traveled as quickly as possible to

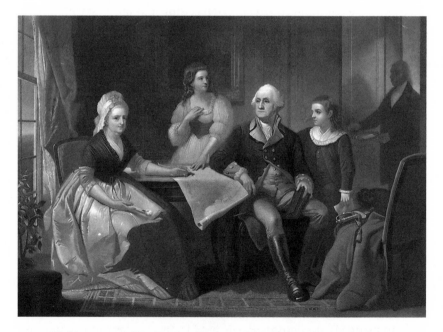

Washington and His Family. George and Martha Washington with grandchildren George Washington Parke Custis and Nelly Custis. (Courtesy Library of Congress)

join him. Washington returned from his victory in the battlefield to visit Jacky but arrived only in time to witness him "breathe his last." John Parke Custis was only twenty-six years old. Martha had now lost the last of her four children to disease, and Washington had certainly thought of both his stepchildren as his own. Subsequently, George and Martha adopted Nelly's two youngest children, Eleanor (Nelly) Parke Custis and George Washington Parke Custis (Wash), and raised them to adulthood.[48] The adoption was driven no doubt by Washington's desire to console Martha for her tragic loss and his own deep affection for the two youngsters, who had often resided for long periods at Mount Vernon. Informal adoption was a common practice at the time, when high mortality rates left many children parentless. Even after Nelly remarried, the two youngest children remained happily with the Washingtons at Mount Vernon, where Martha was in her element successfully nursing them through numerous childhood illnesses, such as measles,[49] which often proved fatal during the era.

Washington as Healer

Medicine continued to play an important part in Washington's life. Like most of the American founders, Washington was very familiar with the medical self-help manuals of the day, and nine medical books graced his library. With the help of his overseers, Washington routinely administered medications and bleeding to his own family and slaves, but called in a physician when necessary for serious ailments on his large plantations. Of course, it was certainly to Washington's economic advantage to keep his slaves in good health, but he seemingly spared no expense to give them the best contemporary treatment available. In 1761, for example, his account lists payment of a year's wages to Dr. James Laurie "for Attendance on all my People in this County,"[50] and he paid a midwife to deliver babies on his estates and called in a surgeon to remove a cataract from the eye of at least one male slave. In 1796, he instructed his overseer that his workers should "want for nothing" in regard to medical attention. As was the case on many large southern plantations, Washington maintained a "hospital" at both Mount Vernon and Fairfax Hall, which served as infirmaries to isolate and treat slaves who were ill, particularly those with infectious diseases, for servants could certainly pass sickness on to the master's immediate family as well as other slaves.[51] Smallpox inoculations were commonly administered to Washington's slaves to prevent them from contracting the dread disease.

In spite of his forward-looking view on smallpox inoculation, however, like most of his contemporaries Washington was also an advocate for the centuries-old heroic measures of bloodletting and purging, sincerely believing that "poisonous" matter in the body had to be evacuated to allow healing. He maintained to one of his plantation overseers that in the case of "pleurisies and all inflammatory disorders accompanied with pain . . . a few days' neglect, or want of bleeding, might render the ailment incurable."[52] At times, he performed the procedure himself on his slaves and liberally administered the popular Peruvian bark for a variety of fevers. When several of his slaves suffered from the effects of lightning that had struck their cabins, he maintained that "with bloodletting they recovered," although it is inconceivable how bleeding could possibly have aided them.[53]

Like most plantations, Mount Vernon was well stocked with herbal remedies and patent medicines such as the cathartics and bark, which contained quinine, to treat malarial fevers. As early as 1759, Washington ordered a large supply of drugs from London, which included not only the ubiquitous jalap and calomel but also rhubarb, laudanum, which was derived from opium and used to relieve pain and aid sleep, smelling salts, and the patent medicine Turlington's Balsam of Life, employed as a preventative tonic health measure.[54] Washington was obviously quite familiar with the use of each medication. He maintained a robust medical kit and placed regular orders for medicinal supplies from the Stabler-Leadbetter Apothecary in Alexandria, Virginia. Like his political contemporaries Jefferson and Franklin, George Washington socialized with a network of physicians, educated himself about medical theory and treatment, and believed in the efficacy of a moderate, balanced, and nutritious diet supplemented by adequate rest and exercise.[55]

Washington's most important contribution to American medicine was in the area of smallpox prevention, and he clearly recognized that there was a beneficial governmental stake in ensuring better health practices. He was an early advocate for smallpox inoculation even prior to his involvement as commander of the army during the Revolutionary War. Unsurprisingly, Washington had railed against early restriction of smallpox inoculation by the Virginia assembly, declaring, "I would rather move for a Law to compel the Masters of Families to inoculate every child born within a certain limited time under Severe Penalties."[56] Washington was apparently prepared to take coercive measures for the sake of public health and would have probably resisted the later popular backlash against mandatory state smallpox vaccination legislation that developed in the late nineteenth and early twentieth century.[57]

In 1760, when Washington was informed that some of the slaves on his Frederick County estate had been stricken with smallpox, he quickly traveled to join them, hired a nurse to look after them, and took precautions to prevent the disease from spreading. As with Jefferson, it is likely that Washington eventually personally inoculated all his own slaves, or at least supervised the procedure. He believed that if proper precautions were taken in diet and preparations, inoculation was both safe and effective. On one occasion Washington observed that "my own People (not less I suppose than between two and three hundred), getting happily through it by following these directions, is no Inconsiderable proof of it."[58]

It is likely that Washington was such a strong advocate of disease prevention and of actively fighting sickness because of his own experience with illness. Over the next years as a member of the Virginia House of Burgesses, in which he served from 1759 to 1774, and as a prosperous gentry-class plantation owner, Washington would continue to experience episodes of serious illness. In 1761, he may have contracted typhoid fever or, more likely, a recurrence of his almost chronic malaria, which once again made him fear his end was near. The resultant fever and weakness left him restricted from his normal activities for the better part of a year. In early summer Martha wrote a friend that her husband "took his vomit—but it did not worke him well today he has begun with the Barke [quinine] & continues it until an ounce is taken."[59] As we have seen, bark was a common treatment for many fevers at the time, but was really only effective for malaria. The next month Washington informed a friend that "I am more than half of the mind to take a trip to England for the recovery of that invaluable blessing—health,"[60] a plan he failed to carry out.

Despite a visit to the Blue Ridge Mountains and Warm Springs for the reputed benefits of water therapy, Washington remained ill for

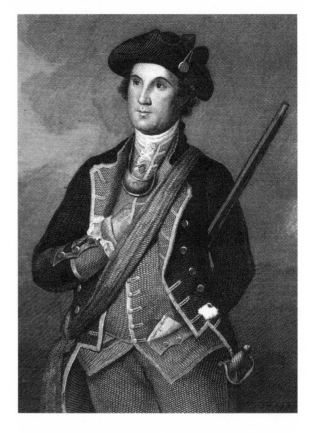

George Washington, 1772. (Courtesy U.S. National Library of Medicine)

about six months and consulted several doctors, including Dr. Rumney, about his troubling state of health. Washington made his first trip to visit the famed mineral springs when he was just sixteen and traveled there again two years later in the company of his ill brother, Lawrence. In 1761, writing from Warm Springs, Washington informed Dr. Charles Green that "[w]e found of both sexes about 250 People at this place, full of all manner of diseases & Complaints; some of which are much benefitted, while others find no relief from the Water's," the latter describing Washington's overall experience, although his initial fever retreated after only one day at the resort.[61] However, in October Washington reported, "I have in appearance been very near my last gasp . . . I fell into a very low and dangerous State . . . but thank God I have now got the better of the disorder and shall soon be restord I hope to perfect health again."[62] Washington finally recovered, but malaria would

be a recurrent challenge in the future. Revolution, however, was looming, and even malaria could stop neither the insurrectionist fever that
afflicted the colonies nor the man who would become commander of
the Continental Army.

Warrior Healer

Although Washington had a long history as a loyal Englishman, repres-
sive British policy in the American colonies gradually turned him into
a revolutionary. He served as a delegate to the Continental Congress in
1774-1775 before being appointed by that body to head the military. Even
in this capacity, Washington's concern for health matters was evident
from the first; one of his first acts as commander-in-chief was to urge
Congress to establish the Medical Department of the Continental Army.

In retrospect, Washington's having contracted smallpox as a teenager
would prove to be a blessing in disguise when he took command of the
army on July 2, 1775. At the time the disease was already wending its
grim path through New England. In light of Washington's medical history, he experienced surprisingly good health during the Revolutionary
War, other than an episode in 1777 when the army wintered at Mor-
ristown, where he contacted a throat infection (quinsy) that left him
weak. The symptoms of this ten-day illness were soothed by a decoction
of molasses and onions solicitously provided by Martha, who had dutifully accompanied her husband to the battlefield camps while he served
as commander. Beginning in 1775, Martha left Mount Vernon to join
her husband annually at his military winter quarters, although she was
generally housed in superior locations at nearby farmhouses. Martha
had always been solicitous of her husband's and children's health and
was frequently torn between family responsibilities back at Mount Vernon and taking her place at her husband's side. However, even under
the most adverse conditions during the eight long years of war, she not
only watched over Washington but personally knitted and sewed for
the troops and nursed the wounded, providing moral support, comfort,
and cheer to the officers and soldiers.[63]

Martha Washington was by no means the only woman who ventured
near the battlefields. Wives of army officers sometimes found hous-
ing near their husbands, and public-minded revolutionary-era women

often tended to sick soldiers and even housed those undergoing small-pox inoculation. Local women also took jobs as nurses and administered medications, attended to the hygiene of "hospitalized" men, and cleaned up after sick patients for meager pay.[64] Martha tended her husband solicitously and later, in 1780, became ill herself while Washington's headquarters were located in New Windsor, New York. Suffering from jaundice and a painful gall bladder attack, she was forced to postpone her planned return to Mount Vernon and spent over a month in bed.[65]

Many of the American soldiers were from the Boston area, but smallpox would soon ignite, threatening the Continental Army up and down the East Coast during the early days of the Revolutionary War. From the start, Washington realized the strong probability of the pestilence spreading among his troops, causing severe illness and death and potentially derailing the fight for independence. He also appears to have had a fairly sophisticated and advanced grasp of public health measures for his era. In his General Orders of July 4, 1775, issued from Cambridge, Massachusetts, Washington emphasized the need for sanitation and that officers were "required and expected to pay diligent Attention to keep their Men neat and clean . . . and inculcate upon them the necessity of cleanliness, as essential to health and service." He ordered that no soldiers be allowed out of camp to go fishing, as he believed "that there may be danger of introducing the small pox into the army."[66] Washington feared that men mingling with Boston citizens might be infected with the epidemic, and he took the threat seriously, introducing sensible measures to reduce contagion.

In a letter written to the president of the American Congress a little over two weeks later he reported, "I have been particularly attentive to the least Symptoms of the Small Pox, hitherto we have been so fortunate, as to have every Person removed so soon, as not only to prevent any Communication, but any Apprehension of Alarm it might give in the Camp. We shall continue the utmost Vigilance against this most dangerous enemy."[67] By December 1775, Washington declared, "If we escape the smallpox in this camp, and the country around about, it will be miraculous." But confronted both with the dangers that could arise from inoculation itself as well as the real threat active smallpox posed for his troops, Washington initially concluded that "variolation was simply too risky," and from his second day as commander, he placed the major emphasis on prevention and strict quarantine when warranted.[68] In early July 1776, Washington still maintained that "if proper precautions are taken, the small-pox may be prevented from spreading."[69]

Smallpox was one of the most feared diseases of the eighteenth century. In the spring of 1776, it wreaked havoc on the American army and killed more soldiers than combat. Smallpox was a camp follower, finding fertile ground for infection during war. As an age-old popular axiom stated, "Where soldiers go, plagues follow." At its peak, smallpox spread like wildfire through the weakened soldiers and crowded army camps, leaving death and devastation in its wake. Many of the army recruits came from rural areas, where they had never been exposed to smallpox, making them especially vulnerable.

As commander, Washington had seen first-hand the tragic effect on both the civilian and the military population, prompting him to urge his wife, Martha, to undergo smallpox inoculation, advice that she finally followed in 1776 in Philadelphia. Washington wrote his brother John from Philadelphia that "Mrs. Washington is now under Innoculation in this City; and will, I expect, have the Small pox favourably, this is the 13th day, and she has very few Pustules; she would have wrote to my Sister but thought it prudent not to do so, notwithstanding there could be but little danger in conveying the Infection in this manner."[70] Martha underwent a three-week quarantine following the procedure, and Washington remained with her for about a week to keep her company in the rooms they had secured in a local lodging inn. Washington's letter demonstrates his familiarity with the course of inoculation versus contracting smallpox the "natural" way. It also reveals the practice at the time of smoking letters to make sure the illness could not be spread through correspondence. Martha's inoculation was successful, and her son Jacky soon wrote to congratulate his mother on the news that "[y]ou were in so fair a Way of getting favorable through the Smalpox:—the small Danger attending that Disorder by Inoculation when the patients follow the Directions of their Physician, has relieved me from much Anxiety."[71]

Long a strong supporter of the controversial smallpox procedure, Washington had previously had his stepson Jacky inoculated in the spring of 1771 in Baltimore without Martha's permission, as she had anxiously blocked an earlier attempt before the young man left for a trip to Europe. However, Martha's own success with inoculation made her more amenable to the procedure and ultimately led her to oversee the inoculation of two of her young nephews in 1777 at Mount Vernon. "I have the very great pleasure of returning,—you your Boys as well as they were when I brought them from Eltham," Martha wrote her sister Nancy. "They have had the smallpox exceedingly light."[72] Sadly, less than a month later Nancy Bassett died suddenly after years of lingering illness.

While Martha handled the inoculation of the family, Washington had to deal with the smallpox issue on a grand scale. Despite his early optimism, neither smallpox prevention nor quarantine had worked effectively among his troops. In 1777 alone, more than one hundred thousand people in North America died as a result of virulent smallpox epidemics. In an effort to halt the spread of the disease, Washington made the controversial decision to have all his soldiers inoculated in that year, which helped sustain the force for the rest of the Revolutionary War. In January, he declared to Dr. William Shippen, then the medical director of the Continental Army, that "[w]e should have more to dread from it [smallpox] than from the Sword of the Enemy."[73] In April, John Adams echoed Washington's thoughts when he wrote his wife, Abigail, that "Disease has destroyed Ten Men for Us where the Sword of the Enemy has killed one." Adams also expressed his hope that the situation would improve as "We have at last, determined a plan for the Sick, and have called into Service the best abilities in Physick and Chirurgery [surgery], that the Continent affords."[74] In his role as commander of the forces, Washington was able to wield his governmental designated powers to mandate health intervention when he felt it benefited the public good. As we will see in future chapters, this was a philosophy that was shared by Franklin, Adams, Jefferson, and Madison.

Still, just weeks later, Washington wavered before the daunting task of inoculating the soldiers en masse, fearing that those undergoing the procedure might spread the pestilence even further. In early February, influenced by Dr. John Morgan, the physician in chief of the American armies, Washington made a final decision to move forward as "[t]he small pox has made such Head in every Quarter that I find it impossible to keep it from spreading thro' the whole Army in the natural way. I have therefore determined, not only to inoculate all the Troops now here, that have not had it, but shall order Docr Shippen to inoculate the Recruits as fast as they come in to Philadelphia."[75] An American congressional commission sent periodic updates on the war to Benjamin Franklin, then in France on behalf of the new American government, and they expressed their satisfaction over the mass inoculation initiated by Washington. Many American leaders, including Franklin and Washington, had shared the unfounded belief that the British deliberately spread the disease to the Continental Army as a strategic measure. The commissioners reported that "[o]ur Troops have been under inoculation from the Small Pox with great success. . . . It will frustrate a Cannibal Scheme of our Enemies who have constantly fought us with that disease by introducing it among our troops."[76]

Although many soldiers were inoculated under Washington's strict orders, it is apparent that a good number also slipped through the cracks, for in the winter of 1777-1778 Washington discovered that three to four thousand of his troops had not undergone the procedure. By January 1778, the campaign to remedy the situation was in full swing. Washington's early involvement in public health resulted in major benefits to the emerging nation. According to historian Elizabeth A. Fenn, who has chronicled the great smallpox epidemics that ravaged America from 1775 to 1782, "Washington's unheralded and little-recognized resolution to inoculate the Continental forces must surely rank among his most important decisions of the war." Moreover, Washington's decision for mass inoculation within the army reflects the first "large-scale, state-sponsored immunization campaign in American history,"[77] making Washington a key player in early American public health endeavors.

Of course, smallpox was far from the only disease that swept through the Continental Army. Crowded conditions in barracks and poor nutrition and sanitation made camps a hospitable environment for illness. Spring saw a rise in throat and respiratory infections, including diphtheria, scarlet fever, pleurisy, and pneumonia, and summer brought another host of diseases that thrived in the heat, such as malaria and dysentery. During the war, the Continental Army was only allotted three hundred pounds of quinine. Many soldiers who were infected with malaria made do with ineffective medicines that left them sick and therefore a source of infection for spreading the parasite that caused the illness.[78] Typhus, which was transmitted by infected lice, venereal diseases, the troublesome skin irritations of scabies, typhoid, and rheumatic fevers that developed into strep infections lurked in army camps as well. Treatments reflected contemporary medical practices, which emphasized purging, bloodletting, bracing diets, and rest. Although soldiers were isolated in medical hospitals for some diseases, common coughs, colds, and sore throats were not considered contagious and so spread rapidly through the barracks.[79]

As we have seen, as a plantation owner Washington was well acquainted with contemporary medical health manuals and had often overseen the medical treatment of his family and slaves. Of course, Washington professed a number of outlandish ideas about illness that circulated in popular and medical circles, such as his advocacy of bleeding for most diseases and the belief that dysentery was caused by new cider. However, he was forward thinking about sources of contagion. He was particularly attuned to the role poor hygiene and nutrition played in the transmission of disease within an army, and he emphasized the need for cleanliness, proper medical care, and a diet that gave vegetables, vinegar, and hearty grains precedence over animal products.

As we will learn in chapter 4, like Jefferson, Washington disliked the use of tobacco, often drank wine socially but not to excess, and advocated moderate eating and adequate rest. When he was not under acute military or political pressure, he attempted to get to sleep by eight o'clock nightly. Washington issued numerous orders and directives aimed at the prevention of disease and the promotion of good health among his troops. In his General Orders of July 14, 1775, the meticulous Washington maintained that "[n]ext to Cleanliness, nothing is more conducive to a Soldiers health, than dressing his provisions in a decent and proper manner."[80] Casualties were to be treated in camp or regimental hospitals by an adequate contingent of army doctors, most of them apprentice-trained rather than university medical school graduates at the time. In addition, camps were to be swept daily and clean clothes, bedding straw, and adequate latrines were considered essential, if not always attainable.

Contrary to Washington's high expectations, the medical department of the Continental Army was often disorganized, despite the efforts of Philadelphian Dr. John Morgan, a protégé of Benjamin Franklin and a graduate of Edinburgh's medical school, who was selected by Congress to serve as the second medical director of the Continental Army.[81] Moreover, fellow Philadelphian and patriot Dr. Benjamin Rush encouraged colonial army doctors to keep camps clean, make sure the soldiers bathed and changed clothes regularly, and ensure that plates and silverware were washed thoroughly after each use. At his own expense, Rush printed an instruction manual for medical officers outlining his recommendations. Despite Washington's goal of setting up encampments in "healthy" areas away from swamps and other "miasmatic" locations, circumstances often dictated camp sites in less than optimum areas. Scurvy was rampant, and with food scarcities during the winter at Valley Forge, for example, the ability to provide fresh fruit and vegetables was practically nonexistent.[82]

Health and Illness in Peacetime

Although Washington stayed remarkably healthy during the Revolutionary War, he still remained worried about, almost fixated on, his many recurrent illnesses. In 1784, at only fifty-two years of age, he pessimistically informed his fellow patriot the Marquis de Lafayette that "I have asked myself as our carriages separate whether that was the last sight I would ever have of you, and though I wanted to answer no, my fears answer yes."[83] Finally, after eight stressful years of war and peace negotiations, with Martha beside him for a total of five, in late December 1783 General Washington was able to return home to his beloved Mount Vernon. The war had aged him considerably, and he found his mansion in disrepair and his finances in disarray. Now a revolutionary hero, he hoped to quietly retire to a tranquil private life of farming and hosting visits for relatives and friends, surrounded by his restructured little family, which now included Martha's two youngest grandchildren and Fanny Bassett, the daughter of her deceased sister, Nancy.

As Washington grew older, he succumbed to many of the not uncommon effects of aging and eventually required full dentures as well as spectacles for deteriorating vision.[84] Diseased and infected gums and teeth, a common ailment at the time before the development of advances in dental care, may have contributed to Washington's uneven health during his lifetime. He began losing his teeth in his midtwenties and did what he could to treat toothaches and sore gums privately at home, a subject mentioned frequently in his diary. His first tooth was probably extracted in 1754, and despite visits to a number of dentists over the years, Washington ultimately lost all his teeth; when he was inaugurated in 1789, only one of his own teeth remained. It was a subject that made him very self-conscious, as he was always very meticulous about his appearance, and he did his utmost to keep the details of his dental problems from the public. Over time, Washington resorted to numerous animal-based teeth and dentures created by the dental practitioners, including some made out of whalebone, elephant ivory, and even walrus tusks that were gold plated. These teeth were combined with a wire dental apparatus to anchor them, and at least one set utilized springs to assist in chewing. One biographer has suggested that Washington even attempted an aborted early dental "transplant," using human teeth he had purchased. They were to have been implanted discreetly by a prominent French dentist, Dr. Jean-Pierre Le Mayeur, who was a supporter of the American Revolution.[85]

Of those who carved dentures for Washington, the famous American artist Charles Willson Peale was probably the most well known, and he produced a set made with cows' teeth anchored in leaden plates. We can only speculate that lead poisoning might have played a part in Washington's many bouts with illness. Difficulty and pain in chewing must have affected his enjoyment of food. John Greenwood from Connecticut had been a soldier in Washington's army, and he produced several sets of dentures for his war hero, including the first in 1789 and the last set Washington wore before he died in 1799.[86]

In addition to dental problems, Washington suffered weaknesses with vision as he aged. As we will see in the next chapter, Washington's fellow patriot Benjamin Franklin, whose ingenious invention of bifocals aided countless Americans, often dispensed glasses for himself and family members. It appears that Washington was also resourceful in acquiring visual aids. During the Revolutionary War, when his eyesight began to deteriorate at the age of forty-six, he tried on the glasses of many army officers stationed at Newburgh until he found the pair that suited him best. He then sent a request to David Rittenhouse of Philadelphia to fill the "prescription." Another infirmity that arrived with age was arthritis, which often was referred to under the vague general name of "rheumatism." Washington suffered a debilitating case of what may have been an episode of rheumatoid arthritis in 1787, when pain in his arms prevented him from moving them above the level of his shoulders.[87]

Despite physical setbacks, the Washingtons became famous for their lavish hospitality after George returned from war, and Mount Vernon soon came to resemble a hotel. Fanny joined the Washington household at the age of fifteen in 1784, and became a beloved surrogate daughter to Martha. The following year Fanny wed Washington's favorite nephew, George Augustine Washington, who suffered from tuberculosis and would die before his thirtieth birthday.[88]

The contagious nature of tuberculosis was not understood at the time, as demonstrated by the fact that the ill George Augustine was allowed to marry Fanny and undertake the taxing job of managing Washington's plantations. Over the next several years George Augustine became debilitated by "consumption," as tuberculosis was also known, and so weakened by lung hemorrhages that he was confined to bed for months before he died in 1793. With Augustine's passing, Martha and George Washington had lost yet another family member who was dear to them. In a letter of condolence to Fanny, Martha admitted, "Tho we were prepared to expect the event by every letter from you—yet we were much shocked to hear that our dear Friend was no more."[89]

Washington's nephew and heir apparent left three small children as well as his young wife, Fanny, who had contracted the wasting disease from her husband. As early as 1788, Martha alluded to Fanny's condition in a letter in which she remarked that "Fanny returned much better of the cough, and a good deal better in health than when she went over the mountains; but not perfectly recovered."[90] Fanny passed away from tuberculosis just three years after George Augustine in 1796, after a brief marriage of less than a year to Tobias Lear. Lear had arrived at Mount Vernon in 1786 as a tutor to the Custis children and became Washington's personal secretary and a close family friend. In the eighteenth century, tuberculosis frequently struck young men and women in their twenties, in the prime of life. Prior to the introduction of an effective antibiotic "cocktail" in the 1940s, it was primarily treated with rest, fresh air, and travel to mountain areas, such as the trip Fanny undertook.[91] Until the mid-twentieth century, tuberculosis was one of the leading causes of death in America, and as we have seen the Washington family appears to have been particularly susceptible to the disease.

Despite personal losses, Martha Washington was in her element back at Mount Vernon, entertaining family and friends and nursing family members when the occasion arose, although she was still plagued from time to time by stomach ailments. The gregarious couple enjoyed many guests at their beautiful home. Mt. Vernon was often updated with improvements and filled with expensive, tasteful furnishings and works of art that befitted a plantation owner of means, but the purchases would eventually strain Washington's finances. In the beginning of 1784, Martha wrote a friend, "My little family are all with me; and have been very well till with in these few days, that they have been taken with the measles.—the worst I hope is over."[92] The couple spent several contented years back at Mount Vernon. However, as we learned, during that period Washington also suffered several health setbacks, including malarial flareups, and dental, vision, and hearing problems. Amid these ailments, he received with mixed feelings the news that he had been named to head the Virginia delegation to the upcoming 1787 convention in Philadelphia that would produce a new constitution. Ultimately, Washington decided to attend, persuaded by friends and his determination to improve on the weaknesses of the Articles of Confederation.

Another bout of malaria in the summer of 1786 brought the telltale fever and chills and required the attention of Dr. Craik, who treated Washington with yet another course of bark. Later in the year inflammations produced by rheumatism resulted in pains in the arms and shoulders that reduced Washington's mobility and required him to wear a sling, and a few years later he contracted pneumonia, one of the common respiratory illnesses that frequently plagued early Americans.[93] In April of 1787, Washington learned that his mother, Mary, was suffering from breast cancer and that his sister, Betty, was critically ill, and he rushed to see them; fortunately both recovered from the immediate crisis. In early 1788, Washington's favorite brother, John Augustine, died suddenly of what Washington referred to as "a fit of gout in the head,"[94] probably a stroke. Martha's family losses also continued to mount. That year both her 75-year-old mother, Frances Dandridge, and her 48-year-old brother, Judge Bartholomew Dandridge, died in the same month, leaving her with only one surviving sibling, her sister Betsy.

To Lead a Healthy New Nation

Under psychological and political stress, Washington left for the Philadelphia convention accompanied by a troubling headache and stomach pains. The former Revolutionary War commander was welcomed warmly by a crowd of admirers and set about his responsibility as a delegate with his customary seriousness and sense of purpose. To no one's surprise, Washington was elected president of the august political gathering, as age and illness had put Franklin, his only serious competitor, out of the running. A quiet but determined supporter of the Constitution, Washington presided over the convention when the pivotal document was unanimously adopted on September 17, 1787. The satisfaction and relief he felt must have improved Washington's mental outlook and stamina, because a visitor to Mount Vernon in October observed, "He is in perfect health and looks almost as well as he did twenty years ago."[95]

Washington had emerged from the protracted Revolutionary War as a popular American and even international hero, so it was not surprising that he was virtually unanimously elected to the nation's highest office. However reluctant Washington was to once again exchange private life for public service, he felt compelled to accept the call to duty and was inaugurated as America's first president on April 30, 1789. Placing the public good above personal interest was an axiom all the founders viewed as critical to the health of the republic. As president, Washington was decisive, dignified, discreet, and civil, even to those with whom he disagreed, but often sensitive to criticism.[96] Martha Washington was even more reluctant than her husband to leave Mount Vernon, but accompanied by her two grandchildren she arrived in New York City several weeks after the ceremonies and became a noted local hostess and supportive partner to her husband.

During the early days of Washington's presidency, when New York City was the seat of the American government, the aging leader became critically ill when he developed an inflamed tumor, or "malignant carbuncle," on his thigh. It was so tender that it made sitting painful, and it was first mistakenly diagnosed as a cutaneous form of anthrax. In reality it probably began as a form of staph infection and developed into a fast-growing abscess that troubled him for three months before it was excised successfully, albeit painfully and without anesthesia, by his physician, Dr. Samuel Bard. Washington's recovery was protracted—six weeks of lying in bed—and so serious that his wife and doctors feared for his life for a time. During his illness, total quiet was recommended, and carriages were banned from traveling on the street outside the president's mansion. Washington appears to have demonstrated his usual stoic yet pessimistic outlook in the face of illness. At one point after he finally healed, Washington alluded to what he believed was his impending demise: "The Want of regular exercise with the cares of office will, I have no doubt, hasten my departure for that country from whence no traveler returns."[97]

Bard had been a Loyalist sympathizer during the war but was then the most prominent and respected physician in New York City. Due to the seriousness of his condition, Washington utilized Bard's expensive professional services because of the doctor's reputation as an outstanding medical man. The combined fees of the university-trained Samuel Bard and his well-known physician father, John Bard, who visited Washington many times at his Manhattan home on Cherry Street, totaled about eighty-four pounds for a three-and-a-half-month period, a princely sum at a time when skilled artisans in London were receiving yearly wages between fifty-five and sixty pounds. When John Bard moved to New York from Philadelphia in 1745, Franklin had described him as "an ingenious Physician and Surgeon."[98] Samuel Bard had graduated from King's College, today's Columbia University, and like so many aspiring colonial doctors, he had traveled to Europe to further his medical education. Bard received his medical degree from the University of Edinburg in the 1760s, as had many of America's leading doctors, including Dr. Rush. Washington's ailment proved to have been an infected abscess rather than a malignancy as all the symptoms, including the high fever and pain Washington had been experiencing, receded after the procedure.[99]

Washington was laid up for six weeks, mostly lying prone on his right side in bed or on a couch to take the pressure off the incision area, but he still managed to project a calm and dignified demeanor to visitors. When he was able to finally venture out for short excursions in his coach, it had to be refitted to allow him to recline. In June, James Madison reported to Jefferson that "[t]he President has been *ill*. His fever terminated in a large anthrax on the upper end of his thigh, which is likely to confine him for some time."[100] Finally, in July Washington was able to report with some relief that "I have my health restored but a feebleness still hangs upon me, and I am yet much incommoded by the incision which was made in a very large and painful tumor on the protuberance of my thigh."[101]

Not long after Washington recovered, his mother, Mary, died at the ripe old age for the time of eighty-one on August 25, 1789. At least

outwardly he appeared to be little affected by the event, other than donning mourning apparel. It is noteworthy that in 1791 a milder version of
the "tumor" on Washington's thigh reoccurred. Secretary of State Jefferson reported to Madison, "The President is indisposed with the same
blind tumour, and in the same place, which he had the year before last
in New York."[102] It was treated in a similar manner to the first, by lancing and draining, once again causing a bout with fever and discomfort
that necessitated rest and again caused Washington some concern over
his lifelong alternations between robust health and serious illness.

Washington had undertaken a regimen of exercise to help promote
his health once his thigh healed, and he must have looked forward to
traveling to Massachusetts in the fall of 1789 in an effort to keep his
finger on the pulse of the nation. However, soon after he recuperated
Washington contracted first an eye infection in the form of conjuncti-
vitis and then pleurisy after an official visit to Boston. The latter turned
out to be part of the influenza epidemic affecting New England at the
time, and it was nicknamed "Washington's flu" in his honor. Fortunately, Washington soon returned to good health, and Franklin, who
greatly admired Washington, sent the president his "affectionate con-
gratulations on the recovery."[103] By the end of 1789, Martha was able
to report that "[t]he Presidents health is quite reestablished by his late
journey—mine is much better than it used to be."[104]

Now that they were in their fifties, some of Washington's and Martha's health issues were simply a reflection of aging, and they were
certainly considered elderly according to the life-expectancy statistics of the era. In 1791, Martha wrote plaintively to her niece Fanny
that although her own immediate family was well, "God only knows
wheather—I shall ever be in tolerable health again." Still, she remained
cheerful and concerned about others. In response to the news that Fanny's son was unwell, she offered the common but naïve advice espoused
by contemporary medical folk wisdom that "[w]orms is the cause of
all complaints in children."[105] Both the president and his first lady, now
grey-haired and with diminished hearing, also required strong reading
glasses for all types of close work, and Washington was wont to complain that his memory was failing. Martha also appears to have been
experiencing her share of dental problems as in the spring of 1794 she
requested that "Mrs Washington will be much obliged to Mr Whitelock

to make for her a set of teeth—to make them something bigger and thicker in the front and a small matter longer. She will be very glad if he will do them as those she has is almost broak."[106]

In the spring of 1790, just before the nation's capital was moved from New York to Philadelphia, Washington contracted yet another serious illness. In early April he recorded simply in his diary that he was "[a]t home all day—unwell,"[107] and friends and family noted his overall uncertain health. A generally lowered resistance may have made him unusually susceptible to the influenza epidemic that was winding through New York, and he even may have contracted the sickness through a visit by Madison, who had recently been taken ill. By May 9th Washington noted that he was "[i]ndisposed with a bad cold."[108] However, his health soon worsened and the cold turned into influenza compounded by pneumonia, with attendant high fever, blood in his sputum, and delirium, and even his hearing and eyesight were adversely affected. Once again, the president feared his end was near and the following month wrote, "I have already within less than a year had two severe attacks, the last worse than the first, a third, more than probably, will put me to sleep with my fathers."[109]

Several physicians, including Dr. Samuel Bard, were called in to treat Washington. Most notably, Dr. John Jones of Philadelphia was summoned amid much secrecy, most probably not to alarm American citizens about the president's precarious state of health. Jones, who had studied in Europe and received his medical degree from the University of Rheims, was Franklin's doctor at the time. Jones later served as the Washingtons' family physician once the seat of American government moved to Philadelphia.[110]

Washington's illness was so severe that not only the president and his wife but also his doctors and many in the government and public felt his days were numbered. One senator among the many well wishers to the president's home observed that "[e]very eye [was] full of tears. His life despaired of."[111] Jefferson articulated the concern of the nation at the peak of Washington's illness when he reported that the president had been "pronounced by two of the three physicians present to be in the act of death. . . . You cannot conceive of the public alarm on this occasion. It proves how much depends on his life."[112] Vice president John Adams and his wife, Abigail, worried that without Washington the fragile unity of the young nation might collapse, leaving an unprepared Adams to step in and fill the breach.[113] However, in mid-May, after reaching a "crisis," Washington began sweating profusely and his fever broke. On the mend, he was advised to take a break from work and exercise, but the conscientious president was determined to continue his duties. In June, with his health improved and finally influenced by the advice to get away, the president felt well enough to share a three-day fishing trip to Sandy Hook, Long Island, with his secretary of state, Jefferson. After a lengthy convalescence in Newport, Rhode Island, characterized by both good and bad days, once again Washington rallied and made a full recovery.[114]

For Martha, Washington's dangerous and life-threatening illness had been a period of intense worry. Once her husband was on the road to recovery in June, she expressed her relief in a letter to her good friend Mercy Otis Warren, a noted patriot and historian who was active in political circles and was the wife of the former paymaster of the Continental Army. "The sevear illness with which the President was attacked some weeks ago absorbed every other consideration, in my care and anxiety for him," she confessed to Mrs. Warren.

> During the President's sickness, the kindness which everybody manifested, and the interest which was universally taken in his fate, were really very affecting to me. He seemed less concerned himself to the event than any other person in ye united states. Happily he is now perfectly recovered and I am restored to my ordinary state of tranquility, and usually good flow of spirits.[115]

In 1790, the nation's capital was relocated, and Martha Washington once again packed up her household to move from New York City to Philadelphia, then America's largest city. Philadelphia at that time was a cosmopolitan, bustling urban center, and the new temporary center of the American government. Despite her numerous obligations as first lady, Martha still fretted about the health of her extended family and most of all about that of her husband, but President Washington appeared to have regained at least some of his strength and energy.

George Washington's serious illness and the pressures of public office had worn him down, and he missed the invigorating outdoor life of Mount Vernon. In early 1791 Senator William Maclay of Pennsylvania described Washington as being "pale . . . almost cadaverous," slow in movement, and remarked that his dentures disturbed his speech, making it "hollow and indistinct." By 1792 Washington had confided to Madison that he felt he might be unfit for the vicissitudes of his administration, which included the growing acrimonious divisions between the Federalists and Republicans and the political fallout from the French Revolution, as his own health was "becoming more sensibly infirm."[116] Certainly the increasing disagreements among Washington's cabinet members, most notably Hamilton and Jefferson, did nothing to ease Washington's mental stress.

However, health issues on a larger scale for the nation's temporary capital would soon appear on the horizon during Washington's second term. Disease again impacted his political life during Philadelphia's terrible yellow fever epidemic of 1793, which as we learned in the introduction began its grim and relentless march in August. Not long before the outbreak, in June, Washington appears to have had a recurrence of malaria. Jefferson reported to Madison that "[t]he President is not well. Little lingering fevers have been hanging about him for a week or ten days, and have affected his looks most remarkably."[117] Washington's familiar indisposition passed, but a significant number of his close acquaintances soon fell ill with the much more serious disease, and as the yellow fever epidemic spread it would impact not only the personal plans of the Washingtons but also those of the young American government. As Washington himself observed, under the threat of disease the government was brought to a virtual standstill, and the office of the president was "[i]n a manner blockaded by the disorder."[118]

Soon all Philadelphia residents, not just those in politics, became acutely aware of the disease, which struck the rich, poor, and prominent political figures indiscriminately. Both Alexander Hamilton, secretary of the treasury at the time, and his wife, Elizabeth, contracted yellow fever but fortunately recovered. Washington made Hamilton a get well gift of six bottles of fine wine, and Martha sent a note to assure the couple that "[t]he President joins me in devoutly wishing Colo Hamilton's recovery."[119] Washington ignored the threats of contagion to his own person and continued carrying out his presidential responsibilities. Clearly Washington felt it was his duty to remain in the nation's capital, but by September 10th a local newspaper reported that "[t]his morning, the PRESIDENT of the United States, set out from town, for Mount Vernon." Although Washington customarily left for Virginia in the fall, that fateful year he set out early, both in an effort to outdistance the sickness and stymied by the lack of governmental workers with whom to run an effective administration. As we have seen, even Washington's political right hand, Hamilton, had been temporarily felled by yellow fever. Washington may have used his wife as a justification for leaving town, informing Lear that

> [i]t was my wish to have continued there longer, but as Mrs. Washington was unwilling to leave me surrounded by the malignant fever wch. prevailed, I could not think of hazarding her and the Children any longer by *my* continuance in the City the house in which we lived being, in a manner, blockaded by the disorder and was becoming every day more and more fatal.[120]

Before he departed Philadelphia, Washington left instructions with his secretary of war, General Henry Knox, to keep him updated on the progress of the yellow fever epidemic and expressed the wish that "you and yours, may escape untouched and, when we meet again, that it may be under circumstances more pleasing than the present." The Washingtons left the city after a short visit with Jefferson, who would soon be following suit and leaving for Monticello. Because of pending foreign affairs, Washington planned only an absence of a few weeks from Philadelphia, but as the yellow fever continued to rage until it gradually disappeared with the advent of colder weather in late November, he postponed his departure from Mount Vernon for a month and a half. During this period, the American government was in disarray, and Washington began to consult Hamilton, Jefferson, and others as to whether Congress could be convened in another place than the official capital. Most of his advisers, including Jefferson, Madison, and Attorney General Edmond Randolph, replied that it was not in the president's constitutional powers to change the venue for Congress.[121]

Although the epidemic continued, Washington again ignored the personal dangers and undertook a convoluted coach journey to Germantown, Pennsylvania, six miles northwest of Philadelphia, where he settled himself temporarily while awaiting the end of the epidemic and the subsequent return of Congress. Jefferson met up with him in Baltimore, and the two men traveled together to Germantown in November and worked together on government business. In October Washington had reported to Madison that Philadelphia was "almost depopulated by removals and deaths."[122] He projected that Congress would be able to meet as scheduled in early December, when it was hoped the epidemic would be a memory of the past. In early November Washington surreptitiously left for Philadelphia and personally inspected the streets on horseback. His presence helped restore a measure of confidence to local residents. Deciding that the health crisis was resolving, Washington continued with plans for December congressional meetings. Members gradually returned piecemeal over the next few weeks, although fear of the yellow fever still hovered over Philadelphia's inhabitants.[123] This is demonstrated clearly in a letter written by Martha Washington as the new year of 1794 began. Back in Philadelphia Martha Washington observed she had

> not the least fear of the yallow fever while the weather is cold some people seems to anticipate its return again in the summer—but I believe they have no cause but that of a glumay disposion [gloomy disposition]— they have suffered so much that it can not be got over soon by those that was in the city—almost every family has lost some of their friends—and black seems to be general dress in the city.

Martha's letter provides us with a poignant and graphic first-hand description of the toll the disease took on Philadelphia's citizens. Less than a month later Martha would complain about her chronic "cholic" but report that "the inhabitants of this city say that Philadelphia was never more healthy than it has been for some months past."[124]

Fortunately, President Washington had avoided the yellow fever that had taken the lives of thousands in Philadelphia, but malaria would still trouble him, and he lost twenty pounds as a result of another episode of the insidious illness in 1794. In a letter to her niece, Martha commented that "I think upon the whole this has been a rather unhealthy winter. . . . Washington is as thin as he can be—but thank god is very well."[125] Later in 1794, a small growth was successfully removed from Washington's cheek, after much anxiety on Martha's part. In August she wrote that "he has had Doctor Tate to look at the spot on his face he makes light of the thing—I hope in god that he well very soon be well of it, the medicine that is given has not the least effect that can be perceived."[126]

Martha Washington continued to keep her finger on the pulse of the health not only of her husband but also of her family and friends. Her social circle served as a microcosm of the health of the nation, and her comments reflect both the mundane and the more serious illnesses that threatened Americans at the time, as well as the misconceptions about how illness was contracted and should be treated. Colds, toothaches, and swollen faces abounded among family members and friends, attributed by Martha to changes in the weather, including daily rain. Even the death of a friend who left "two little girls to lement her loss" was laid at the door of "bad air." In the spring of 1794, smallpox also raced through Richmond, Virginia: "Am exceedingly sorry to hear that the small pox has been so fatal in Richmond and that they have lost so many of the inhabitants," Martha commiserated. "I heard Mrs. Coles say that more than two hundred had died some time ago, want of care—I should think, or proper care, must be the reason of it, the season was bad which made against them."[127]

By the time Washington's physician, Dr. Craik, and his wife, Merrianne, lost a son in 1794, Martha had already witnessed the death of all four of her children, an occurrence only too common in late-eighteenth-century America. Martha mourned with "pore Mrs Craik I am truly sorry for her—I was told that her son was a very amiable youth." However, she appears to have been compelled to offer practical advice based on her own experience: "as she has several good children left she should endevour to reconcile herself to the loss of one however hard it may be."[128] Fanny, Martha's surrogate daughter, continued to be the recipient of her aunt's motherly advice (probably often unappreciated!) on the upbringing, health, and diet of children. In the fall of 1794 Martha cautioned Fanny that

this is the season for children to have complaints of different kinds and as you let your children eat . . . as they will—I am not surprised that a delicate child like Fayette is sick for certain it is that children should not eat every thing they will. . . . I hope it will be soon that you will see it or that child will suffer very much in his health.

Just a few weeks later Martha was still fretting over Fanny's children and also shared her concern that the hot weather in Philadelphia had prompted rumors about yellow fever. Her letter emphasized the common belief in what was often termed the "sickly months" and the efficacy of a change of location away from "malignant" air to foster good health. Martha expressed her hope that "the cool weather will carry off fevors of every kind; sore throats (probably diphtheria) among the children has been fatal in many cases, many have died with the complaint,"[129] reflecting that common childhood illnesses at the time often resulted in death, leaving virtually no household untouched.

Martha's greatest concern, however, was reserved for her husband. In the spring of 1794, Washington went horseback riding and sprained his back as he tried to avoid an accident. Martha unburdened herself to Fanny, lamenting,

> I have been so unhappy about the Presdt that I did not know what to do with myself—he tells me in his letter of Wednesday that he is better and that he will soon be able to return . . . if he is not getting better my dear Fanny don't let me be deceived . . . if he is likely to be confined at Mount Vernon longer than was expected I will get into the stage or get stage horses and come down emidately.

Two weeks later, Martha's anxiety was still palpable:

> The President arrived here on Monday a good deal fatagued with his ride—I fear he got some cold, it rained all day on satterday and he rode in the rain and was wet . . . I very much fear that it [the shoulder strain] will be a troublesome complaint to him for some time or perhaps as long as he lives he will feel it at times.[130]

Although very few letters between Martha and George Washington survive, Martha's correspondence with her niece provides us with a window into not only the lives of the first couple but also the degree to which health and illness occupied a prominent role in their thinking. The rich exchange of information came to an abrupt close in March of 1796 with the death of Fanny, then only in her twenties. Fanny's husband, Tobias Lear, had kept the president and first lady abreast of her decline from consumption, but as Martha asserted, "Your former letters prepared us for the stroke, which that of the 25th announced; But it has fallen heavily notwithstanding." Martha's next words reflect her deep religious belief in the wisdom of Providence that helped sustain her during her greatest trials in losing loved ones, an outlook she shared with both Abigail Adams and Dolley Madison. "It is the nature of humanity to mourn for the loss of our friends; and the more we loved them, the more poignant is our grief," she consoled Lear. However, Martha continued, "It is part of the precepts of religion and Philosophy, to consider the Dispensations of Providence as wise, immutable, uncontroulable; of course, that it is our duty to submit with as little repining . . . but nature will, not withstanding, endulge, for a while, it sorrows."[131]

Tobias Lear went on to a third marriage, this time to another of the Washington's nieces, Frances Henley, also nicknamed Fanny. In a letter dated November 22, 1797, Martha wrote that she hoped that Fanny had arrived safely at her parents' home as Martha was anxious that travel and cold would have a negative impact on her health. It is also clear that Martha was contemplating her own demise: "I hope if I live till next [year] you may find time to come [visit]. . . . The General and myself are well . . . Washington is with us he will spend this winter hear with us He is in good health." Two summers later, Martha "was so very sick lately . . . and concluded my time had come, and that I should be taken first," but with Dr. Craik's ministrations, she recovered.[132] In the winter of 1800, she confided morosely to a friend that after an "uncommon sickly autumn . . . I have always one complaint or another—I never expect to be well as long as I live in this world."[133]

The General's Last Gasp

On March 4, 1797, George Washington formally completed his second term as president, and despite growing political divisions within the infant government between Federalists and Republicans, he was clearly regarded as a revered leader, who remained highly popular with the American public. He looked forward to his retirement at his beloved home at Mount Vernon, but sadly he was only able to spend two years on the plantation before his death at the end of 1799. In the summer of 1798, he suffered an episode of ague and fever that was typical of

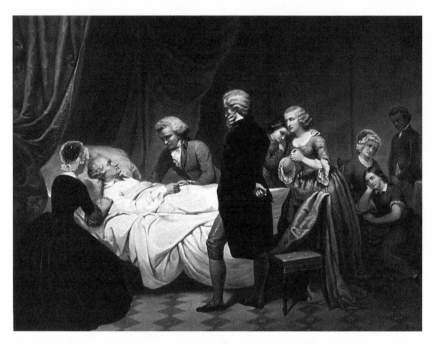

Life of George Washington. Idealized depiction of Washington on his
deathbed surrounded by family and friends. (Courtesy U.S. National
Library of Medicine)

malaria but recovered fully after losing a good deal of weight. In the
fall of 1799, not only did Martha contract a debilitating fever, but Washington's younger brother, Charles, also died. In December, Washington
experienced his own last and fatal sickness. The cause of Washington's
death, after only about twenty-four hours of illness, has attracted the
attention of numerous historians and physicians, with the ensuing controversy commencing immediately after his demise. Perhaps the most
important aspect of the president's final illness is that it was emblematic
of the limitations of contemporary medicine during the colonial and
early national period in America.

The basic facts of Washington's last days are well known, and much of
the information comes from the account written by Tobias Lear. Despite
hail and snow, on December 12, 1799, the former president conducted his
regular inspection of his plantation on horseback, returning to Mount
Vernon in the midafternoon. He attended dinner in his wet clothing,

and by the next morning he developed a severe sore throat. Although we know today that throat infections are not caused by either cold or wet weather, years of chronic illness had undoubtedly compromised the aging Washington's immune system, and fatigue may have made him more susceptible to contracting an infection. In any case, he went out in the snow again to mark some trees for future chopping, and by nightfall he was hoarse and had difficulty speaking, but stoically refused any medication to help alleviate his symptoms. According to Lear, Washington said, "You know I never take anything for a cold. Let it go as it came."[134]

During the night his discomfort grew. There is a question as to whether he woke his wife, Martha, during the night, but by morning he was clearly worse, with paroxysmal chills, referred to as "ague," and difficulty breathing. While Martha and Lear waited for Dr. Craik to arrive, they offered Washington what they thought was a soothing drink of molasses, butter, and vinegar. But in his critical state, he was unable to swallow the treacle-like concoction, nearly suffocating. Like so many of his contemporaries at the time, physicians and lay people alike, Washington viewed bloodletting as a panacea for most ills. Even before Dr. Craik arrived, Washington had ordered his overseer to take about fourteen ounces of blood and another local physician, Dr. Gustavus Richard Brown, was sent for to offer his expert assistance.[135]

Once Dr. Craik arrived, he applied a hot compress to Washington's neck for the throat infection, drew even more blood, administered a purge, and tried to get the retired president to gargle sage tea and vinegar. This all proved to no avail, however, as by this time the former president's throat had swelled to such a degree that his windpipe was closing up, making breathing more and more difficult. Faced with a dire situation, Craik called in another eminent local physician, Dr. Elisa Cullen Dick, who arrived midafternoon, followed by Dr. Brown. Dick argued against further bleeding because of Washington's weak pulse, but Craik and Brown prevailed and performed yet a fourth bleeding. Martha Washington, who had anxiously remained close to her husband's sickbed the entire last day of his life, also opposed further bleeding of her husband in his weakened state. But the two doctors were desperate to save their long-time friend and beloved leader. Craik and Washington had been especially close, and the always-generous Washington had even paid for the education of some of Craik's children. In addition to bleeding, calomel and antimony tartar were administered as laxatives. By this time Washington was so weak and resigned to his death that he dictated his final will to his overseer, graciously thanked his doctors, and requested them to let him die peacefully. In considerable distress and pain, he managed to maintain his calm and dignity. According to Lear, Washington declared, "I find I am going, my breath can not last long. I believed from the first that the disorder would prove fatal."[136]

Still, the physicians clung to the hope that they could save the former president. Dr. Dick even suggested a tracheotomy to open the air passage, a procedure he had only performed once previously, but it was rejected by Dr. Craik as too dangerous. We know that early American physicians had some experience with tracheotomies. For example, in a letter written in 1751, Franklin referred to the illness of the rector of the Philadelphia Academy, whose serious case of throat "Quinsey" forced the man's doctors "to open his Windpipe, and introduce a leaden Pipe for him to breath thro."[137] Washington died quietly at 10:00 p.m. on December 14, 1799, at the age of sixty-seven as the momentous eighteenth century was winding to a close. Increasingly frail and grief-stricken, Martha Washington declined to attend her husband's simple funeral at Mount Vernon.

Of the many discussions of the cause of Washington's final illness, the explanation offered by modern-day physician Dr. Michael Cheathan appears the most complete and sensible in the light of what we know from a contemporary vantage point. Cheathan has concluded that an initial strep or staph throat infection led to adult acute epiglottis, which resulted in near suffocation, and that the repeated bleedings— over half of Washington's circulating blood—and the other heroic measures led to septic shock, ultimately causing his death. Today, modern medicine would have probably treated the initial infection with antibiotics, unavailable at the time, and a tracheotomy in extreme nonresponsive cases, a highly dangerous procedure during Washington's era, particularly without reliable anesthesia. However, given Washington's age, delay in seeking treatment, and the limitations of medicine during the period, there was little else his three doctors could have done to prolong his life.[138] The course of Washington's illness is highly instructive of the manner in which a relatively minor illness could lead to dire consequences. Ironically, a strong man who had survived numerous life-threatening illnesses and danger on the battlefield died from what began as a simple throat infection.

Martha Washington died quietly three years later on May 22, 1802, at the age of seventy-one after a three-week illness of "bilious" fever and jaundice connected to her recurrent stomach ailments. She had been treated by the Washingtons' old friend and long-time physician, the by-now-elderly Dr. Craik. For forty years she had stood beside George Washington in war and peace as a supportive and loving companion, one who entertained and charmed her husband's friends and political associates. Martha had survived into what was then considered advanced old age, as the life expectancy of early American women at the time was the early fifties, for those who had not already been carried off in their twenties and thirties by complications of pregnancy and childbirth. She had outlived two husbands, all four of her children, and her seven siblings, yet took comfort in her last days in her grandchildren and many nieces and nephews.

Dr. Benjamin Rush noted Washington's death in 1799 in his diary.

This day died, universally lamented, General Washington His disease was Cynanche Trachialis. It proved fatal in 14 hours. He was patient and resigned in his illness. He said his will was made, his private affairs settled, and his public business but two days behind. He wished his physicians to enable him to die easy. Congress instituted public honors in his memory. The whole United States mourned for him as a father.[139]

Washington's death unsettled the country and sent the public into mourning. As many as four thousand Americans attended the official congressional memorial service in Philadelphia. Abigail Adams reflected popular sentiment when she wrote to her sister that "[n]o Man ever lived, more deservedly beloved and Respected."[140]

Generations of biographers have praised Washington for his military prowess, his strong leadership capabilities, and the sacrifices he made on behalf of the new nation and the American people, but his contributions to the advancement of medicine and public health in early America have been largely overlooked. For Washington, controlling smallpox among his troops and providing them with more healthful living conditions was one of his most challenging battles. Indeed, because

Washington's most prominent role regarding public health was related to his military career, particularly as the commander of the Revolutionary War army, he might well be considered a "warrior healer." Washington never attained the high level of scientific medical understanding exhibited by Franklin and Jefferson, which will be examined in upcoming chapters, but he had a solid fundamental understanding of medicine for his era. In his roles as commander, plantation owner, and president, he appreciated both the value of preventative health measures and the need for prompt medical intervention for sickness using the best contemporary tools available at the time.

2

Benjamin Franklin

A Founding Father of American Medicine

[Exercise] is of the greatest importance to prevent
disease, since the cure of them by physic is so
precarious.

—*Benjamin Franklin to William Franklin, August 19, 1772*

Merging Medical Science, Philanthropy, and Civic Leadership

Benjamin Franklin has become an iconic figure in American history as
a highly versatile and visible revolutionary leader and statesman, skillful
diplomat, sage writer, successful businessman, and innovative scientist,
but few today realize that this multidimensional Renaissance man was
also a pivotal player in the development of medicine in early America.
An avid student of the Enlightenment, Franklin focused his prodigious
intellect on the use of reason to advance progress for the benefit of civili-
zation. Scientific curiosity that emphasized observation and experimentation, coupled with pragmatic benevolence, drove Franklin's work on
disease prevention, health care, and the broader subject of medicine, one
of his chief interests. Franklin embodied a pioneering scientific approach
to medicine in America, which was complemented by his roles as a civic
leader and philanthropist, as well as his successful career as a printer and
publisher. That unique combination enabled Franklin not only to develop
his own medical theories and conduct scientific medical experiments but
also to disseminate medical information to a wide American audience.

If Franklin professed a religious credo, it was one that focused on
good works as the essence of religiosity. As he wrote to a friend in

1753, "I mean real good Works, Works of Kindness, Charity, Mercy, and Publick Spirit."[1] Early on, Franklin arrived at the firm conviction that government, whether municipal, state, or, eventually, federal, had a pivotal role to play alongside concerned individual citizens in promoting health and reducing sickness and disease, a commitment he shared with all the founders in this study. Indeed, the founding of the Pennsylvania Hospital, in which Franklin played so key a creative and fundraising role, was financed by a combination of government funds from the colonial legislature and private contributions. The hospital has been lauded as "a testimony to both the charity of the citizens and

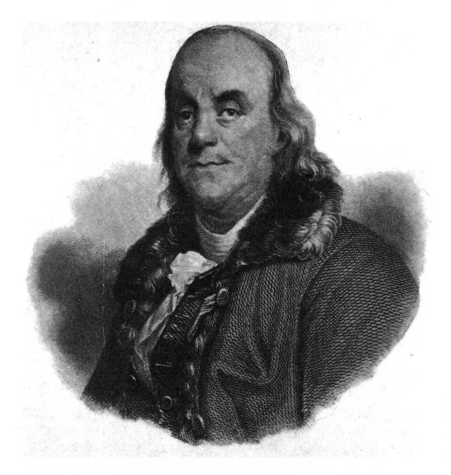

Portrait of Benjamin Franklin. (Courtesy U.S. National Library of Medicine)

the professional aspirations of the profession." It certainly advanced the practice of medicine by allowing medical students to witness and participate in actual everyday hospital activities, while at the same time aiding the sick, particularly those with little means.[2] Moreover, hospitals provided the "opening wedge" for national government involvement in the public health arena.[3]

When Franklin decided to retire from active business at the age of forty-two to concentrate on intellectual and charitable undertakings, his mother, Abiah Folger Franklin, expressed her disapproval. Franklin famously informed her in 1750, "I would rather have it said, *he lived usefully*, than, *He died rich.*"[4] The quintessential civic leader, in 1727 at the age of only twenty-one, he established a Philadelphia club for "mutual improvement" known as the Junto, which was organized to share knowledge and promote good citizenship and communal responsibility. As the leader of the Junto, Franklin would go on to play a central role in establishing a local public subscription library, a fire company, a voluntary militia, a postal service, and the learned American Philosophical Society for scientific inquiry. In 1751, Franklin was elected to the Pennsylvania Assembly, ushering in almost forty years of service as a public official. Perhaps most importantly, as noted, Franklin was the moving force behind the founding of the voluntary public charitable hospital in 1752, as well as the Philadelphia college academy (which became the University of Pennsylvania) and helped establish America's first medical school there in 1765.

As a disciple of the Enlightenment, Franklin venerated abstract knowledge, science, and discovery for its own sake and to satisfy his curious mind. Indeed, one author has designated him "the first scientific American."[5] Franklin faithfully adhered to the principles of emerging scientific method laid down by Isaac Newton and Francis Bacon, which emphasized objective experimentation, observation, and careful and accurate documentation of results. Stanley Finger, one of the few biographers to concentrate on Franklin's role in medicine, noted that what distinguished him from most other medical "practitioners" of his era was his "scientific approach to medicine from early on until his dying day."[6]

Franklin's scientific interests were wide and far reaching. In terms of disease, he explored not only prevention and cure but also how the body functioned, including respiration, perspiration, and blood circulation, subjects he discussed quite knowledgeably at length in the 1740s through correspondence with the well-known New York physician Dr. Cadwallader Colden. However, Franklin's interest in medicine, illness, and what made for good health had a primarily practical and egalitarian underpinning: the public good. Indeed, Franklin biographer Walter Isaacson has maintained that "the essence of Franklin is that he was a civic-minded man," and that his central vision was "an American identity based on the virtues and values of the middle class," which he hoped to bolster.[7]

Franklin's Early Years and Health

Benjamin Franklin, who was born in Boston on January 6, 1706, was the youngest son of the seventeen children that English-born candle maker Josiah Franklin fathered over two marriages. Unlike his famous revolutionary-era contemporaries John Adams and Thomas Jefferson, Franklin did not attend college, as his father was "burdened," as he put it, with supporting his large brood. Although he was an outstanding student, Franklin's formal schooling ended at the age of ten, when he began working in his father's candle shop.[8] Both George Washington and Franklin were largely self-educated, but Washington's intellectual breadth never approached the genius level of Franklin.

Franklin's truncated education did not stop him from becoming a highly knowledgeable scholar and later receiving honorary degrees in 1753 from both Harvard and Yale universities in America and numerous European awards, including the prestigious British Copley Award, in recognition of his many scientific accomplishments. Moreover, though Franklin never earned a medical degree, he was elected a member of several medical societies in recognition of his expertise, and many of his physician friends welcomed his insights regarding sickness and health. Franklin made his first trip to Scotland in 1759, when the University of Saint Andrews conferred the title of "Doctor" on him in recognition of his world-wide reputation as a pioneer of electricity experiments, and in 1768, Franklin was elected the first president of the American Philosophical Society, which gathered together the leading intellectual lights of the era.[9]

At the age of twelve, Franklin became an apprentice to his brother James, a Massachusetts printer. Benjamin not only learned the printing trade from James but also demonstrated his literary talent and gained experience as a contributor to and sometimes editor of his brother's *New England Courant*. He also may have acquired lifelong immunity to small-pox by surviving the notorious Boston epidemic of 1721. However, Benjamin chafed under James's strict hand and ran away to New York before settling in 1723 in Philadelphia, where he worked for another printer, Samuel Keimer. Philadelphia was then a town of only about three thousand residents but was poised to become a great commercial center.

It is interesting to note that even at this young age, Franklin had an interest in and knowledge of popular medicine and ideas about healthful living. Throughout his life, he was a voracious reader, exploring books on natural philosophy (science), history, and health. He is known to have possessed a copy of *Way to Health, Long Life, and Happiness*, authored by Thomas Tyron in the seventeenth century, which undoubtedly influenced his ideas about moderation in eating. When the eighteen-year-old Franklin became ill on the journey to Philadelphia in 1723, he recalled that "I found myself very feverish and went to bed; but having read somewhere that cold water drank plentifully was good for a fever, I followed the prescription . . . my fever left me, and in the morning . . . I proceeded on my journey."[10]

In 1724, with the encouragement of Pennsylvania governor William Keith, Franklin was persuaded to leave Philadelphia and travel to England aboard the *London Hope* to broaden his horizons and purchase printing equipment. This was the first of eight cross-Atlantic voyages Franklin would make in his lifetime. However, Keith reneged on his promise to extend letters of credit for Franklin, and the disillusioned young man only found work as a compositor in a printing shop. Still, Franklin became a master printer in London, and at the same time he became a popular local figure and achieved modest fame for his daredevil swimming demonstrations. Two years later, when a merchant named Denham encouraged him to return to Philadelphia and offered him a job in his shop, Franklin readily agreed. Franklin's return journey was taxing on his health, and he arrived in America in a weakened state. Despite his frailty, he began working for Denham, for whom he expressed affection, noting that the older man "counseled me as a father." Indeed, Franklin speculated that he and Denham would have continued their partnership happily if not for an undefined illness that struck his mentor. Denham died, but left Franklin a modest bequest by canceling the debt of the cost of his voyage.

At about the same time, Franklin also fell victim to one of the many sicknesses of the era. "In the beginning of February, 1727, when I had just passed my twenty-first year, we both were taken ill. My distemper was a pleurisy, which very nearly carried me off. I suffered a good deal, gave up the point in my own mind, and I was at the time rather disappointed when I found myself recovering."[11] In his typical wry writing style, Franklin demonstrated that lung infections were often life-threatening at the time, and even a strong young man was not immune to the ravages of disease. Later, in 1735, when Franklin was in his late twenties, he suffered another severe bout of pneumonia, and the resulting infection and ruptured abscess in one lung left him prone to severe colds as he grew older. Probably more people in colonial America died as a result of complications from common respiratory infections than the more highly publicized occurrences of epidemics such as smallpox.[12]

Franklin's Role in the American Smallpox Campaign

Thwarted in his aspirations as a merchant, Franklin returned for a short-lived stint at Keimer's printing shop. The two would later become bitter rivals when Franklin purchased a local newspaper and established his own shop from which he launched *The Pennsylvania Gazette*, a popular forum for his political, social, and health viewpoints. In 1732, he also initiated his famous *Poor Richard's Almanac*. Franklin was always receptive to new ideas. One of his most valuable medical contributions was his ardent support of the then-controversial use of smallpox inoculation to prevent a virulent case of the disease. As we saw in chapter 1, smallpox was a vicious disease that produced flu-like symptoms such as fever and chills and often severe internal damage, followed by flat red spots that evolved to oozing pustules, leaving mild to severe scarring in those who survived. The mortality rate for smallpox at the time was around 25 percent of those who contracted the infection.[13]

As we have learned, using the matter from a smallpox pustule to immunize a healthy person against a virulent attack—that is, inoculation—was first introduced in the American colonies in Boston in 1721.

Its primary proponent was the famous Massachusetts clergyman Cotton Mather, who had lost several family members to the disease following a major outbreak that year that killed almost 10 percent of the city's inhabitants. Mather learned about the practice from his black slave who had been successfully inoculated back in Africa. The procedure was initially far from universally accepted, as a small number of those inoculated still contracted severe, sometimes fatal, cases of smallpox, and the individuals who received the live virus could still spread the disease if they did not remain isolated until the transmission period passed. For many years the medical establishment remained firmly opposed to its use until the safer method of cowpox vaccination was perfected in the late eighteenth century.[14] Ironically, although Benjamin Franklin would become a vocal advocate for inoculation, his brother James's *New England Courant* had been sharply critical of Mather's support of the procedure in 1721 because of his concern about the potential of dangerous side effects.

The threat of smallpox was a constant fear in the lives of most colonial Americans. In 1731, Franklin reported a Philadelphia epidemic "which raged violently while it lasted," and that fifty people had been inoculated through variolation, but only one person, the child of the doctor who performed the inoculations, died.[15] The tragic loss of Franklin's own son, Frances (Franky) Folger Franklin, in 1736 as a result of naturally acquired smallpox was a primary factor in his ardent support of inoculation. Franky was the son of Franklin and Deborah (Debby) Read Franklin, the woman who became his common-law wife in 1730. Deborah's widowed mother was a well-known domestic healer who sold salves for scabies and other troublesome skin conditions, and Franklin often advertised her potions in the *Pennsylvania Gazette*. William Franklin, two years older than Franky, was Benjamin's acknowledged illegitimate son, and Deborah raised him as her own, although she does not appear to have been overly fond of the boy. In 1742, Deborah and Franklin also became the parents of a daughter, Sally (Sarah), who was successfully inoculated at the age of four.

Franklin had intended to have Frances inoculated but had unfortunately postponed the procedure because the child was ill with a common stomach ailment. Franklin recalled his young son's death graphically in his autobiography:

A fine boy of four years old, by the smallpox, taking him the common way [naturally acquired]. I long regretted him, and still regret that I had not given it to him by inoculation. This I mention for the sake of parents who omit that operation, on the supposition that they should never forgive themselves, if a child died under it, my example showing that the regret may be the same either way and therefore the safer should be chosen.[16]

Later, when Franklin's grandson Benjamin Franklin Bache was born in 1769, he immediately instructed his daughter, Sally, to make sure the baby received a smallpox inoculation as soon as it was practical to do so.[17]

For many years thereafter, Franklin dutifully recorded statistics on outbreaks of smallpox throughout the colonies in an effort to demonstrate that smallpox acquired by inoculation was safer than that received in the "natural" way. In 1759, Franklin collaborated with the English physician William Heberden on a pamphlet that promoted inoculation accompanied by simple instructions. Franklin not only contributed a preface, which contained statistics from a recent Boston epidemic, but paid for fifteen hundred copies to be distributed free of charge to American physicians, community leaders, and the working poor.[18] It is likely that George Washington, who was well read about medical matters and admired Franklin, was influenced by Franklin's and Heberden's work in his early support of smallpox inoculation among his troops. Franklin understood realistically that "the practice of Inoculation always divided the people into parties, some contending warmly for it, and the others against it," but he used rational evidence and his persuasive powers to demonstrate the great benefits of the procedure.[19]

Franklin, who retired from his lucrative printing business in his early forties, was sufficiently wealthy to be able to ignore the not inconsiderable cost of inoculation, but the fee was out of the reach of most workingmen with families. Probably inspired by the tragic loss of his young son, coupled with his keen sense of civic responsibility, Franklin played a part in providing free inoculation for poor children in Philadelphia by helping to raise funds for the project.[20] Franklin's friend and America's foremost physician, Dr. Benjamin Rush, was among the local physicians who volunteered their services.[21]

Franklin's Key Role in America's First Public Hospital

Franklin's unwavering support and pivotal role in the founding of the first colonial public hospital, the Philadelphia Hospital, which expanded free medical care for the working poor, is a prime example of the manner in which his civic and medical commitments intertwined. Early hospitals were focused on the poor, for those who could afford the preferred type of care through the services of a private physician brought doctors to their homes for treatment. Formerly, the Almshouse in Philadelphia had performed the public health function of a hospital, but its services were limited to local residents who could prove pauperism or when quarantine was deemed necessary for people who arrived on incoming ships.[22]

Local Philadelphia physician Dr. Thomas Bond enlisted Franklin's support of a new, expanded project, which would also serve as a practical training ground for medical students and budding physicians, an aspect that clearly appealed to Franklin's pragmatic nature. Moreover, Franklin was one of Philadelphia's leading boosters, and he realized that a "healthy" city would attract residents who could contribute to its economic growth and prosperity. Franklin's public call for financial support and his astute fundraising campaign, which in 1751 introduced the concept of matching funds for the Pennsylvania Hospital project, was innovative. As Franklin put it, "I not only subscribed to it myself, but engag'd heartily in the design procuring subscriptions from others."[23] Later in 1767, when Franklin was living in London, he lent his assistance to the development of a medical library at the hospital. He wrote to Dr. Cadwallader Evans, then serving as a physician to the Philadelphia Hospital, that "I am pleased with your scheme of a Medical Library at the Hospital, and I fancy I can procure you some donations among my medical friends here."[24]

Franklin served a six-year term as a manager of the hospital, where he had the opportunity to observe patients and diseases first-hand. On June 30, 1755, he was unanimously elected president of the board. The hospital project embodied Franklin's underlying philosophy on the subject of civic virtue and health: "The good particular men may do separately in relieving the sick is small compared with what they may do collectively."[25] Later, in 1754, in *Some Account of the Pennsylvania Hospital,* Franklin would report with satisfaction that through the

"Endeavours of skilful Physicians and Surgeons, [the patients'] Diseases May be Cured and Removed . . . discharged sound and hearty."[26] The Pennsylvania Hospital admitted some private patients but concentrated primarily on the impoverished sick in need of charitable assistance, and it was the first health institution in the American colonies to offer care for the mentally ill.

Dispensing Medical Advice

At times, Franklin acted as both an informal medical "practitioner" and a disseminator of medical information. This is clearly revealed in a letter he wrote his parents, Josiah and Abiah Franklin, in 1747:

> I apprehend I am too busy in prescribing, and meddling in the Dr.'s sphere, when any of you complain of ails in your letters; but as I always employ a physician myself when any disorder arises in my family and submit implicitly to his orders in every Thing, so I hope you consider my advice, when I give any, only as a mark of my good will.

Franklin then went on to discuss a variety of popular herbal remedies for the treatment of kidney stones and sediment in the urinary tract that could be used for the benefit of family members, settling on "moderate Use of them [salts]" as the best remedy. He even recommended "Chinese Ginseng," popularly touted today for its health-giving properties.[27] In 1756, Franklin wrote his wife, Deborah, that he had assisted in improving the health of an ill friend when they traveled together. He first arranged to have his companion "blooded" to treat a fever and pain in his side, then wrapped him up warmly in the coach to make him more comfortable and provided camomile tea on their arrival at their destination of Newcastle.[28]

Franklin often discussed health issues in correspondence with family members in other colonies in an effort to learn how public health there compared with his local conditions. In October 1747, he asked his mother "what kind of sickness you have had in Boston this summer," reporting that in Philadelphia, "Besides the measles and flux, which have carried off many children, we have lost some grown persons, by what we call the *Yellow Fever*."[29] In other words, life was Franklin's laboratory, and he welcomed information and freely espoused theories about virtually every disease and its treatment. Another instructive example of his wide-reaching medical interests is his appreciation for the efficacy of citrus fruits in promoting the health of the American colonists and sailors by preventing scurvy and other ills. In one instance, in a letter to his fellow colonist Richard Jackson in Rhode Island, Franklin mixed politics with health issues as he decried the proposed Stamp Act as well as the seizure of a Portuguese ship bearing lemons, maintaining, "In our hot Summers they [lemons] are necessary to our Health." The following year Jackson and Franklin would travel to England on behalf of the colonies to state their case against the Stamp Act.[30]

Franklin's interest in medicine led him to examine and speculate about a variety of illnesses. Some of Franklin's medical ideas, such as how colds were acquired and spread, were surprisingly advanced, while others, such as the advocacy of a common garden weed to treat cancer, appear ludicrous to us today. In Franklin's time, physicians viewed disease as arising from conditions within the body, primarily as an imbalance of humors, but Franklin understood that colds, for example, were transmitted from person to person, and that people who suffered from lack of exercise, poor nutrition, or lack of sleep might be more susceptible to illness. He also observed that sponge bathing with water or alcohol could help reduce fevers, a procedure that many pediatricians still recommend today. As Franklin, donning his medical hat, wrote from London to Dr. Rush in 1773,

I have long been satisfy'd from Observations, that besides the general Colds now termed *Influenza's*, which may possibly spread by Contagion as well as by a particular Quality of Air, People often catch Cold from one another when shut up together in small close Rooms, Coaches, &c. and when sitting near and conversing so as to breathe in each other's Transpiration.[31]

Although Franklin left extensive notes for a proposed article on contracting colds, he never completed the undertaking, but he always advocated proper ventilation in hospitals as well as private homes.[32]

Franklin espoused opinions not only on everyday illnesses but also on those that were comparatively rare but life-threatening. For example, most of Franklin's views on cancer were admittedly far-fetched, but indicate that he gave serious thought to the etiology of diseases and that he attempted to hold contemporary treatments up to the rigors of scientific evidence. In 1731, he was very concerned to hear that his sister Mary Franklin Homes had been diagnosed with breast cancer. Only twenty-five at the time, Franklin passed on medical advice to another sister, Jane Franklin Mecom:

> I know a cancer in the breast is often thought incurable; yet we have here in town [Philadelphia] a kind of shell made of some wood, cut at a proper time, by some man of great skill (as they say), which has done wonders in that disease among us, being worn for some time on the breast. I am not apt to be superstitiously fond of believing such things, but the instances are so well attested as sufficiently to convince the most incredulous.[33]

Over twenty years later, contemporary understanding of cancer treatment had not progressed much. As we learned, Franklin had long carried on an active correspondence with Dr. Colden, in which they discussed medical articles and theories. As late as 1752 the two men, who were by then respected medical authorities, appeared to give credence to an especially outlandish proposal for cancer treatment. Franklin wrote Colden that "I am heartily glad to hear more Instances of Success of the Poke Weed, in the Cure of that horrible Evil to the Human Body, a Cancer,"[34] demonstrating that even leading minds of the era could be misled.

Colden and Franklin displayed a more progressive understanding of medicine when they turned to the causes of endemic fevers and epidemics. Colden had studied the incidence of yellow fever in New York City, and in 1743 published a treatise that combined the age-old theories of noxious air with more forward-thinking ideas on sanitation. Colden pointed to miasmas generated by unsanitary conditions and foul water as the key source of the spread of the illness.[35] Of course, we know today that yellow fever is transmitted by infected mosquitoes, but they did indeed breed in open fresh-water receptacles such as uncovered cisterns, and they thrived in the crowded hot environments of urban centers in the South. In 1745, Franklin informed Colden that he owned a copy of Dr. Mitchel's *Tract on Yellow Fever*, which he would happily share with his friend.[36] This is especially noteworthy because Franklin would later pass on this pamphlet to Dr. Benjamin Rush, who was influenced by Mitchel's ideas when he treated yellow fever victims during the notorious 1793 epidemic in Philadelphia.

Using Print to Spread the Gospel of Good Health

Not only did Franklin conduct medical experiments and serve as a medical practitioner from time to time, but through his *Poor Richard's Almanac* and *The Pennsylvania Gazette*, he was a consummate popularizer who helped to disseminate scientific and medical information and influence public opinion about the treatment of sickness and the quest for good health. In the 1742 edition of *Poor Richard*, Franklin outlined a detailed "Rules of Health and Long Life, and to preserve from Malignant Fevers, and Sickness in general," which emphasized careful attention to a strict and temperate diet and appropriate exercise. It is interesting to note that Franklin maintained that such a regimen not only helped to prevent illness but had mental benefits as well, since it "preserves the Memory, it helps the Understanding."[37]

Franklin bought *The Pennsylvania* Gazette in 1729 and used it to provide information about a variety of epidemics and illnesses, including the common cold. As early as 1730, Franklin ran a short article about a smallpox outbreak in New England, with statistics about mortality rates that favorably reflected the efficacy of inoculation for hundreds of people.[38] Decades later, in 1751, he provided a clear explanation of the design and use of the microscope, which was beginning to reveal the presence of "animalcules," an intimation of the discovery of microbes to come in the next century.

In 1755, another important article appeared about Gaol Fever, known to us as typhus, a virulent "Distemper," as Franklin put it, and one that we know today is spread from person to person through infected lice. Franklin had learned a great deal about the disease from his close friend Dr. John Pringle, the eminent Scottish physician who had written extensively about the illness in the early 1750s. Franklin attributed the spread of Gaol Fever in America primarily to former prisoners and other passengers arriving on crowded ships. "It is said that several of our People lost their Lives last Year by purchasing Dutch [indentured]

Servants out of Sickly Ships, and bringing them into their Houses." Franklin warned that until strict laws were instituted to quarantine ill passengers, Americans should be extremely cautious as to "how they buy the Plague, and bring it home to their families."[39] In advocating legislation, Franklin was reflecting his recognition that the state had an important role to play in fostering public health and protecting citizens from contagious epidemics.

As Franklin put it in his *Autobiography*, he considered his newspaper and especially the *Almanac* "a proper vehicle for conveying instruction among the common people, who bought scarce other books."[40] As we will see in the upcoming chapters on Jefferson, the two men shared the view that Americans could play a key role in ably managing their own health and that educating people in all walks of life about good medical practices and treatment benefited the country as a whole. *Poor Richard* was filled with advice and remedies, aimed at a popular audience, about treating or preventing a variety of everyday diseases and promoting health. It was one of the most successful almanacs in America, with an annual circulation of about ten thousand copies. In an era when most people could not afford the services of a trained physician and health care took place primarily in the home, publications such as Franklin's often filled the gap, both espousing prevention and pointing out the role of the individual in achieving good health.[41]

This was probably the same impetus behind Franklin's decision in 1734 to reprint and sell at the modest price of one shilling Dr. John Tennent's popular book, *Every Man His Own Doctor; or, The Poor Planter's Physician*. In the afterword to the book, Franklin not only added advice on recent updates in medical practice concerning the treatment of pleurisy with rattlesnake root but also offered a surprisingly forward-looking caution about what we would today consider mental health issues. "But while we are solicitous about the Health of the Body," he wrote, "let us not forget, that there are also *Diseases of the Mind*, which concern us no less to be thoroughly cured of."[42] Nearly two decades later, Franklin republished another home-health-aid volume, a botanical primer book by Thomas Short titled *Medicina Britannica*. Franklin's work in the field of printing helped make Philadelphia not only the early publishing capital of America but also a prolific source of affordable health education for laypeople.

Although Franklin was well read in medical treatises, often supported new medical treatments, and developed lasting networks of friendship and intellectual exchanges with numerous physicians both in America and abroad, he steadfastly preached preventative moderation above medical intervention. In Europe, he would meet many of the leading scholars and scientists of the Enlightenment. The 1742 edition of the *Almanac* offered Franklin's underlying Enlightenment rationalist philosophy: "Wouldst thou enjoy a long Life, a healthy Body, and a vigorous Mind? Labour. . . . Bring the Appetite into Subjection to Reason," he staunchly proclaimed.[43] Franklin's prescription for long life proved to be personally successful, for he lived to be eighty-four. Although he was troubled by colds, gout, and kidney stones, he only rarely suffered from prolonged serious illness and regularly exercised by walking, lifting weights, and swimming even into old age. In 1773, he informed a friend that "[t]he exercise of swimming is one of the most healthy and agreeable in the world," recommending it as an aid to sleeping during hot nights and even as a cure for stomach upsets.[44]

Franklin frequently shared his medical knowledge with friends and relatives. In 1750, for example, he advised the Reverend Samuel Johnson that in regards to his case of malaria,

If you have not been us'd to the Fever and Ague, let me give you one Caution. Don't imagine yourself thoroughly cur'd, and so omit the Use of the Bark [quinine] too soon. Remember to take the preventing Doses faithfully. Tis an old Saying, That an Ounce of Prevention is worth a Pound of Cure, and certainly a true one, with regards to the Bark.[45]

Franklin exerted a profound influence in the area of health on many early Americans, and George Washington, who admired Franklin, was probably influenced not only by the latter's advocacy of smallpox inoculation but by his praise of the quinine-based bark as well.

In the previous year's edition of *Poor Richard's Almanac*, Franklin had praised the bark as "that famous specific for the cure of intermitting fevers, agues." He noted that the medication had fallen out of favor for many years, but he was pleased that it was now held "in high esteem, daily gaining ground, and overcoming by the success attending it the prejudices that were once . . . universal against the use of it." In the light of today's renewed interest in herbal treatment, it is interesting to note that Franklin presciently predicted that "some other valuable old medicines have been disused . . . and may in time be advantageously revived again, to the benefit of mankind."[46] In his letter to Johnson, Franklin also reported that "[t]he Small Pox [in Philadelphia] spreads apace, and is now in all quarters. Yet as we have only Children who have it, and our Doctors inoculate apace."[47] Franklin's words reflect his familiarity with the medical issues of the day, and it was certainly true that pregnant women, babies, and the elderly were most vulnerable to smallpox.

Preventative Health and Experimental Treatment

Although Franklin clearly believed in the efficacy of medical intervention when necessary, his preventative triad for good health emphasized fresh air, exercise, and a moderate diet, a regimen advocated by modern medicine today. Franklin was almost manic about proper ventilation, and he sent John Adams into distress when the two roomed together in New Jersey during revolutionary days, when he insisted that their window be left open to let in the cold night air. In his diary, Adams noted wryly that "[t]he Doctor then began an harangue, upon Air and cold and Respiration and Perspiration, which I was so much amused that I soon fell asleep."[48] As we learned in the previously cited letter to Dr. Rush, long before germ theory was developed, Franklin seems to have intuitively understood that many common illnesses such as colds and influenza were spread by close contact and that fresh air could mitigate the transfer of sickness. Later, while living in London in 1773, Franklin would reiterate his belief that fresh air, even cold air, did not produce rheumatism or other illnesses. In his typical tongue-in-cheek style he observed, "But as this [opinion] is Heresy here, and perhaps may be so with you, I only whisper it, and expect you to keep my Secret. Our Physicians have begun to discover that fresh Air is good for People in the Small Pox and other Fevers. I hope in time they will find out that it does no harm to People in Health."[49]

More unusually, Franklin practiced a daily ritual of cold air baths and reported to his French translator, the eminent Paris physician Dr. Barbeu-Dubourg, "I rise almost every morning and sit in my chamber without any clothes whatever, half an hour or an hour, according to the season, whether reading or writing . . . I shall therefore call it for the future a *bracing* or tonic bath."[50] Though Franklin sometimes lapsed in the face of temptation, he was also at times a vegetarian and advocated moderate eating habits. He had a clear understanding that certain foods aggravated his gout, and he critically once declared that people ate "twice as much as nature requires." He also recommended walking and especially swimming as excellent forms of exercise and as an aid to cleanliness, remaining an active swimmer well into his seventies.[51]

Franklin is known to nearly all schoolchildren for his famous kite experiments with electricity and the invention of the popular lightning rod, but few people are aware of the innovative electrical medical experiments he conducted or that he first speculated electricity might be used effectively to treat epilepsy, palsy (Parkinson's disease), and paralysis. To his credit as a "natural philosopher," or scientist as we term it today, Franklin was always open to new ideas, but never manipulated the results of his experiments to justify a theory. He was skeptical of reported miraculous cures following electrical shocks administered to the deaf, blind, and paralyzed reported from remote locations in mid-eighteenth-century Europe. However, desperate American would-be patients soon came knocking at his door and, propelled by his sympathetic nature as much as his natural curiosity, Franklin felt compelled to try to help them. For example, Franklin treated an old paralyzed Philadelphia scholar who had been an early mentor, as well as offering advice to Jonathan Belcher, the colonial governor of New Jersey, who suffered from palsy. Repeated electric shocks involving bottles and wires were administered three times daily to both men, but neither patient experienced any notable or lasting improvement.[52]

On the other hand, in 1752 Franklin apparently had some success with a young woman who suffered from convulsions, who remained free of her affliction for at least a few years after electrical treatment was initiated and who lived to an old age. After several years of medical experiments involving electricity, Franklin concluded that any improvement in cases of paralysis or palsy were temporary at best but still held out hope for the use of electricity in treating depression. As a result of his sensitive, sophisticated understanding of the human mind, he offered an explanation for instances of improvement that relied on psychosomatic underpinnings and cited the cause as "spirits given by hope of success."[53] In other words, Franklin was attuned to what we now refer to as "the placebo effect."[54]

Despite Franklin's very limited success with "medical electricity," and even though electro-shock therapy for the mentally ill did not begin in earnest until the nineteenth century, some have viewed him as a pioneer in the field. With his friend the progressive Dutch physician Jan Ingenhousz, Franklin experimented with using electricity applied directly to the head to cure depression, or melancholia as it was then known. Through a series of unintended experimental accidents, both Franklin and Ingenhousz learned that people could survive intense shocks, and Franklin was encouraged enough by the possibility of the efficacy of electrical shocks in the mentally ill to advise further clinical trials, perhaps influencing others later to continue their initial work.[55] Today, the use of electricity for mental illness is making the news, with a number of medical experts lauding its benefits in treating depression. In 2012, researchers successfully utilized deep brain stimulation through direct application of electrodes to treat depression and halt tremors in more than one hundred thousand patients with Parkinson's disease, seemingly demonstrating that Franklin's work conducted centuries ago had the potential for success given the right technology.[56]

Two of Franklin's most well-known and effective contributions to medicine were his development of an improved flexible urinary catheter and the invention of bifocal glasses. Practical need drove the catheter project, which was based on a European model. Franklin's brother John, who lived in Boston and was often ill and in pain, asked if it was possible to come up with a device to help him urinate more easily. With the help of a local silversmith, Franklin designed the first American catheter, a thin silver flexible tube, which could be inserted and withdrawn with relative ease.

Franklin's letter to his brother describing the catheter reflects not only the workings of Benjamin's creative mind and his scientific reliance on experimentation but also how determined he was to see a project through once it was conceived. In December 1752, Franklin wrote, "Reflecting yesterday on your desire to have a flexible catheter, a thought struck into my mind how one might probably be made . . . I went immediately to the silversmith's and gave directions for making one (sitting by till it was finished) that it might be ready for this post." Franklin went on to say he was concerned the "machine" might be too unwieldy for easy use and offered suggestions for adjustments. He concluded by acknowledging that "[e]xperience is necessary for the right using of all new tools or instruments, and that will perhaps suggest some improvements to this instrument as well as better direct the manner of using it."[57]

Bifocal glasses were also born out of practicality. The latter eliminated the necessity for people to carry two pairs of glasses as they juggled the need to augment their eyesight for both close reading and seeing at a distance. Many of the pictures we have of Franklin depict him wearing the newfangled spectacles. In 1775, Franklin sent his friend the English economist George Whatley a drawing of bifocals and explained how he invented them.

> I . . . had formerly two pairs of spectacles, which I shifted occasionally, as in traveling I sometimes read, and often wanted to regard the prospects. Finding this change troublesome, and not always sufficiently ready, I had the glasses cut, and half of each kind associated in the same circles. . . . By this means, as I wear my spectacles constantly, I have only to move my eyes up or down, as I want to see distinctly far or near, the proper glasses always ready.[58]

Franklin also often dispensed general advice about the use of eyeglasses to friends and family members. In 1771, Franklin sent his favorite sister, Jane Mecom, "a pair of every size of glasses from 1 to 13. To suit yourself, take out a pair at a time, and hold one of the glasses first against one eye, and then against the other, looking on some small print." Franklin continued with specific instructions on how to carefully choose the best "prescription," noting that both eyes seldom were identical in terms of vision. He concluded by generously offering, "[W]hen you have suited yourself, keep the higher numbers for future use as your eyes may grow older; and oblige your friends with the others."[59] Franklin's method of determining the strength of the glasses is much like the procedure optometrists follow today, albeit with much more sophisticated machinery for calculating and calibrating the patient's needs.

Although we generally think of Franklin as short and having a rotund body, in reality as a young man he was robust, stood about five feet ten inches tall, and actually maintained a muscular physique due in no small part to his emphasis on exercise. Like his good friend Jefferson, Franklin recognized the need for regular exercise among college students immersed in intense study. He recommended that the students at the Academy of Philadelphia, which he helped found and where he served as the first chairman of the Board of Trustees, "be frequently exercis'd in Running, Leaping, Wrestling and Swimming." Unsurprisingly, the practical Franklin emphasized that students be taught "useful" knowledge, and he also recommended a temperate diet, which was "plainly" and "frugally" prepared.[60]

In a letter to his son William in 1772, Franklin strongly applauded the young man's resolve to undertake a rigorous exercise program. What is more remarkable is that Franklin appears to have understood the concept of burning calories and that the more vigorous the exercise, the higher the impact and ultimate benefit. He related this concept to the level of "warmth" a particular exercise produced in the body and opined that "there is more exercise . . . in one mile's walking on foot than in five on horseback; to which I may add that there is more in walking one mile up and down stairs, than in five on a level floor."[61]

Diplomatic Medicine on the European Continent

At the age of seventy, Franklin risked the loss of his comfortable and successful lifestyle as he joined an uncertain revolution with his fellow patriots. The self-made civic and business leader was the eldest of the group, which included Jefferson, thirty-seven years his junior, and Adams, twenty-nine years younger than Franklin. Although Franklin had been a staunch supporter of the British Empire through the early 1760s, his "Americanization," as historian Gordon Woods has aptly described it, moved him quickly toward the American cause.[62] From 1752 to 1762, Franklin was stationed in London as a colonial agent with the goal of limiting the proprietary power of the Penn family in Pennsylvania. He returned to America in 1762 and until 1764 oversaw the development of the colonial postal system. Franklin sailed to England in 1764 to promote Pennsylvania's interests and witnessed first-hand the dangers of royal government, being especially outraged by the Stamp Act of 1765 imposed on the American colonies. In 1775, his service in England came to an unhappy end when he was chastised by the British government for alleged traitorous political intrigues. Upon his return to America, he became a leading vocal member of the Philadelphia Continental Congress and pivotal in the drafting of the Declaration of Independence.

In late 1776, Franklin was named the first minister on behalf of the United States to France, where he would develop crucial French financial and military support for the new American nation and where he resided until returning to the United States in 1785. We learn much about Franklin's personal health in Europe through his extensive correspondence with his wife, Deborah, who declined to accompany Franklin on any of his voyages across the ocean. Although they were separated for inordinately long periods of time, he wrote her regularly and with some affection, addressing her as "My dear Child" and frequently sending her lavish gifts.

In Franklin's day, the 3,000-mile hazardous sea journey across the Atlantic took four to six weeks, and he arrived in Paris on December 21, 1776.[63] The rough winter crossing on the *Reprise* took a toll on Franklin, resulting in boils, a skin rash, and loss of weight as a result of poor food aboard ship. The fear of being captured during the voyage and hanged by the British may have contributed to the seventy-year-old Franklin's weakness as he disembarked with his two young grandsons, who had accompanied him on the journey. However, once on land Franklin overcame his illness and became an effective, engaging spokesman on behalf of America and the toast of the glittering Paris society, navigating numerous treaties, including the momentous Treaty of Peace with Britain in 1783, formally negotiated on May 12, 1784. In France, Franklin was particularly popular with the ladies, and one of the many inventions of his creative mind, a glass musical instrument he called the armonica, became the rage. Franklin's sparkling charm captivated the French, but the amiable Franklin certainly had his detractors among his fellow Americans. Although fellow revolutionary John Adams and his wife, Abigail, respected Franklin's many accomplishments, while they were stationed together in Europe the Adamses often disapproved of what they considered Franklin's frivolity and fondness for high society.[64]

At his residence in Passy, France, even in his seventies Franklin enjoyed relatively good health. However, psoriasis, which he referred to as "scruff," spread from his head to most of his body, causing itching and scaling, and troubled him on and off for many years.[65] Franklin's careful description of the symptoms of his psoriasis reveals his acute powers of observation in regard to illness. Writing to his sister in 1779, Franklin reported in his usual optimistic vein that "I continue to enjoy, Thanks To God, a greater Share of Health and Strength than falls to the Lot of many at my Age. I have, indeed, sometimes moderate Fits of the Gout; but I think it is not settled among the Physicians whether that is a Disease or a Remedy."[66] A journal Franklin kept to record the state of his health from 1778 through the beginning of 1780, on the eve of his seventy-fifth birthday, reveals the progress of his chronic illnesses, particularly gout and psoriasis; however, he maintained that prior to his early seventies he "enjoy'd continu'd Health for nearly 20 Years."[67]

In addition to being a skilled diplomat and negotiator both in France and in England, Franklin's engaging personality and reputation as a man of science made him a welcome guest in French salons and English intellectual circles, where he was viewed as a symbol of political and scientific progress. Most famously, his systematic experiments had proved that lighting was similar to static electricity. Honorary degrees and memberships in scientific and medical societies were frequently bestowed upon him. Physicians on both sides of the Atlantic were among his many admirers, and his opinions on medical matters were often sought. Dr. John Fothergill, the Edinburgh-educated Quaker physician who served as Franklin's personal doctor while he resided in England, discussed his own experience with gout with Franklin, obviously agreeing that he was knowledgeable about medical matters.[68] Franklin also shared an interest in medical and sanitation reform with Sir John Pringle, and at times they traveled together through Europe by coach.[69]

As further evidence of Franklin's transatlantic medical reputation, he was often invited to meetings of the Société Royale de Médicine while he was in Paris. In a 1781 letter to its secretary, physician Félix Vicq d'Azy, Franklin thanked him for a number of medical reports that had been distributed at a meeting he was unable to attend and promised to forward them "to different Parts of America." Franklin also provided the doctor with anecdotal reports about whether infection could be transmitted through the remains of those long dead. Franklin concluded in his usual prudent scientific manner that "[a]s we do not yet know with Certainty how long the Power of Infection may in some Bodies be retained, it seems well in such Cases to be cautious till farther Light shall be obtained."[70]

In France, Franklin also encountered many famous European philosophers such as the English writer David Hume and the leading French *philosophes*, Voltaire and Diderot, who were impressed with Franklin's wide-ranging knowledge and wit. Franklin crossed paths with Dr. Pierre Cabanis, the progressive French physician who would do much in the future to reform and modernize medicine in his country. The two men certainly discussed medical issues, and Cabanis would eventually prove the worthlessness of bleeding as a medical practice. As we will learn in chapter 4, Cabanis also exhibited a strong influence on Jefferson's progressive ideas about medicine.

Although Franklin rarely criticized doctors and "Physic" as strongly as his fellow American Jefferson, he maintained a healthy skepticism about contemporary medicine. From London in 1772, he wrote his old friend Dr. Bond back in Philadelphia that "I suspect there is more valuable knowledge in Physic to be learnt from the honest candid Observations of an old Practitioner . . . who by Experience has discovered the Inefficacy of most Remedies and Modes of Practice, than from all the formal Lectures of all the Universities upon Earth."[71] On the other hand, he was always open-minded about suggestions for new medications and procedures, as long as their claimed efficacy was backed up by sound and verifiable experimentation. Franklin became a mentor to a number of America's preeminent budding physicians studying in Europe, including Benjamin Rush, John Morgan, William Shippen, and Caspar Wistar, with whom he exchanged ideas about medical treatment. He had encouraged them to study in Scotland, where he had been impressed with the quality of the country's medical schools, and many dedicated their dissertations or treatises to him.[72]

While Franklin resided in France, the touted wonders of Dr. Franz Anton Mesmer's "animal magnetism" was the talk of Paris. Mesmer believed that magnetic fluid fields were present in all living beings and that if they were out of balance, disease resulted. He claimed to have successfully treated patients with magnetic rods that manipulated these supposed fields into better alignment, so they could be restored to good health.

In early 1784, even before Franklin had the opportunity to observe the procedure first-hand, he gave his opinion on "the cures performed by Comus and Mesmer. . . . As to the animal magnetism so much talked of, I am totally unacquainted with it, and must doubt its existence till I can see or feel some effect on it." He went on to describe patients who he felt were hypochondriacs and to explain why, from a psychological perspective, such "useless" remedies might have an unintended positive effect.

> There are in every great rich city a number of persons who are never in health, because they are fond of medicines and always taking them, whereby they derange the natural functions, and hurt their constitutions. If these people can be persuaded to forbear their drugs in expectation of being cured by only the physician's finger or an iron rod pointing at them, they may possible find good effects though they mistake the cause.[73]

In other words, if people had great faith in their physicians and their healing powers, a positive mental outlook would speed them on the road to recovery, especially if the malady was psychosomatic in origin.

In 1784, the 78-year-old Franklin was appointed by King Louis XVI to serve on a three-man commission to evaluate Mesmer's claims. It appears that Mesmer employed some form of hypnotism on the patients, which may have temporarily persuaded them that they had experienced an improvement in health, further supporting Franklin's supposition. An experimental demonstration took place at Franklin's house in Passy and proved that Mesmer's theory was scientifically unfounded. In the subsequent report on Mesmer's clinical work, Franklin rejected the fanciful medical claims, but presciently offered clues on the role of psychology and the power of suggestion on the mind in the successful healing of the body.[74]

Franklin's Personal Health in England and France

During his long periods of residence in Europe, Franklin often took annual trips "to preserve his health," as he put it. Writing from London in the summer of 1766, for example, he informed the Committee of Correspondence of the Pennsylvania Assembly back in America that "In June . . . I acquainted you that I was about to make a Journey for the Establishment of my Health." He continued with a description of partaking of the restorative waters at Pyrmont as well as "relying more on the Air and Exercise of Traveling" as he toured Germany and Holland. He happily reported that he returned from his trip "well and hearty, my Journey having perfectly answered its Intention." In 1772, he was still taking long summer jaunts, which provided him with "Daily Exercise in the open air to recover and Establish my health."[75]

Franklin's letters reveal that in addition to flareups of gout, a form of arthritis that is characterized by high levels of uric acid, and stones in the urinary tract, he was for a long time plagued by psoriasis and frequent head and chest colds. We now know that gout and psoriasis are often medically related. Beginning his stay in London in 1757, Franklin endured nearly two months of repeated sickness, characterized by several bouts with colds and "intermitting fever" that often confined him to bed as he became adapted to the climate and built up some resistance to circulating illnesses. Franklin was treated by Dr. Fothergill, who in addition to bleeding Franklin from the head, ordered strict rest and "forbid me the use of pen and ink." Franklin also resorted to his favorite medicine, bark (quinine), to the point that "I took so much bark in various ways that I began to abhor it." After many weeks of illness, Franklin was "seized one morning with a vomiting and purging," which inextricably finally placed him on the road to recovery and prompted the firm hope that "my seasoning is over, and that I shall enjoy better health during the rest of my stay in England."[76]

For the most part, over the ensuing years Franklin treated episodes of a variety of illnesses with exercise, increased exposure to fresh air, and moderation in diet. But he did sometimes fall back on emetics or the popular age-old medical practices of bleeding and blistering. Franklin seemed to gain relief from being "cupped," as bleeding was also called, and we might wonder why the sensible and medically sophisticated Franklin found the procedure helpful, as there is no medical explanation. Given Franklin's reliance on scientific proof and his often forward-thinking medical theories, it is surprising that he was willing to so often subject himself to bloodletting for a variety of illnesses. He was undoubtedly influenced in this area by many of the physicians who served as close friends, and for whom he had developed a loyal respect.

As we have seen, bleeding had for centuries been a mainstay of medical treatment and many physicians of the Edinburgh school of medicine, such as William Cullen and his student Dr. Rush, evidenced a strong belief in its efficacy. Perhaps, as Franklin had pointed out in judging the validity of Mesmer's theory of animal magnetism, *belief* in the efficacy of a treatment and confidence in a particular doctor often produced a positive psychological state that promoted healing. Franklin died before the infamous yellow fever epidemic of 1793, before he could witness the fact that, as we have seen, Rush's reliance on heroic bleeding did nothing to stem the devastation brought on by the disease.

For colds, Franklin staunchly continued to recommend the use of quinine as a tonic and maintained, "I have found by a good deal of Experience, that three or four Doses of Bark taken on the first Symptoms of a Cold, will generally put it by."[77] For other ills such as insomnia and several attacks of "giddiness" (dizzy spells), he consulted his doctor. For one such episode Dr. Fothergill prescribed thirty grams of a powder of Contrayerva, an herbal remedy derived from a plant root. According to Franklin, it provided him with a good night's sleep without the aftereffects of headache produced by the Hartshorn Drops he had taken in the past. However, the following morning he still experienced "a Giddiness and Swimming in my Head . . . which makes me stagger a little . . . hear a humming Noise in my head, and seem now and then to see little faint twinkling lights,"[78] perhaps an indication of what today we would term a migraine headache.

In February 1760, Franklin reported to Deborah that he had "been much indispos'd with an Epidemical Cold . . . but being cupp'd [bled] by Dr. Fothergills's Advice, and parting with 8 Ounces of Blood from the Back of my Head, find my self better." The next month he informed Deborah he had recovered from another attack of giddiness, but "I have been cupp'd blooded, physick'd and at last blister'd for it; and it seems now quite remov'd; but by those Operations and very spare Living, I am grown a little thin, which I do not dislike."[79] The latter remark reflected his understanding that being overweight was not conducive to good health and that heroic medical measures understandably often resulted in weakness. In 1765, Franklin wrote, "I have generally had my Health pretty well lately, except a Fit of the Gout, which confin'd me about a Fortnight, and my Foot is still tender. I am advis'd to spend a Week or two at Bath,"[80] presumably for the reputed curative powers of the resort's healing waters.

As the years passed, Franklin's gout was still an issue, but in 1768 he declared to his wife, "I am now, and have been all this Winter, in very good Health, Thanks to God. I only once felt a little Admonition as if a Fit of the Gout would have attack'd me, but it did not. Whether sick or well, I am ever, my dear Debby Your affectionate Husband."[81] That fall, he informed Deborah that in October he had left London to visit friends in the English countryside for a few days to "breathe a little fresh air" but had not taken his usual summer journey because he had enjoyed unusually good health, "a greater Share of which I believe few enjoy at my time of Life."[82] Franklin was only in his early sixties at the time, but his musings reflect that he had already passed the average life expectancy of the era and that sixty was considered elderly by contemporary standards.

A few years later, Franklin was revisited by both dizziness and gout, coupled with a severe throat infection. He described his health woes at length to Deborah but ended on an upbeat note:

> I had from Christmas to Easter a disagreeable Giddiness hanging about me, which however did not hinder me from being about and doing Business. . . . In the Easter Holidays . . . I was taken with a Sore Throat, and came home half-strangled. From Monday till Friday I could swallow nothing but Barley Water and the like. I was bled largely and purged two or three times. On Friday came on a Fit of the Gout, from which I had been free Five Years. Immediately, the Inflammation and Swelling in my Throat disappeared; my Foot swelled greatly, and I was confined about three Weeks; since I am perfectly well, the Giddiness and every other disagreeable Symptom having quite left me.[83]

In 1772, he again reported painful gout to Deborah: "I wrote to you . . . that I was pretty well recovered of my Gout, but it return'd upon me that Day, and has handled me pretty severely for some Nights past, tho' now I am something better."[84] Gout continued to be one of his primary physical complaints for the remainder of his life.

Deborah died in late 1774 after a series of debilitating strokes while Franklin was still representing the colonies in London. By then, after so many years of separation, the Franklins appear to have settled into a rather perfunctory relationship. If the news of his wife's demise saddened him deeply, Franklin never displayed any outward grief, but it did prompt him to leave Europe after his ten-year stay to oversee the affairs Deborah had managed during his long absence. On the eve of the American Revolution, Franklin returned to Philadelphia, where he was elected to the Second Continental Congress, but later in 1777, during perilous times during the Revolutionary War, he was once again dispatched to Europe as an envoy to France to garner political and economic support.

On his return, the charismatic Franklin remained an extremely popular figure in France, but despite his protestations to family members of only moderate attacks, recurrent bouts of gout and stones continued to plague the aging diplomat, and during his last years in Europe he was eager to return home. Franklin had thrived in the heady intellectual and cultural atmosphere of the French salons, sponsored by aristocratic men and women, but they often featured gargantuan meals with over a dozen courses. Like the *philosophes* Franklin so admired, he found that theories of moderation and abstinence were hard to follow in the face of tempting excess. No doubt his rich French diet, which often included large portions of red meat and wine, aggravated his chronic medical conditions. We know now that Franklin's three chief complaints, gout, bladder stones, and psoriasis, are related and may have had a genetic component. In 1780, Franklin penned his humorously famous "Dialogue between Franklin and the Gout," in which he playfully chastised himself for drinking large quantities of the Madeira wine of which he was so fond, eating "too freely," and not getting enough exercise.[85] That fall Franklin was often confined to bed as the result of one of his most severe gout attacks, and his essay was sent in an exchange of letters with his good friend in France, the aristocratic and cultured Madame Brillion, who was then suffering from the effects of severe depression.

The classic essay reveals that Franklin had a good medical understanding of what provoked gout but was also well aware of his only-too-human tendency to rationalize his lapses. Franklin often returned to his own professed emphasis on moderation when prompted by pain and discomfort. Earlier in the year, Franklin had also discussed his recurrent gout with British surgeon Alexander Small, with whom he shared a strong belief in the efficacy of proper ventilation for health. Franklin informed Small that he had obtained some relief by extending his foot outside of the bedcovers while sleeping. Although Franklin, always a careful and honest empirical scientist, maintained that the method helped him, he concluded, "But this method requires to be confirmed by more experiments, before one can conscientiously recommend it."[86]

Regardless of his physical ailments, Franklin's sense of humor remained undiminished. From France he wrote American patriot John Temple in the summer of 1781 that "[t]hanks to God I still enjoy Health and good Spirits, tho' the English News writers have thought fit to kill me several times in their Prints. It must at last be true that I am dead; but that Article hitherto has been, as their Papers phrase it, *premature.*"[87] A few years later Franklin would tell his good friend the economist and an officer of London's Foundling Hospital, George Whatley, that

> I must agree with you that the Gout is bad, and that the Stone is worse. I am happy not having them both together; and I join you in your Prayer that you may live till you die without either. . . . I have some reason to wish that in a future State [the afterlife] I may not only be as well as I was, but a little better.

Franklin proceeded to describe the care of foundlings in France, noting with approval that nurses were required to be licensed to attest to their good health so that they would not be a source of contagion to the infants.[88]

Despite their significant differences in political style and personality, Franklin's reputation as a "medical man" was appreciated by his fellow diplomat John Adams, who, as we learned, took a clearly pragmatic approach to the subject of health and medicine. In 1781, Adams was in The Hague to negotiate commercial agreements on behalf of the United States when he fell seriously ill. When Franklin heard he was sick, he sent Adams his best wishes for a speedy recovery as well as advice about taking "the Bark" to reduce fever. Adams dutifully thanked Franklin "for your Advice as a Physician, which I have ventured to follow."[89] Even though Adams did not always approve of what he considered Franklin's inappropriate behavior, it is clear that Adams followed the progress of Franklin's health as well.

In a letter written in October 1782 to Abigail Adams in America, John informed her that "Dr. Franklin has been a long time much indisposed, as I lately heard with the Gout and Strangury [stones]."[90] Similarly, in his diary at the time Adams, who often dined with the elderly statesman, noted that due to his ailments Franklin "was infirm . . . and could not Sleep," but just two weeks later Adams noted, "[H]e is getting better. The Gout left him weak. But he begins to sit, at Table."[91] Later, after joining her husband in France, Abigail Adams would witness the aging Franklin's continued ailments first-hand. In December 1784, she wrote her sister Mary Cranch that "Dr. Franklin is much afflicted with his disorder, which prevents his going abroad, unless when the weather will permit him to walk."[92]

That Franklin suffered from stones in the urinary tract was certainly true, but at that point in his life, in his late seventies, he seems to have regarded it as more of an annoyance than a serious disorder. To his old friend Mary Stevenson Hewson, the daughter of his former landlady in England, he admitted, "I have been lately ill with a Fit of Gout, if that may indeed be called a Disease," but he maintained, "I rather suspect it to be a Remedy; since I always find my Health and Vigour of Mind improv'd after the Fit is over."[93] Later in the year, the stone became more troublesome, and Franklin wrote the Comte De Vergennes that "[b]eing now disabled by the Stone, which in the easiest Carriage gives me Pain, wounds my Bladder, and occasions me to make bloody Urine, I find I can no longer pay my Devoirs personally at Versailles."[94]

The procedure of cutting for bladder stones, lithotomy, was common in seventeenth- and eighteenth-century surgery, indicating how widespread the affliction was at the time. Since the operation itself was often quite painful and sometimes produced serious side effects such as incontinence and impotence, healers experimented with alternative treatments to dissolve the stone, including injections of alkaline fluids or ingestion of herbal extracts.[95] In early 1784, Franklin openly discussed his ailment in great detail in a letter written to the American patriot John Jay:

> It is true, as you have heard, that I have the stone, but not that I had thoughts of being cut for it. It is as yet very tolerable. It gives me no pain but when in a carriage on the pavement, or when I make some sudden quick movement. If I can prevent its growing larger, which I hope to do by abstemious living and gentle exercise, I can go on pretty comfortably with it to the end of my journey, which can now be of no great distance. I am cheerful, enjoy the company of my friends, sleep well, have sufficient

appetite, and my stomach performs well its functions. The latter is very material to the preservation of my health. I therefore take no drugs, lest I should disorder it. You may judge that my disease is not very grievious, since I am more afraid of the medicines than of the malady.[96]

Franklin's words underscore his underlying commitment to moderation and the healing powers of nature, as well as his skepticism of medicine—all health viewpoints he shared with his close friend and admirer Jefferson.

Despite his health problems, overall Franklin was in relatively good shape for one his age, and he retained a positive attitude. Perhaps his good friend, the French physician Cabanis, divined the source of Franklin's creative energy and stamina. In recalling Franklin, Cabanis observed that Franklin possessed the "art of living in the best fashion for himself and others . . . he would eat, sleep, and work whenever he saw fit, according to his needs."[97] In other words, Franklin lived an extraordinarily full and busy life, but he was not so regimented that he could not enjoy himself. In a letter to Adams, Jefferson later recalled that when he himself was stationed in France, he had informed a bishop with whom he was dining at Versailles that Franklin's "Health is very robust, his Spirits cheerful, and his Intellect as bright as ever."[98] Yet, when Jefferson first visited Franklin in Passy, he noted that the elderly diplomat was housebound with a kidney stone as well as gout.[99]

Home, Sweet Philadelphia

As much as Franklin was invigorated by his long stays in Europe on behalf of the American government—a total of eight years in France and sixteen in England—he longed to return home as encroaching age took its toll. Along with Adams and Jay, Franklin's signature graced the 1783 Treaty of Paris, but there were still details to be worked out with England and vital commercial treaties to be negotiated with the assistance of Adams and Jefferson. Franklin finally set out for America on July 12, 1785, in the company of the two grandsons who had accompanied him to Paris (Franklin had virtually adopted his estranged son William's son Temple as his own), after he was feted at several grand dinners in his honor. Before he left, several English physicians reviewed Franklin's case history of a "stone in the bladder," concluding that although it some-times made urination difficult, it was a "*Tolerable* Malady," which could be controlled by medication to help dissolve the stone, supplemented by mild exercise and a careful diet. Surgery was not recommended for someone of Franklin's advanced age. Franklin was cautioned by one of the doctors that at the age of seventy-nine, "it is high time to lay aside all business,"[100] certainly not a piece of advice that Franklin took to heart.

Franklin's voyage home from France was not without challenges pre-sented by bad weather and wind, but the trip gave him the opportunity to think, write, and even design a few new inventions without politi-cal distractions. In a lengthy treatise Franklin composed on board con-cerning the construction of chimneys, he veered off to one of his favor-ite subjects—the benefits of fresh air.

> Some are as much afraid of fresh Air as Persons in the Hydrophobia are of fresh Water. I myself had formerly this Prejudice, this *Aerophobia*, as I now account it, and reading the suppos'd dangerous Effects of cool Air, I consider'd it as an Enemy. . . . Experience has convinced me of my Error. I now look upon fresh Air as a Friend. I even sleep with an open Win-dow. I am persuaded that no common Air from without, is so unwhole-some as the Air within a close Room, that has been often breath'd and not changed.[101]

Franklin's emphasis on fresh air had also served as the impetus behind his invention of the Franklin stove, which provided a better way to heat rooms and reduce the lung-irritating soot and smoke; many of his improved chimney designs over the years; and his advice for greater ventilation in schools and hospitals.

In his diary, Franklin noted his first view in many years of "dear Philadelphia!" The ship cast anchor, but because of the usual precau-tion to avoid epidemics, the passengers were required "to wait for the health officer, who having made his visit, and finding no sickness, gave us leave to land." While this may have been inconvenient, Franklin undoubtedly approved of the health procedure since it was a sugges-tion he had offered many years previously. Franklin's arrival in Phila-delphia was greeted with cheers and festivity "by a crowd of people with huzzas," as he put it.[102] Without delay, Franklin soon resumed his active participation in American government as the elected "president," or governor, of Pennsylvania in 1785-1786, as well as pursuing his keen interest in medical science. Indeed, although he retired from active business as a comparatively young man, he never withdrew from his commitment to scientific inquiry. Perhaps Franklin's greatest contribution to medicine was his emphasis on preventative health, and many of his theories remain sound today. In an entertaining essay written in 1786, titled "The Art of Procuring Pleasing Dreams," Franklin skillfully wove together psychology and his strong belief in the benefits of exercise, moderate eating habits, and fresh air.

The main point of Franklin's essay was that good health and a relaxed mind and body promoted sound sleep and undisturbed dreams. According to Franklin, exercise should precede meals as an aid to digestion and to the development of natural sleep patterns. Furthermore, he observed that "[i]n general, mankind, since the improvement of cookery, eat about twice as much as nature requires." Franklin also appreciated the benefits of drinking water over alcoholic beverages, unusual in an age when heavy drinking of beer and hard liquor was far from uncommon. Like his friend Jefferson, however, he continued to enjoy "light" wines. It takes little imagination to predict how Franklin would have reacted to America's addiction today to high-calorie fast foods.

Franklin also reiterated his long-held belief that the circulation of fresh air, even during the night, was essential to good health because it dispelled elements of disease. While knowledge of the role of germs in spreading disease was a century in the future, Franklin espoused at least an embryonic theoretical concept of how colds and disease were transmitted. In his typical playfully humorous style, he wrote,

> Physicians, after having for ages contended that the sick should not be indulged with fresh air, have at length discovered that it may do them good. It is therefore to be hoped that they may in time discover likewise, that it is not hurtful to those who are in health, and that we may be then cured of the *aerophobia*, that at present distresses weak minds.[103]

Franklin's long friendship with Dr. Rush reveals that even in old age his interest in medical matters was still keen. In Rush's diary entries between the summer and late fall of 1786, he recorded several conversations with "Doctor Franklin." During one visit Franklin discussed the ill effects of tobacco use, which he believed caused hand tremors, and "declared he had never snuffed, chewed, or smoked." Later in the year Franklin reported to Rush that his old friend the physician "John Pringle once told him 92 fevers out of 100 cured themselves, 4 were cured by Art, and 4 proved fatal," underscoring both Franklin's many interactions with prominent physicians and his fervent belief in nature over the intervention of doctors and medicines.[104]

Always curious about cause and effect in relation to disease, in 1787 Franklin wrote a long discourse to British politician Benjamin Vaughan, in which he provided many examples of the "bad effects of lead taken inwardly." Poisoning as a result of lead pipes used in the processing of beverages such as cider was common in eighteenth-century America. In his essay, Franklin recalled that when he was a boy in Boston it was found that lead used in the process of making rum caused stomachaches called "dry gripes." As a young printer in London, Franklin had also observed that lead used in typesetting caused pain in his hands and that another more experienced printer informed him that hand problems were more probably caused by ingesting small particles of lead while eating food with improperly washed hands after handling type.

Centuries before lead in paint was outlawed in America, Franklin understood that it could cause serious health problems, and as an example he described the story of a European family who was sickened because their water was collected via a leaded roof. Finally, Franklin wrote Vaughan that while he was living in Paris, he had visited a hospital where *Colica Picotonum* (dry bellyache) or colic and gastritis, as we would term it today, was treated and had examined a list of patients. He was not surprised to discover that almost all the patients had worked with lead in some way in the course of their jobs! "You will see . . . that the opinion of this mischievous effect from lead is at least above sixty years old," Franklin concluded.[105]

In his last years, Franklin resided in his enlarged and remodeled spacious Philadelphia home on Market Street, happily surrounded by family members, including his daughter, son-in-law, and six grandchildren. In 1786, he informed his friend Jonathan Shipley that "[m]y health and spirits continue thanks to God, as when you saw me. The only complaint I then had does not grow worse, and is tolerable. I still have enjoyment in the company of my friends; and being easy in my circumstances have many reasons to like living." In his wry style Franklin also alluded to his death and to a "growing curiosity to be acquainted with some other," remarking that he could "cheerfully, with filial confidence, resign my spirit to the conduct of that great and good parent of mankind."[106] His words reflect his underlying optimism as well as his belief in an afterlife and a benevolent creator.

A moderate lifestyle helped to minimize distress from his chronic gout and kidney stone, but the latter continued to grow larger and more troublesome, to the point that he could feel the stone shifting when lying down. However, a letter to a friend and former neighbor in France reveals that he not only retained his belief in the health-giving properties of moderation and exercise but also maintained a cheerful and optimistic outlook that would see him through his last years. "I live temperately," Franklin maintained, and

drink no wine, and use daily the exercise of the dumb-bell, I flatter myself that the stone is kept from augmenting so much as it might otherwise do, and that I may still continue to find it tolerable. People who live long, who will drink the cup of life to the very bottom, must expect to meet with some of the usual dregs.[107]

Still, when the Constitutional Convention met in Philadelphia in May 1787, the 81-year-old Franklin had to miss the opening day and forgo his desire to personally nominate George Washington as its chairman due to a flareup of his kidney stones. Despite his pain, Franklin insisted on being present during the subsequent meeting days, even though it is said that he had to be carried to the meeting hall in a sedan chair from his home a block away.[108] Not long after, Franklin confessed to a friend, "I am now past 81 Years of Age, and therefore tho' still in tolerable Health cannot expect to survive much longer."[109] The following year Franklin was attacked by an even more severe case of gout, and although his pain was moderate he exhibited "swelling in both feet, which at last appeared also in both knees, and then in my hands." Curiously, this attack of gout seems to have put an end to the psoriasis that had affected him on and off for nearly fourteen years. Though the swelling receded, he concluded, "I am on the whole much weaker than when it began to leave me. But possibly that may be the effect of age, for I am now near eighty-three, the age of commencing decrepitude."[110]

In his last year, Franklin's health deteriorated appreciably, and like his friend Jefferson, he resorted in old age to regular doses of laudanum to dull his pain and allow him to rest. In the fall of 1789, he informed a friend in France that "I have a long time been afflicted with almost constant and grievous pain, to combat which I have been obliged to have recourse to opium, which indeed has afforded me some ease from time to time, but then it has taken away my appetite and so impeded my digestion that I am become totally emaciated."[111] His mental powers remained sharp, but he found it increasingly difficult to complete his memoirs, which we know as *The Autobiography of Benjamin Franklin*. Franklin's discomfort forced him to dictate his words to his grandson, as "[o]pium gives me ease when I am attacked by pain, and by the use of it I still make life at least tolerable. Not being able to bear sitting to write, I now make use of the hand of one of my grandsons, dictating to him from my bed."[112]

In the fall of 1789, Franklin also summoned the energy to write to congratulate his admired friend and the new nation's first president, George Washington, on his recovery from illness. Washington's reply is evidence of their warm relationship, his deep appreciation for his revolutionary compatriot, and his realization that Franklin was living out his last days in discomfort, with little that contemporary medicine could do to ease his pain. "Would to God, my dear Sir," Washington wrote to Franklin,

[t]hat I could congratulate you upon the removal of that excruciating pain under which you labour! And that your existence might close with as much ease to yourself, as its continuance has been beneficial to our Country and useful to mankind! . . . But this cannot be, and you have within yourself the only resource to which we can confidently apply for relief: a *Philosophic mind*.[113]

Despite increasing disability, in his final months Franklin continued to enjoy the company of friends. The year before his death he informed a friend, "I have as much Health and Chearfulness as can well be expected at my Age, now 83. Hitherto this long Life has been tolerably happy." He concluded that if he had the opportunity to relive his life, he would be well satisfied, only he would wish to do "what Authors do in a second edition of their Works, correct some of my Errata."[114] Less than a year before, Franklin had mused,

> I have not of much reason to boast of it [health]. . . . However, when I consider how many more terrible [maladies] the human Body is liable to, I think myself well off that I have only three incurable ones, the Gout, the Stone, and Old Age; and those not withstanding, I enjoy many comfortable Intervals, in which I forget all my ills, and amuse myself in Reading or Writing, or in conversation with Friends, joking, laughing, and telling merry Stories, and when you first knew me, as a young Man about Fifty.[115]

Franklin's words were echoed by Jefferson. Writing to a mutual friend in France, Jefferson described the state of Franklin's health after a recent visit: "I found . . . Franklin in his bed, cheerful and free from pain, but still in his bed. He took a lively interest in the details I gave him of your [French] revolution. I observed his face often flushed in the course of it. He is much emaciated."[116]

In his memoirs, Jefferson also recalled his last visit with his hero Franklin in Philadelphia. Of the American founders, these two were most similar in their scientific approach to medicine and their emphasis on disease prevention. After a lively discussion over the fate of many of their acquaintances in France, who were now experiencing the "perilous" convulsions of the French Revolution, Franklin entrusted Jefferson with a fragment of his autobiography. "I called on the venerable and beloved Franklin," he wrote, and "[h]e was then on the bed of sickness, from which he never arose."[117] After Franklin's death, Jefferson wrote a mutual friend in France that

> [t]he good old Dr. Franklin, so long an ornament of our country, and I may say of the world, has at length closed an eminent career. He died of the 17th instant, of an imposthume of the lungs, which having suppurated and burst, he had not the strength to throw off the matter, and was suffocated by it. His illness of this impostume was of sixteen days.[118]

Without the intervention of modern antibiotics, chest infections could often prove fatal at the time, especially in the elderly.

As Jefferson had described, the immediate cause of Franklin's death on April 17, 1790, at the age of eighty-four was failure of his lungs as a result of a systemic infection related to pleurisy. Dr. Rush recorded the event in his diary, and Rush's description reveals the limits of medical understanding at the time. "Last evening at 11 o'clock died the venerable Dr. Franklin," Rush wrote.

> He had been reduced by the stone in his bladder, but died finally of a pleurisy which terminated in an abscess in his lungs from which he discharged matter a few days before his death. This pleurisy was caught by lying with his window open. He possessed his reason to the last day of his life, but spoke nothing of his future existence or expectation beyond the grave.[119]

Adams, with whom Franklin had long debated the benefits of fresh air for colds, wrote in his diary that the cause of Franklin's death was sitting "for some hours at a Window, with the cool Air blowing upon him."[120] Knowing Franklin's firm belief in the efficacy of fresh air in the prevention of illness, we can speculate that he would have been amused and perhaps a good deal irritated by Rush's and Adams's connection between Franklin's illness and an open window. More likely, the long years of repeated episodes of gout and the large bladder stone made Franklin increasingly immobile, wore his body down, and compromised his immune system.[121]

Notions of patient confidentiality and privacy in Franklin's time were far removed from their state today, and his private physician published a detailed description of Franklin's last days in the April 21, 1790, edition of *The Pennsylvania Gazette*. "The stone, with which he had been afflicted for several years," Franklin's doctor wrote,

> had for the last twelve months confined him chiefly to his bed; and during the extremely painful paroxysms, he was obliged to take large doses of laudanum to mitigate his tortures—still in the intervals of pain, he not only amused himself with reading and conversing cheerfully with his family and a few friends who visited him, but was often employed in doing business of a public as well as a private nature.[122]

The article confirms our impression of Franklin in his last days, still mentally alert, cheerful, but wracked with increasing pain.

The physician reported in his article that about two weeks before his demise, Franklin contracted a fever, which developed into "a cough and laborious breathing." A slight improvement gave the Franklin family hope, but in the end a liquid-filled abscess apparently burst in his lungs, ultimately causing respiratory failure and "a calm lethargic state," which probably reflected that Franklin had become comatose. According to the attending doctor, "On the 17th instant, about eleven o'clock at night, he quietly expired, closing a long and useful life of eighty-four years and three months."[123] An astounding number of people—over twenty thousand—attended the funeral of one of the most admired and revered men of his era.

As we have seen, as a long-time supporter of the Philadelphia Hospital, Franklin had a knack for fundraising that literally enabled the institution to open its doors. Leading physicians welcomed him into medical societies and engaged in frequent discussions with the erudite politician, scientist, and philosopher. During his long lifetime, Franklin amassed a wide and eclectic library and collected medical books and equipment along with volumes on history, philosophy, and science, and counted the great French philosopher Voltaire as his admiring friend. One visitor to Franklin's home in 1787 described a "glass machine" on display that exhibited "the circulation of the blood in the arteries and veins of the human body." Franklin built his own "little machine" based on a model he had seen in Boston.[124]

Benjamin Franklin's brain had hummed with creativity throughout his long life. We are fortunate that a good deal of that energy was directed toward the art of healing. Franklin was considered one of the leading scientists in the world during his lifetime, and during the revolutionary era he was widely venerated for his contributions to our understanding of nature and science, especially his work with electricity. Not only did he revolutionize America, but he revolutionized science, and today contemporary science historians "still refer to the mid-eighteenth century as the Age of Franklin."[125]

If Franklin's role in the areas of health and illness was not quite as visible or dramatic as his political role, it was still certainly central to the advancement of medicine in America, despite his being "merely" a layman. As one writer put it, he not only helped shape medicine in colonial America and the young nation, but earned the respect of those "involved in the healing arts throughout the world."[126] Franklin was an especially keen observer of his surroundings. His views on diet, exercise, and moderation helped guide Americans of his day, and his practical bent provided the impetus for the invention of such widely used items as bifocals and the urinary catheter. Franklin's ideas about how colds are transmitted, theories about lead poisoning and treatment of gout, still ring true today, and he even speculated on the connection between mental attitude and sickness and healing. Many of his medical predictions came to pass. Finally, his work on documenting statistics on smallpox epidemics, his support of smallpox inoculation, and his central role in establishing America's first hospital and medical school, reflect his underlying concern for the health of the budding nation, certainly a focus he shared with Washington, Adams, Jefferson, and Madison.

3

Abigail and John Adams

Partners in Sickness and Health

My anxiety for your welfare will never leave me
but with my parting Breath, tis more important to
me than all this world contains besides.
—*Abigail Adams to John Adams, July 21, 1776*

Take great care of your health which is precious to
me beyond all Calculation.
—*John Adams to Abigail Adams, November 8, 1794*

Abigail's Early Health

Abigail Smith Adams, born on November 11, 1744, in Weymouth, Massachusetts, was no stranger to illness, so it is not surprising that the subject of health and disease occupied such a prominent place in her life. Recurrent childhood illnesses, especially rheumatic fever, which would also later haunt her as an adult, kept Abigail from attending school in her home town. As a determined but delicate young woman, she also suffered periodically from insomnia and headaches, which also troubled her in later years. Weymouth was then a small town with a population of about twelve hundred, located about fourteen miles from Boston. A variety of epidemics were rampant in Weymouth when Abigail was growing up, including throat distemper (diphtheria), smallpox, pleurisy, and other viral and bacterial infections. Her uncle, Cotton Tufts, was a well-respected local doctor who treated Abigail during the course of many early sicknesses. Her mother, Elizabeth Quincy Smith, appears to have been especially overprotective of the sometimes frail Abigail and probably wanted to keep her isolated from the general population by schooling her at home.[1] Her parents' concerns were not unfounded. In 1751, when Abigail was only six, a serious diphtheria epidemic broke out in Weymouth, killing one in eight people, and it took a particularly high toll among children. Abigail's father, Pastor William Smith, kept a diary during the time that recorded the loss in only three months of thirty residents, including twenty-one children.[2] As we have seen in the previous chapters, in Abigail's day it was commonplace to be surrounded by illness and death on an almost daily basis.

Abigail's mother made sure her daughters were raised to be capable wives and mothers,[3] and it is clear that illness and healing were not the only factors in homeschooling them. As was common at the time, her parents did not subscribe to the notion of advanced education for women, and both Mary and Elizabeth, the other two Smith daughters, also learned to read and write at the parsonage. However, all three became highly articulate, literate women, and they also learned how to treat many common illnesses at home using a store of medicinal tonics and herbs. Abigail was descended from respected prominent Puritan stock and raised in a highly devout family. Although the young Abigail did not attend school, her father, a well-to-do prominent local liberal Congregational minister, and her mother, born into a well-known Massachusetts political merchant family, also made sure that her voracious appetite for reading and knowledge was well fed in both religious and secular subjects. Thus, Abigail and her sisters were educated at home and probably in a manner superior to most New England females of the era. Moreover, as a pastor's wife, Elizabeth Smith also served as a role model for all three of her daughters as a female community leader. She kept her finger on the pulse of the health of congregation members, visited the sick regularly, and offered nursing care and home remedies when needed.[4]

Health, Pragmatic Medicine, and the Newlywed Couple

After a two-year engagement, on October 25, 1764, Abigail Smith married John Adams, future revolutionary leader and American president. It was a union initially opposed by her parents, especially by Abigail's mother,

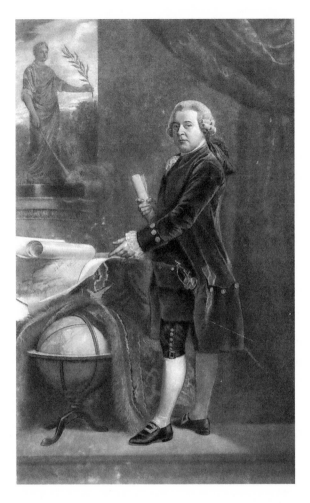

Engraving of John
Adams from an Origi-
nal Painting by Gilbert
Stuart. (Courtesy
Library of Congress)

who did not care much for the fiercely intelligent but brash, talkative
young lawyer whose status and prospects she deemed beneath her daughter's social station. When she wed, the slim, petite Abigail was nineteen
years old; John was nine years her senior and at around five feet six inches
tall, half a foot taller than Abigail and already on the road to stoutness.
Adams was born in Braintree, Massachusetts, on October 30, 1735. From
the beginning Abigail kept the brilliant and principled but sometimes
vain, prickly, and erratic John grounded, and her natural serenity and
optimism were a strong influence on taming his often mercurial temperament. As historian Joseph J. Ellis put it, Abigail provided John's "ballast."[5]

By all accounts their long marriage of almost sixty years was a loving and enduring partnership, attested to by well over a thousand affectionate letters. Illness was a constant in their life together, and in the voluminous correspondence between the couple, rare was the letter that did not contain references to the sickness or state of health of family and community members. Abigail's concern for John's health and welfare was foreshadowed during their days of courtship. She may have had a premonition that in the future extreme stress could play havoc with John's health, and in her perceived role as primary helpmate, she would always strive to mitigate such situations through unfailing moral support. In a letter to John dated April 8, 1764, Abigail admonished John to take care: "I am very fearful that you will not when left to your own management follow your directions—but let her who tenderly cares for you both in Sickness and Health, intreet you to be careful of that Health upon which depends the happiness of Your A. Smith."[6]

In an earlier letter, Abigail had expressed relief that her anxiety about John's planned inoculation for smallpox had disappeared following her uncle Tufts's assurance that Dr. Perkins, the physician who would conduct the procedure, was highly respected and knowledgeable. John quickly replied that her letter had put his "Heart at ease," as he made arrangements to isolate himself for several weeks to prevent spread of the disease after taking "the modern way of Inoculation."[7] The two ways to acquire immunity to smallpox at the time were either by variolation (using live human variola virus) or by contracting it naturally, which carried a much higher mortality rate. Smallpox had struck fear in the hearts of humans for millennia, and colonial Americans were no exception. As we have seen, John's great-uncle, Dr. Zabdiel Boylston, and the influential New England clergyman Reverend Cotton Mather had been early advocates for smallpox inoculation in Boston during the terrible epidemic of 1721.

In 1761, John's mother, herself ill at the time, lost her seventy-year-old husband, John Adams Senior, through a contagious disease. In his autobiography Adams recalled that both his parents were "seized . . . with the violent Fever, a kind of Influenza, or an Epidemick which carried off Seventeen Aged People in our Neighbourhood."[8] This personal health crisis may have exacerbated Mrs. Adams's fear that she would lose her son as well in a smallpox epidemic if he was not inoculated. Boylston's support and earlier example undoubtedly played a part in her son's undergoing the still contested and potentially dangerous procedure. In his autobiography Adams later observed, "This Distemper [smallpox] was very terrible even by Innoculation at that time. . . . My Physicians dreaded it, and prepared me, by a milk Diet and a Course of Mercurial Preparations, till they reduced me very low before they performed the operation." The preparation itself could cause troublesome side effects. As Adams recalled, "every tooth in my head became so loose. . . . By such means they conquered the Small Pox." The loose teeth were probably the result of some degree of mercury poisoning, and Adams attributed later dental problems in old age to the earlier procedure.[9]

New England was then the region with the strictest restrictions against inoculation, but many cities in the colonies had imposed rules to govern the controversial procedure. Regulations were set locally by law in Boston, and Massachusetts was the first colony to establish an effective quarantine system.[10] Although Boston had adopted a law against inoculation, in the light of a new smallpox outbreak of "naturally" acquired cases in 1764, numerous daring souls like John Adams ignored the prohibition. Nearly seven hundred cases of smallpox in the spring of 1764 resulted in 124 deaths, and inoculation became more attractive. Many trained doctors as well as medical quacks in Boston advertised their services, sometimes with outlandish claims. For example, one newspaper advertisement noted that an "experienced," newly arrived irregular practitioner from Constantinople had inoculated "about 50,000 people without losing a Single Patient. He requires not the least Preparation Regimen or Confinement. Ladies and Gentlemen who wish to be inoculated need only acquaint him with how many Pimples they choose and he makes the exact number of Punctures with His Needles which produces the Eruptions."[11]

Of course, the sensible John Adams had chosen a reputable physician, but the ad underscores the lack of regulation in regard to medical practitioners at the time and the degree to which charlatans often competed with trained physicians. Due to the quarantine following his inoculation, Abigail and John were separated for over a month, and he remained isolated in Boston with his brother and some other friends who had undergone the procedure at his uncle's house. The goal of inoculation against the *Variola major* virus was to acquire immunity from the most dangerous form of smallpox. It generally produced a mild case, but those who were inoculated were contagious, and some contracted a serious form that in rare cases even resulted in death. It was this latter concern that prompted Elizabeth Smith to forbid her daughter Abigail from undergoing inoculation, and it was not until 1776, when she was a married woman and mother of four, that Abigail would receive the immunization.

Soon John Adams penned a long letter to his fiancée from Boston that focused almost exclusively on his personal experience with prevention of one of the greatest scourges of the age. All his letters to Abigail during the quarantine period were double "smoked" to insure that the smallpox virus would not be transmitted to her. It was recommended that those undergoing inoculation undertake an elaborate week-long preparation that included medications such as the purgative calomel (mercury) and abstention from eating certain foods, including meat. Additionally, most were instructed to take ipecac just prior to the procedure to induce vomiting to cleanse the body. Adams followed this regimen. His musings provide us with a graphic description (punctuated with typical bits of his caustic humor) about the inoculation process from a patient's point of view:

> Dr Perkins demanded my left Arm and Dr Warren my Brothers. They took their Launcetts and with their Points divided the skin for about a Quarter of an Inch and just suffering the Blood to appear, buried a Thread about a Quarter of an Inch long in the Channell. A little Lint was then laid over the scratch and a Piece of a Ragg pressed on, and then a Bandage bound over all. . . . The Doctors have left us Pills red and black to take Night and Morning. But they looked very sagaciously and importantly at us, and ordered my Brother, larger Doses than me, on Account of the Differences in our Constitutions.[12]

John's account seems to corroborate that he believed the potential benefits of inoculation outweighed the risks. His concern for the health of the wider local community was a factor as well. He concluded the letter by asking Abigail's father to pray for his good health as "when We are undertaking any Thing of Consequence as the small Pox, undoubtedly tho, I have not the Least Apprehension at all of what is called Danger."[13] John broke out with the anticipated pustules but escaped any serious consequences from the procedure other than the temporary dental problems. Overall, he experienced a remarkably easy recovery, as he declared to Abigail: "None of the Race of Adam, ever passed the small Pox, with fewer Pains, Achs, Qualms, or with less smart than I have done."[14]

After marriage the couple settled into a modest-sized saltbox cottage on the sixty-acre family farm. John had inherited the property from his father, a moderately successful local farmer and respected community leader, and it was located in Braintree, about five miles from Abigail's more impressive family home in Weymouth. John's widowed mother, Susanna, lived close by, just down the road in the house where John had been raised. Abigail admired and became close to her caring but sometimes domineering mother-in-law and was later very solicitous in tending her in old age. Abigail's literary and intellectual horizons further widened as she availed herself of her husband's extensive library. She developed into an uncommonly accomplished and well-read woman who was not afraid to express her strong opinions. To his credit John, in turn, was inclined to listen and take his wife's views seriously.

John Adams's parents, both intelligent individuals who taught their own children to read at an early age,[15] wanted their eldest son to enter the prestigious ministry, but instead John had followed his own inclinations and become a lawyer, considered an inferior occupation at the time. It is thought he once considered becoming a physician,[16] and during a stint as a teacher Adams boarded with a doctor and studied his medical library, perhaps a contributing factor in his forward-looking support of smallpox inoculation and affinity for medical matters.[17]

The only New Englander among the founders in this study, John Adams brought his pragmatic nature to bear on his medical views. For Adams, on both a personal and a public level, the goal of medicine was a practical one: to provide good care and employ the most up-to-date treatments and medications to cure or prevent illness. As we learned above, as an early advocate of smallpox inoculation he weighed the evidence before deciding that the benefits of the procedure trumped the potential danger. Although Adams never attained the sophisticated scientific understanding of medicine displayed by both Franklin and Jefferson, his commonsense approach made him an advocate for community as well as personal health. By no stretch of the imagination could Adams be considered a scientist on the level of Franklin, or even Jefferson, but he was certainly interested in the biological sciences and was an impressive intellect in his own right. As a college-educated man with a degree in law from Harvard, who was raised during the Age of Reason, Adams surely had a grasp of fundamental contemporary scientific thought.[18]

Toward the Revolution

The Adams family moved to Boston for several years beginning in 1768 before returning to Braintree in 1771 so that they could see more of one another, be closer to John's growing law practice, and take a more active role in the political affairs leading to the American Revolution and the War for Independence. According to Massachusetts governor Hutchinson, John's busy law practice and health precluded him from the early and extensive involvement in public affairs displayed by his cousin Sam Adams.[19] However, John and Abigail were keenly interested in the unfolding events, and they each read several newspapers daily to keep abreast of developments. Both were equally incensed with Britain's encroachment on liberty in the colonies and increasingly felt that separation from the Mother Country was both desirable and inevitable. From the beginning of John's political involvement Abigail served as an able adviser and sounding board.

Despite the progress of John's career, these were stressful years for the couple. Until his midthirties, John Adams enjoyed remarkably good health, other than the usual assortment of minor indispositions that affect all humans. However, as he grew older political and emotional stresses may have played a role in some of his rare but more serious ailments. During the early 1770s, Adams took a controversial step in defending the British soldiers charged in the Boston Massacre, witnessed the heartbreaking death of his young daughter, Susanna, and also played a key role as a member of the Massachusetts assembly just as increasingly unpopular British measures fueled colonial protest. In February of 1771, Adams appears to have suffered a "collapse," characterized by weakness, anxiety, and "Pain in my Breast and complaint in my Lungs." In the somewhat exaggerated and histrionic fashion Adams was sometimes reduced to in a health crisis, he noted in his diary that he had spent "a most unhappy Night—never in more misery, in my whole life." Whatever the real cause of his sickness, which "seriously threatened my Life," it kept him away from pressing work for months, and on the advice of his physician, he even traveled to Connecticut to visit the mineral springs to improve his health.[20] The return to Braintree in 1771 may indeed have been prompted in part by health concerns and the feeling that a hiatus from politics would restore his former health. As John wrote to a relative, "I must avoid Politicks . . . or I should soon have shaken off this mortal body."[21]

In the late 1990s, historian John Ferling and physician Lewis E. Braverman speculated that this episode and two later serious illnesses experienced by John Adams may have been caused by thyrotoxicosis, a disease of the thyroid. They postulated that in periods of extreme stress Adam's underlying thyroid condition was exacerbated and latent symptoms became more pronounced, producing depression, irritability, confusion, and even a goiter.[22] A thyroid condition is certainly a plausible *possible* explanation for Adams's intermittent health "breakdowns." However, to put his illnesses in perspective, we must acknowledge that the terms "breakdown" and "collapse" were often used as catchall phrases at the time to describe periods of a wide variety of debilitating illness. The times were indeed perilous and stressful. Adams's fellow founding fathers James Madison and Thomas Jefferson, for example, often succumbed to what they and their contemporaries described as "collapses." As we will see in the next chapter, Madison's latent malaria and epilepsy flared up in times of political upheaval, and Jefferson suffered from notorious debilitating headaches when confronted with intense political or emotional agitation.

Abigail certainly worried about John's health but generally took a more stoic attitude than her husband in the face of life's infinite challenges. During the long periods when John was absent from their Braintree or Boston homes, Abigail supervised the running of the farm and household and oversaw the raising of their children. She also became an adept businesswoman and manager. In periods of crisis, some of them political but many of them tied to issues of illness, Abigail was left on her own without the close proximity of her husband for support. During one of John's absences Abigail and her eldest son, John Quincy, witnessed the memorable and terrifying Battle of Bunker Hill on their own from a position near their Boston house. As John became more involved in the growing rift between England and the colonies in 1774 as one of four Massachusetts representatives in the Philadelphia Continental Congress, absences of six months at a time were not uncommon.[23]

Both John and Abigail shared in the sacrifice, propelled by a sense of duty in the service of their country. Indeed, like their fellow revolutionists the Washingtons, Franklin, Jefferson, and the Madisons, the Adamses subscribed to a political ideology and moral philosophy that emphasized devotion to the common good. As John put it succinctly, "Public Virtue is the only Foundation of Republics."[24] Abigail was content in her traditional roles as wife and mother, so assuming the responsibility for the farm and all business matters was a task she took on reluctantly.[25] Yet her strong religious beliefs emphasized charitable deeds, and on one level her commitment to independence and the new republic reflected her willingness to often forgo private inclinations for the benefit of the public good. The exchange of letters, even though mail delivery could be unreliable and excruciatingly slow, was the lifeline that held John and Abigail Adams tethered together during their frequent, often lengthy physical separations. After twelve years of marriage Abigail once regretfully speculated that "we have not lived together more than six."[26]

At times while each awaited a letter containing much anticipated news about the health of one another or their children that failed to arrive for weeks or even months, Abigail's and John's anxiety became palpable. It is to their credit that despite their worries they carried on their political, parental, and household duties in an admirable fashion. Although she is most often referenced as the wife of one American president and the mother of another, Abigail Adams was a highly accomplished woman and talented writer in her own right, well versed in the political and social issues of the day. Her letters are gracefully written, full of interesting details and observations that allow us a firsthand glimpse into her world, including contemporary medicine.[27]

Dr. Benjamin Rush described Abigail Adams with affection and admiration. "Mrs. Adams," he wrote in his autobiography, "in point of talent, knowledge, virtue, and female accomplishments was in every respect fitted to be the friend and companion of her husband in all his different and successive stations, of private citizen, member of Congress, foreign minister, Vice President and President of the United States."[28] Perhaps more remarkable for the era was the contemporary assessment of Abigail's intellectual capabilities offered on the occasion of a eulogy delivered by a friend of John's after the former president's burial in 1826: "[John Adams] found in her a mind as powerful and capacious as his own."[29] A prolific, articulate, and observant letter writer, Abigail wrote missives that provide us with frank reflections about the ways illness affected individuals in America from the mid-eighteenth to the early nineteenth century. As Abigail herself once put it on the eve of the Revolution, "My pen is always freer than my tongue. I have wrote many things to you [John] that I suppose I never could have talked."[30]

Health, Illness, and the Adams Family

John and Abigail Adams became the parents of six children, but only four survived childhood. Their eldest child and only surviving daughter, born in 1765, was named Abigail after her mother but was always affectionately referred to as Nabby. She was a chubby, healthy, and active baby, although when she contracted whooping cough as an infant, she quickly passed it on to Abigail.[31] John Quincy arrived in 1767, followed by Susanna in 1768. Sadly, the baby, Suky, as she was nicknamed, died at the age of only fourteen months of unknown causes, and we have no record of the undoubtedly painful reaction to her death by her parents. In 1770, a second son, Charles, was born, followed by their third son, Thomas, in 1772. Five years later, in 1777, Abigail gave birth to a still-born daughter they named Elizabeth.

The life of Abigail Adams demonstrates that women during the era took a prominent role in healing and the practice of "domestic" medicine. In the absence of hospitals, or before hospitals were viewed as safe and desirable environments for the ill, aiding the sick or those in childbirth became a community responsibility, with local women stepping in to offer assistance with nursing care, comfort, and food. In other words, medical care was often provided by women in private homes, and many became prominent lay practitioners.[32] Indeed, Abigail's mother was clearly influenced by an American colonial tradition that regarded providing for the sick and needy as a religious obligation of a wife of a clergyman in pursuit of the public good.[33] Following their mother's example, Abigail and her sisters faithfully nursed and watched over neighbors and family members through innumerable illnesses, extending their female network and sharing medical knowledge and their storehouse of medicinal compounds and remedies. On one level it was Abigail's modest, although important, step into the area of public health care.

The typical birth pattern for fertile women during the era was generally eighteen-month to two-year intervals. Most women carried out their normal chores during pregnancy, but childbirth itself was considered an illness, demanding special attention from a social network of supportive female family members and friends, who often took over some of the new mother's household tasks to provide a respite after her physical ordeal.[34] Abigail's mother and her sister, Mary, assisted with the birth of Abigail's children, reflecting that colonial women often desired the comforting "circle of female support" during childbirth. Midwives commonly delivered and helped care for babies in this period, but by the end of the century physicians were edging out midwives among the middle and upper classes by equating medical delivery with scientific progress and offering medicinal potions to ease labor pains.[35] The move toward the use of "learned" doctors also reflected the undermining of traditional social relations and the increased emphasis on discrete private family units rather than reliance on the psychological and emotional supporting bonds formerly provided by the community of local women.[36]

The transformation from the almost exclusive use of midwives to physicians was often not a positive one for new mothers. It has been demonstrated that maternal mortality rates as a result of childbirth actually rose with exclusive "male management," which had been kept relatively low at a rate of less than 4 percent under the cooperative ministrations of skilled midwives assisted only rarely by doctors in the late eighteenth century.[37] A study of the comparative stillbirth rates for Martha Ballard, an experienced and busy midwife who delivered 814 babies between 1785 and 1812, reveals that she exhibited the lowest number in comparison to several doctors and to the overall rate in other New England towns of the era. Ballard's rate of maternal mortality was also considerably lower when compared to those at the time in London and Dublin.[38] Doctors coming to a birth could bring the promise of comfort and safety through pain-relieving drugs and the newest obstetrical technology, but their intervention often unwittingly carried contagion from the germs of infectious patients they had previously attended or danger from the overenthusiastic use of forceps.[39]

In the fall of 1774, the Adamses moved once again to Boston before later returning to the family farm in Braintree in June 1776. In response to the notorious Boston Tea Party, England had imposed the Coercive Act on Massachusetts to bring the colony to heel. John's law practice in Boston was adversely affected. In a letter to Abigail back in Braintree, he provided an account of one of his many colds, "the most obstinate and threatening one, I ever had in my life," mixed in with comments on his lack of business and the political tensions between England and the colonies. "We live my dear Soul, in an age of Tryal," he wrote, and signed his missive "with great Anxiety for your health," as he had learned from Abigail's father that she too had contracted a cold.[40]

Attending the Continental Congress

In August 1774, John left Boston to attend the Continental Congress in Philadelphia, where he remained until October when it adjourned. In September, Abigail wrote John that she was distressed not to have had a letter from him in five weeks and that she longed to hear he was safe, but "I enjoy better health than I have done these 2 years."[41] As the political crisis intensified Abigail was increasingly willing to sacrifice for the good of the colonies and was proud of John's growing role in the political crisis, as she believed that "the fate of Empires depend upon your wisdom." But that did not prevent her from worrying about his real or imaginary illnesses. "The anxiety I suffered from not hearing one syllable from you for more than five weeks . . . agitated me more than I have been. . . . I feard much for your Health when you went away," she wrote in June 1775. "I must intreat you to be careful as you can consistant with the Duty you owe our Country. That consideration alone prevaild with me to consent to your departure, in a time so perilous and hazardous to your family— and with a body so infirm as to require the tenderest care and Nursing."[42]

During John's four years as a delegate to the Continental Congress, health issues would plague him repeatedly. Writing from Philadelphia in the spring of 1775, John noted that he had experienced ocular problems but ended by giving Abigail a somewhat reassuring update on his health: "I have had a very disagreeable Time of it. My Health and especially my Eyes have been so very bad, that I have not been so fit for Business." John certainly tended to be melodramatic about his health at times and also a bit of a complainer, but a visit to two local doctors seemed to improve his conditions, as "Dr. Young has made a kind of a Cure of my health and Dr. Church of my Eyes."[43]

John, who had a tendency to hypochondria, certainly took his ailments very seriously. Back in Massachusetts following the outbreak of war with England in the spring of 1775, Adams fell ill with fever and other "allarming" symptoms that caused him to delay his departure for Philadelphia. During 1775 and 1776, he complained intermittently of ill health, including periods of depression, painful eyes, sweating, tremors, and skin rashes, and at one point when the Declaration of Independence was being composed and debated he declared, "I am always unwell."[44] Although they acknowledge that even Adams himself realized he was undergoing extreme stress, these episodes were once again attributed by Ferling and Braverman to a presumed thyroid condition, which can flare up from a latent state in periods of undue psychological strain.[45] However, it is impossible to confirm that specific diagnosis, and certainly the symptoms are not inconsistent with patients who exhibit extreme anxiety alone.

Abigail Adams as Family Healer and Patient

Although John was often away from the family, he was a doting father and always tried to keep abreast of his children's activities. While he was absent during the Revolution, Abigail not only faced heightened responsibilities and the challenges of work and motherhood but the trauma of war and the specter of disease. Both British and American troops made Boston a strategic military location, and the presence of the armies fueled the spread of disease. During one of John's frequent absences, the Boston area was struck by a widespread epidemic of virulent dysentery in 1775. Fever, uncontrollable bouts of stomach cramps, and bloody diarrhea characterized dysentery and often left victims weak and helpless. During the era no specific effective cure for the illness was available and the mechanism of contagion was poorly understood. As a result, hundreds died and thousands were affected. Abigail reported from Braintree that many of her neighbors were ill or dying and "such is the distress of the Neighbourhood that I can scarcly find a well person to assist me in looking after the sick. . . . So sickly and so

Mortal a time the oldest Man does not remember."[46] Abigail's family, servants, and farmhands were not spared, and her mother, Elizabeth, came to help her daughter cope with a sick household. The first to be stricken was Isaac Copeland, a hired hand on the Adams farm, and a few days later even thirty-year-old Abigail found herself weakened by the bacterial ailment.

Before Abigail could recover, two-year-old Thomas and two serving girls were also severely afflicted, and then her 54-year-old mother succumbed as well. Abigail was exhausted from round-the-clock nursing of her young son, caring for her mother, and cleaning up after her young maidservant Patty. In a letter to her husband Abigail wearily reported, "Our House is an hospital in every part, and what with my own weakness and distress of mind for my family I have been unhappy enough."[47] The family apparently had at least a rudimentary understanding of contagion and the value of a disinfectant, perhaps acquired through her reading of Dr. William Buchan's popular self-help book *Domestic Medicine*, and Abigail and the servants worked doggedly to mitigate the spread of disease by "cleaning it [the house] with hot vinegar."[48]

Abigail mustered what little energy she had to tend to her family and begged John to send her rhubarb root, nutmeg, cloves, and cinnamon, which she used as medicinal aids to brew simples and cordials as "so much sickness has occasioned a scarcity of medicine."[49] Like so many colonial women, Abigail was a fairly skilled herbalist. Many years later, for example, she recommended a variety of home remedies to aid her ill niece, who had recently given birth. "A Bath of Hot Herbs was the most salutary means made use for me," she suggested. "A poultice of Camomile flowers is also very good. . . . Painful experience would teach me upon the very first chill, to apply a white Bread poultice because those cold fits are always succeeded by a fever and complaints of the Breast always follow."[50] In 1799, she advised her sister Elizabeth Shaw Peabody to take "elixir vitrol, the bark [quinine]" to treat the symptoms of menopause.[51]

Abigail and her young children survived the 1775 dysentery epidemic, but sadly the maidservant Patty and Elizabeth Smith died, demonstrating how what is today generally considered an uncomfortable but treatable illness could devastate a population without the capability of intravenous hydration and nutrition and antibiotics. Certainly dysentery was a specter that hovered over soldiers in the revolutionary militias at the time and spread quickly among troops in the close quarters. As we learned in the previous chapter about Washington, diseases such as dysentery and smallpox rivaled the British as the cause of mortality among those who served in the Continental Army. John's youngest brother, Elihu Adams, was serving as a captain in the militia when he contracted dysentery and died in August of 1775, leaving a young widow and three children.

Abigail was heartbroken at the loss of the beloved mother who had shown her such affection throughout her childhood and adult life. "Have pitty upon me," Abigail entreated her husband after Elizabeth Smith died. "How can I tell you o my (bursting heart) that my Dear Mother has Left me. . . . 'Tis a dreadful time with the whole province. Sickness and death are in almost every family."[52] Although she had often chafed under Elizabeth's close watch when she was younger, as a wife and mother Abigail came to appreciate her mother's sincere attention and the sad reality that extreme concern about the health of one's family was not unfounded during the era. Abigail's words also underscore that against the backdrop of the horrors of war lurked the ever-present threat of disease. "The desolation of war is not so distressing as the havoc made by the pestilence," Abigail maintained.[53]

John's reply to Abigail reflects the grim reality of mortality rates during the period. After reiterating that he hoped that Abigail's firm religious faith would help sustain her, John observed, "If We live long ourselves We must bury our Parents and all our Elder Relations and many of those who are younger. I have lost a Parent, a Child and a Brother, and each of them left a lasting Impression on my Mind."[54] Weakened by the dysentery epidemic, Abigail was soon troubled by a severe cold as well as a flareup of rheumatism and jaundice, and she informed John that many other dysentery victims "are now afflicted both with the Jaundice and Rhumatism, some it has left in Hecticks [recurrent fevers] some in Dropsies [edema]."[55]

As a forceful advocate for independence, John Adams became one of the leaders of the Congress and one of its most effective public speakers, often overwhelming the members with his "oratorical energy" and frequently volcanic delivery.[56] On her own in Braintree in the momentous year of 1776, Abigail continued to be preoccupied with health issues within her family and the larger community while running the farm and household. March brought scarlet fever to their son Thomas. In April she wrote John with sadness that "I have been attending the sick chamber of our Neighbor Trot whose affliction I most sensibly feel but cannot describe, stripped of two lovely children in one week" due to a "Canker [scarlet] fever." At the same time her niece Betsy Cranch had been seriously sick with the disorder and another local child was fatally ill. "Many grown persons are now sick with it, in this street 5. It rages much in other Towns." Mumps also hovered over the area, striking Isaac, their farm hand, and Abigail revealed that she feared it would soon infect her children as well, and "My Heart Trembles with anxiety for them."[57]

To add to the general distress John's brother's youngest child died of convulsive fits in the same month, and Nabby, John, and Charles contracted the mumps but recovered without any serious effects.[58] Abigail's letters reveal that colonial Americans experienced epidemics on at least a regular seasonal if not a monthly basis. With few effective disease-specific medical resources to treat these numerous diseases, neighbors provided what assistance they could to aid one another. This volunteer health network was supplemented by advice and sometimes patent medicines from traditional physicians and the use of herbal remedies to ease symptoms provided by "irregular healers" or handed down from generation to generation within families.

In the summer of 1776, with John still in Philadelphia and preoccupied with developing political events and the drafting and details surrounding the adoption of the Declaration of Independence, Abigail was left to cope with yet new health battles on the home front back in Braintree and Boston. Like her husband John, Abigail's response to health issues was generally a pragmatic one in which she tried to level-headedly educate herself about treatments and follow those that had proven most successful. Just months after young Thomas recovered from scarlet fever in March,[59] another, even more serious disease threatened the family, and indeed most Americans. From 1775 to 1782, smallpox was endemic in North America, and New England was especially hard hit. In June 1776, a virulent smallpox epidemic struck Boston, infecting thousands, and numerous local residents and visitors rushed to be inoculated at a group of homes that became temporary smallpox clinics.

John Adams was keenly aware of the situation in Boston as well as the potential of the disease to devastate the Continental Army. In June he wrote his wife from Philadelphia with concern, "The small Pox! The small Pox! What shall we do with it?" and concluded that it was "[t]en times more terrible than Britons, Canadians, and Indians together."[60] Like General Washington, Adams understood that disease thrived in the close quarters of army bases and advised one Continental Army colonel that soldiers needed exercise, sanitation, and cleanliness because that regimen "preserves their health and hardens their bodies against disease."[61]

In early July, while the Continental Congress was in frenzied session as it edged toward independence, the Boston ban against smallpox inoculation was lifted for nearly two weeks. Abigail, who like her husband John followed developments in health prevention closely, had long desired that she and her family be inoculated against the dread disease. However, until then she had abided by her mother's insistence that they not be subjected to the potential danger of immunization. In July 1776, just a week after the Declaration of Independence was adopted, Abigail left Braintree for Boston and the hospitality of her Uncle Isaac Smith's mansion so that her four children—and another thirteen family members and servants—could be inoculated. With the threat of smallpox looming so imminently, like thousands of other Bostonians, Abigail was taking advantage of the temporary cessation of the local prohibition. Under Abigail's talented pen the seriousness of the disease and the fear it aroused in the public, as well as what it was like to be inoculated, are graphically portrayed. "I yesterday arrived and was with all 4 of our Little ones inoculated for the small pox," she wrote to John. "Our little ones stood the operation Manfully. . . . Such a spirit of inoculation never before took place; the Town and every House in it, . . . are as full as they can hold. God Grant that we may all go comfortably thro the Distemper. The Phisick [medication] part is bad enough I know."[62]

By the next day Abigail reported to John that "[t]he Little folks are very sick and puke every morning but after that they are comfortable." Although the threat of a smallpox epidemic was widespread and real, Abigail's letter reveals that popular acceptance of inoculation was still controversial, confirming Franklin's earlier observation that the procedure always divided early Americans. Commenting on the devastation wrought in Canada by the disease, she observed, "In many Towns, Already around Boston the Selectmen have granted Liberty [permission] for inoculation. I hope the Necessity is now fully seen." In this instance Abigail clearly supported a strong role for government in the health arena. At the end of the letter Abigail managed to sneak in a "medicinal" request for the then politically controversial tea, noting, "A Little India herb would have been mighty agreeable now."[63]

Meanwhile, John alternated between worry over the fate of his family and the increasing reality of widespread debilitating and virulent smallpox within the Continental Army, poised for battle. "The Small Pox," John reported to Abigail anxiously, "has done Us more harm than British armies, Canadians, Indians, Negroes, Hannoverians, Hessians, and all the rest," and he placed the blame for the American retreat from Quebec on the disease.[64] Under heightened emotional stress over the final break with England, the unremitting pressure of work, and anxiety over his family, John's own health suffered. He declared that he was subject to jangled nerves, fevers, eye inflammations, and the prospect of an imminent collapse if he did not receive a leave of absence to travel to Massachusetts, but he was unable to return until fall.[65]

Because of the tense political situation, inoculation for Abigail and her children had been a more harrowing ordeal than John Adams had experienced during the procedure shortly before his marriage. However, on July 18th, while the children were in various stages of recovery, Abigail was able to personally witness the momentous public reading of the Declaration of Independence at the Massachusetts Statehouse, thrilled that she and especially her husband had had a central role in launching the colonies on the road to liberty. Although Americans at the time understood that people who underwent inoculation were potentially contagious, the ten- to fourteen-day incubation period may not yet have been strictly understood, for the recently inoculated Abigail joined the crowd. Despite the political news, the health of her family remained paramount in Abigail's mind, and she wrote John in Philadelphia, "Nabby has been very ill, but the Eruptions begin to make its appearance upon her, and upon Johnny. Tommy is so well that the Dr inoculated him again to day fearing it had not taken. Charly has no complaints yet, tho his arm has been very soar."[66]

From afar John worried about the possible side effects of the inoculation for his family and admonished them to get plenty of fresh air. He also sent Abigail's doctor instructions compiled by Dr. Rush, Philadelphia's leading physician, about administering the procedure. In

Boston the physicians recommended the use of calomel to aid its success. During the eighteenth century the poisonous qualities of mercury were unknown, but in hindsight its deleterious effects appear to have left Abigail extremely weak and fatigued.[67] Certainly the entire process could be quite uncomfortable and sometimes produced a massive amount of itchy pustules. In 1772, a young college student who traveled to New York City from Providence to undergo inoculation recorded that he broke out with about three to four hundred pocks but felt that the benefits of inoculation far outweighed the discomforts.[68]

The first inoculation successfully produced the desired pustules in Abigail and her son John Quincy, but Nabby, Charles, and Thomas had to be reinoculated, as did many of those who had undergone the procedure in Boston that summer. Abigail and John Adams were relieved when Thomas and Nabby finally displayed the lesions, even though Nabby's case produced a spectacular mass of the pustules and fear that scars might mar her appearance. As Abigail put it in her letter to John, "Nabby has enough of the small Pox for all the family beside." John's advice to Nabby, his "Speckled Beauty," as he termed her, would be to keep out of the sun to avoid permanently damaging her face. Their fears were not unrealistic, as most people who contracted smallpox and survived were left scarred for life, but Nabby appears to have escaped severe disfigurement. Abigail also strongly expressed her ever-present fervent wish of seeing her husband soon. Always concerned about possible overwork on John's part, she urged him to return to Braintree from Philadelphia as "Your Health I think requires your immediate return."[69]

In the absence of reliable scientific testing to ascertain if one had actually acquired the desired immunity to smallpox, many people were lured into a false sense of security, only to fall dangerously ill when future epidemics broke out. Abigail reported that "[t]he Town instead of being clear of this distemper are now in the height of it, hundreds having it in the Natural way through the deceitfulness of inoculation."[70] Abigail's words reflect that initial smallpox inoculations during that summer failed at an alarming rate, and many had to undergo a second inoculation to be properly protected. Abigail's good common sense and innate practical nature made her cautious, and her decision to subject her children to further rounds of the immunization helped to ensure that they would not become smallpox victims. Six-year-old Charles

Adams would prove especially resistant to inoculation and in the end contracted the disease the "natural way," through physical contagion from another smallpox victim. Frail by nature, Charles became violently ill, and Abigail nursed him anxiously for many days, extending her stay in Boston to nearly two months. Learning of his symptoms John would share her fear and distress, but by the first week in September their young son was weak but according to Abigail recovering with the aid of "the Bark," and she was expressing regret that she had needlessly worried her husband. With evident relief Abigail ended her letter reporting that in the Boston area, "Tis Here a very General time of Health."[71]

In the fall of 1776, Adams was finally given a several-month respite from his duties in the Continental Congress, and he eagerly traveled home from Philadelphia to be reunited with his growing family. Abigail became pregnant with their sixth child during the visit, but John was in Philadelphia when she delivered a stillborn daughter in the summer of 1777, and she endured the sorrow of the baby's death without him by her side. Anesthesia for childbirth or even for major surgery were unheard of at the time, and it was not until 1846 that the first operation using ether was performed in America, in Boston. The couple's commitment to the ideals of the Revolution and the sacrifice involved in building the new nation took a heavy toll on their personal lives. Although Abigail had felt in good health for most of the pregnancy, just days before the birth she had a premonition that all was not well with the fetus after she endured a "shaking fit."[72]

John Adams shared Abigail's anxiety and lamented the fact that because of his political and governmental responsibilities in times of crisis he was often absent and could not offer his support in person:

My mind is again Anxious, and my Heart in Pain for my Dearest Friend. Three Times, have I felt, the most distressing Sympathy with my Partner, without being able to afford her any Kind of Solace, or Assistance. When, the Family was sick of the Dissentery, and so many of our Friends died of it. When you all had the small Pox. . . . Oh that I could, be near . . . that I could take from my dearest, a share of her Distress, or relieve her of the whole.[73]

Abigail's emotional support from her husband from afar and her fervent religious beliefs were certainly some comfort to her. Regardless of their personal religious beliefs, America's founders almost uniformly adopted a stoic attitude toward sickness and death and bore their sorrows with fortitude. Though Abigail was heartbroken at the death of the "dear Infant," which occurred on July 11, 1777, she poignantly invited her husband to "[j]oin with me my dearest Friend in Gratitude to Heaven, that a life I know you value [her own], has been spaired and carried thro Distress and danger altho the dear Infant is numberd with its ancestors."[74] The perfectly formed baby may have died as a result of a tangled umbilical cord that had cut off her oxygen supply, a condition that could not have been diagnosed before birth at the time. Despite emotional distress and physical exhaustion, Abigail was grateful that her own life had been spared and was apparently ready to move on and return to caring for her remaining children.

John responded with thanks that "Providence has preserved to me a Life that is dearer to me than all other Blessings in the World." Yet, the loss of the infant was a cruel blow to John, and his words are filled with poignancy: "Is it not unaccountable, that one should feel so strong an Affection for an Infant, that one has never seen, nor shall see?"[75] Despite Abigail's brave front and willingness to sacrifice for the new country, John's absence during the birth was clearly felt. She wrote rather wistfully to her husband that the children would have benefited from the "joint instruction" of both parents and that "[t]is almost fourteen years since we were united, but not more than half that time we had of happiness of living together."[76] It is interesting to note that John's very apparent sadness and anxiety during this family loss did not trigger any new health crisis for him, calling into question a diagnosis of a thyroid ailment that became exacerbated in periods of stress. In fact, in September of 1777, he was able to report to Abigail that "[my] Health is as good as common."[77]

Abigail's fortitude in the face of the second tragic death of one of her children is a reminder of the high rate of infant and maternal mortality in that period. It also demonstrates her own strong religious faith and that of John, which taught them that pain, sickness, and death were to be accepted with stoicism and resignation as the will of God. Many years later, when Abigail comforted Thomas Jefferson after the death of his adult daughter, Maria Jefferson Eppes, she spelled out clearly her religious views on the challenge of the loss of a loved one in a heartfelt letter: "I have tasted the bitter cup, and bow with reverence, and humility before the great dispenser of it, without whose permission, and over ruling providence, not a sparrow falls to the ground."[78]

Health, Sickness, and Diplomacy in Europe

After so many prolonged separations, both John and Abigail were undoubtedly relieved when he returned to Braintree in November 1777, poised to resume his law career and a normal family life. But Adams's return to private life was short-lived, as in the same month he was appointed by Congress to officially serve as a joint commissioner to France, ushering in a ten-year period of diplomatic service abroad on behalf of the United States. In February of 1778, accompanied by his ten-year-old son, John Quincy, John Adams set sail on a rough six-week voyage to France to join Arthur Lee and Benjamin Franklin as part of a three-man commission. Abigail, who feared ocean voyages, remained behind to care for the other children and supervise the farm.

Franklin's and Adams's temperaments could not have been more dissimilar and did not always make for an amiable political and diplomatic partnership. Nor was Adams enamored of the opulent Parisian society, which he considered dissolute and immoral, once his initial excitement wore off. In mid-September 1778, Congress officially appointed Franklin as sole minister to the court of Louis XVI, and Adams received the news with mixed feelings. This first stay in Europe lasted a relatively short eighteen months, and to Abigail's relief John returned to Boston in the summer of 1779, when he began work on a new Massachusetts state constitution as the elected representative from Braintree. The hiatus back in America was again short-lived, however, for in October Congress assigned Adams a new diplomatic task. In November 1779, and this time accompanied by sons John Quincy and Charles, John returned to France as American minister to negotiate peace and commerce with England. This turned out to be somewhat premature as the war did not go well for the Americans in 1780. It would not be until after the Battle of Yorktown in late 1781 that Great Britain would view the war as lost, and Adams did little to endear himself to either Franklin or French diplomats while he marked time during yet another period of stress. Congress ended up removing John as minister plenipotentiary in France, and instead he became a member of a five-man delegation to negotiate a peace settlement and promote America's interests in Europe.

It was Adams himself who decided that his mission while he waited would be to garner financial and moral support for American independence in the Netherlands. In late 1780, he relocated to a canal house in Amsterdam, and over the next several years John served as minister plenipotentiary and eventually achieved great success in his economic diplomacy. At first he reported, "I have hitherto preserved my Health in this damp Air better than I expected. So have all of Us, but Charles who has had a tertian [a fever that spiked on the third day, such as in the case of malaria] fever but is better."[79] According to Ferling and Braverman, however, the stress related to diplomatic intrigues in France that might have damaged Adams's political fortunes brought about another resurgence of their speculated "probable hyperthyroidism," causing weakness, irritability, paranoia, and a possible neck goiter. Indeed, they attribute his sometimes crusty behavior and irascibility during his lifetime, particularly in stressful situations, to his "thyroid malady."[80]

Whatever the real medical cause, although he was basically a robust man, John's health did suffer in the damp, humid climate, and he contracted an undisclosed "ague," probably one of the many infectious fevers that circulated in the eighteenth century in both Europe and America. His illness, what he termed a "nervous fever of a dangerous kind," became so severe that he apparently lapsed in and out of consciousness and lay near death: "For five or six days I was lost, and so insensible to the Operations of the Physicians and surgeons, as to have lost my memory of them."[81] Without Abigail at his side John always seemed more susceptible to illness, and he was probably made vulnerable to disease by exhaustion and depressed spirits after learning that he had lost his initial diplomatic commission.

Since Adams responded to the administration of quinine through Peruvian Bark, he had probably fallen victim to typhus or, more likely, acute malaria, easily spread by mosquitoes in the heat of the European summer. As we learned in the introduction, quinine was one of the few effective medications known to physicians in the eighteenth century. For the next few years he complained intermittently of ill health and weakness, possibly a result of a thyroid problem but more likely the lingering effects of malaria or another type of infection that, once contracted, could resurface numerous times in a person's lifetime. This seem a more likely scenario than an ongoing thyroid condition, as John's own secretary and others in his Amsterdam household were also stricken with a similar bout of illness and fever, one being "almost shaken to pieces."[82] Moreover, many of the symptoms that John experienced off and on over the ensuing years, such as weakness, swelling, eye irritations, skin rashes, fatigue, and insomnia, were also exhibited by Abigail as she aged!

Benjamin Franklin, Adams's fellow American minister in Europe, was aware that Adams had been seriously ill. In a letter dated October 5, 1781, Franklin congratulated Adams "on your Recovery. I hope this Seasoning will be the means of securing your future Health, by accommodating your Constitution to the Air of that Country." When Franklin, who as we have seen was highly familiar with health issues, referred to "seasoning," he no doubt meant the period of adjustment that contemporary medical men felt was necessary to develop some immunity to "malignant air" found in a new locale. In his next letter to Adams the following week, Franklin offered medical advice in addition to good wishes: "I hope your health is fully established. I doubt not but you have the Advice of skillful Physicians, otherwise I should presume to offer mine, which would be, though you find yourself well, to take a few Doses of Bark, by way of fortifying your Constitution, & preventing a Return of your Fever."[83]

Adams's reply demonstrated that though he sometimes vehemently disagreed with Franklin's diplomacy and disliked the older man's more ostentatious lifestyle, he respected Franklin's medical opinion: "I thank your Excellency for your advice as a Physician, which I have ventured to follow, though I had taken very largely of the Bark in my illness by the Advice of Dr. Osterdyke, a very able Physician at the head of his Profession in this Town." Adams concluded that "I am still very far from being a Man in Health and capable of going through much business."[84] Indeed, he was weak after his health crisis, his recovery was prolonged, and he did not return to his normally highly active schedule for some months.

Following his success in the Netherlands, where Adams signed an economic agreement in 1782, Adams was later redispatched to France to help negotiate a peace treaty with England. In Paris he succumbed to a virulent influenza epidemic circulating in the city but recovered in a relatively short time. He actually took a positive view of the illness and informed Abigail back in America that "I have had another Fever, which brought me low, but as it has carried off certain Pains and Lameness the Relicks of the Amsterdam Distemper, I am persuaded it will do me, much good."[85] After a series of tension-producing complications, the peace treaty was finally consummated and ready for his final signature in the fall of 1783. Abigail clearly recognized the connection between stressful situations and John's health, but although John repeatedly entreated her to join him, she still dithered over traveling to Europe. "The State of your health gives me great anxiety, and the delay of your return increases it . . . the Scenes of anxiety through which you have past, are enough to rack the firmest constitution, and debilitate the strongest faculties," she opined in October of 1783.[86]

While John Adams was in Europe with their sons John Quincy and Charles, Abigail certainly worried from afar. At the same time, she proved a most capable businesswoman and built up a thriving enterprise in Massachusetts, selling imported trimmings for women's fashion supplied by her husband from France. Still, the unreliability of the mail often kept her in the dark about her husband's and sons' health and whereabouts for months at a time and provoked anxiety as well as loneliness. In 1781, fourteen-year-old John Quincy was sent to Russia as an assistant to Francis Dana, secretary of the American delegation, and Charles was sent home to America due to homesickness and ill health. Increasingly delicate, Charles had been subject to several bouts of sickness in Europe, and his trip home was prolonged due to illness. Understandably, Abigail was relieved to have him back under her watchful eye.

Abigail Sails to Europe

Fear of the long, potentially dangerous sea voyage and concerns for her other children and her father, William Smith, in Braintree had long made Abigail reluctant to join her husband in Europe. But finally Abigail concluded that their current separation, which had stretched over four years, was untenable. Although she was terrified by the thought of crossing the ocean, Abigail gathered her courage and even hoped that she would be "benefitted by my voyage as my Health has been very infirm and I have just recoverd from a slow fever."[87]

Abigail and Nabby sailed from Boston on June 18, 1784, accompanied by two servants. From almost the moment she set foot on ship Abigail became wretchedly ill with seasickness, as did the entire party, albeit to differing degrees. Abigail was prostrated for ten days, and in her journal she recorded that "[t]o Those who have never been at Sea or experienced this dispiriting malady tis impossible to discribe it, the Nausia arising from the smell of the Ship, the continual rolling, tossing and tumbling contribute to keep up this Disorder, and when once it seazeis a person it levels Sex and condition."[88] The dampness of the ship also aggravated her rheumatism, and to her sister, Mary Cranch, Abigail described her seasickness as the "most disheartening . . . malady" and reported, "[W]e crawled on deck when able." The party landed on July 20th. "Heaven be praised, I have landed safely upon the British coast," Abigail proclaimed in relief.[89]

John Quincy was dispatched by his father from The Hague to meet his mother and sister, and John Adams joined the family in England in August. Once land was firmly beneath her feet and she had recovered from the rigors of the voyage, Abigail and John traveled to France with their son, daughter, and servants and settled into a luxurious, spacious home in the Paris suburbs in Auteuil on the banks of the Seine. Abigail noted that the repeated attacks of fever John had endured in Europe obliged him to live in the countryside, where the air was reputed to be healthier. At first Abigail disapproved of much that she found in the pleasure-loving French society, especially the luxurious excesses of the royal court, and evidence of Parisian immorality assaulted her at every turn. Though she professed to enjoy French plays, she complained that they often left her with a headache.[90] Over time Abigail began to appreciate aspects of French culture and developed several close friendships while she resided in the country, including one with American diplomat Thomas Jefferson, whom she viewed as a highly cultured man and delightful conversationalist. When the Adamses left France for England, Abigail told Mary that "I shall really regret to leave Mr. Jefferson; he is one of the choice ones of the earth."[91]

The presence of numerous servants to take care of housework reduced Abigail's physical activity, and the rutted and often flooded French local roads discouraged the formerly slender Abigail from taking her regular walks. As a result, she complained in 1784 to her sister Elizabeth Shaw

back in America that "I suffer through want of exercise, and grow too fat."
Two years later the problem had grown in proportion as she informed
her other sister, Mary Cranch, that "[t]is true I enjoy good health but am
larger than both my sisters compounded! Mr. Adams keeps pace with
me."[92] As always, she fretted over her husband's complaints of ill health,
but John apparently was strong enough to take his daily exercise despite
the rough streets, as Abigail reported that "Mr. Adams makes it his constant practice to walk several miles every day, without which he would
not be able to preserve his health, which at best is but infirm."[93] Apparently concern about obesity is not only a modern phenomenon, as Abigail would later warn her son John Quincy that "[a]s you and I are both
inclined to corpulence we should be attentive to exercise."[94]

After John was elected the first American minister to England in
1785, John Quincy returned to America for college, and John, Abigail,
and Nabby relocated to a fine home in an elegant neighborhood in London. Abigail had spent only eight months in France, but would reside
in England for three years. Understandably, the English did not enthusiastically welcome the couple who had played such a pivotal role in the
American Revolution. Still, the court of St. James was more to Abigail's
liking than the French court had been, and she was relieved to be able
to converse in English, as her command of French had been rudimentary at best. Moreover, in England Nabby would meet and marry William Smith in 1786, and at the time both her parents were pleased with
the match to the promising young man, then secretary to the American legion. In 1787, the young couple became the parents of John and
Abigail's first grandchild. Shortly after Nabby's wedding, Abigail sickened with one of the vague but serious illnesses that punctuated her life.
Though she first diagnosed herself with her old nemesis, rheumatism,
her English physician diagnosed a "bellious [stomach] complaint" and
she was sent to Bath to seek the curative powers of the waters at the
famed health spa. Abigail seems to have led a busy social life in Bath,
but any cure was short-lived. By the next summer she was still unwell
and the Adamses, accompanied by their daughter Nabby and new
grandson, traveled for Abigail's health to Devon, where she was introduced to the wonders of swimming.[95]

Like the other American founders and especially her good friend
Jefferson, Abigail clearly understood the connection among physical

exercise, good health, and weight control. Echoing Thomas Jefferson's advice to his nephew, in November 1786 Abigail emphasized the importance of exercise when she wrote to her son, now enrolled in the study of law at Harvard, "I hope you will not apply so constantly to your Studies to injure your Health; exercise is very necessary for you."[96] A year later she was still cautioning against overwork and advised him to exercise as a bulwark against ill health, maintaining that "[m]oderation in all things is conducive to human happiness . . . our Bodies are framed of such materials as to require constant exercise to keep them in repair, to Brace the Nerves and give vigor to the Animal functions."[97]

Despite recurrent ill health Abigail would outlive many of the members of her family. In the fall of 1783, Abigail's father, Parson Smith, died as a result of a serious urinary tract disorder. Prostate enlargement and similar ailments were common at the time in elderly males, and as we learned in the previous chapter, Benjamin Franklin's invention of a flexible urinary catheter had provided relief for some. Abigail had once referred to rheumatism as "our [Smith] family infirmity."[98] She could have just as well included both tuberculosis, which would strike her sister Mary Cranch and several of her nieces (Mary's daughter Betsy died of consumption at age eighteen; Elizabeth Peabody's daughter, a second Betsy, passed away in her late forties), and alcoholism, which proved the downfall of several of the men in her family. Of course, until Koch's discovery of the tuberculosis bacillus in 1882 medical wisdom viewed the disease as a hereditary illness rather than a communicable infectious disease. In the fall of 1787, Abigail was informed that her brother William, just forty years old, had died of jaundice of the liver, the result of years of heavy drinking. Later, alcoholism would be the main factor leading to the death of her beloved son Charles, and Thomas Adams's bouts with excessive drinking would also damage both his health and his career as a lawyer.

Unlike Jefferson, Abigail and John appear to have been early advocates for the radical practice of bleeding and mistakenly believed that the procedure was helpful for inflammations and headaches since contemporary medicine often asserted that these conditions arose from an imbalance resulting from an "excess of blood" that was too thick in the body. From London in January of 1787, for example, Abigail advised her son John Quincy "upon the approach of Spring to lose some Blood. The

Headacks and flushing in your face with which you used to be troubled was occasiond by too great a Quantity of Blood in your Head."[99]

Indeed, it appears that bleeding, blistering, and purging were Abigail's recommended panacea for many ills. Why would Abigail Adams, who was progressive in her thinking concerning politics, women's rights, and education, cling to these primitive medical procedures? It appears even more puzzling in light of the fact that John and Abigail had enthusiastically embraced smallpox inoculation when it was still considered an innovative but dangerous undertaking. First, we must recall that at the time purging and bleeding were considered by most leading medical practitioners as advanced therapeutic procedures, and the Adamses' outlook on bleeding reflects the ongoing conflict in the medical profession. We know that Abigail was a staunch admirer of Dr. William Buchan's *Domestic Medicine*, and Buchan, a leader in the Edinburgh school of medicine, relied heavily on bloodletting. In addition, both John and Abigail seem to have had a far greater respect for contemporary physicians than skeptics Jefferson or Franklin, perhaps because of the Adamses' great affection for two noted Boston physicians, Abigail's uncle, Dr. Cotton Tufts, and Dr. Benjamin Waterhouse, who would treat Abigail in her last illness.

Moreover, Abigail had an even higher regard for the preeminent physician Dr. Benjamin Rush, who was her doctor while Adams later served as vice president in Philadelphia when it was the nation's capital. Of course, bleeding was nearly always Rush's first recommendation in the face of illness, one as we have seen that proved singularly unsuccessful during the notorious yellow fever epidemic in 1793. In 1798, Abigail would consult Rush on behalf of her consumptive niece back in Boston, and Rush concluded that the pain in the young woman's side was the result of an abscess that would have healed had she been bled and blistered. Abigail despaired that Betsy was too far gone to improve, but concluded that she hoped "my friends will conquer the aversion to the Lancet, which I believe is not used sufficiently early in inflamitory diseases."[100]

Although Rush's reputation had suffered in the aftermath of Philadelphia's momentous yellow fever epidemics of 1793 and 1797, John Adams had remained a loyal friend. To help address Rush's economic woes, during his presidency Adams appointed Rush to head the United States Mint to augment the income from the doctor's diminished medical

heat, & heat to cold, or want of proper attention to their clothing. I think it ought to be a subject of investigation by the Medical Society.[104]

Abigail's views on the causes of tuberculosis were common at the time, reflecting the emphasis on the role of "malignant" air, or an unhealthy climate, in fostering disease. However, her recommendation that the Boston Medical Society investigate demonstrates her familiarity with emerging scientific inquiry and reveals that for a layperson she was quite knowledgeable about medicine at the time.

In 1790, Abigail contracted another one of her many mysterious fevers, what was probably a severe case of rheumatoid arthritis or the flu, also known as distemper at the time. To Mary Cranch, she wrote, "I have had the severest attack of the Rhumatism attended with a violent fever which I have had in several years."[105] Just a month later Abigail informed her sister with a characteristic touch of humor that "[t]he disorder termed the Influenza has prevaild with much violence & in many places been very mortal, particularly upon Long Island. Not a Creature has escaped in our Family except its Head [John], and I compounded to have a double share myself rather than he should have it at all."[106] The most famous victim of the New York flu epidemic was President George Washington. Abigail revealed that "[h]e has been in a most dangerous state . . . I dreaded his death." Abigail's concern was twofold: she feared for the future of the country if its leader perished, and she was just as concerned that her husband would have to assume the "highest Post." As we learned earlier, Washington recovered, but ten days later the epidemic still raged in New York, "and almost every Body throughout the whole city are laboring under it." At the time, several Adams family members were in various stages of sickness and recovery. Abigail liberally dosed them with one of her favored remedies, purging through "Tarter Emeticks,"[107] which probably accomplished nothing more than weakening the patients further.

Once the temporary seat of the federal government was relocated to Philadelphia, John and Abigail Adams moved there in November 1790. Abigail's health, always precarious, deteriorated further, perhaps affected adversely by menopause and the stress of packing up furniture and boxes of household items. While still in New York in late October, she was overcome with "shaking" fits, severe head and back pain, and the most violent fever I ever felt. It quite made me delirious. No rest for 5 Nights & days. It settled into a Regular intermitting Fever. The Dr. after having repeatedly puked me, gave me James's powders, but with very little effect. I began upon the Bark . . . and it has appeared to have put an end to my fever, but I am very low and weak.

From a modern perspective it is no wonder that inducing vomiting did nothing to reduce Abigail's fever. James's Powder, named after the English physician who had first patented the medicine in 1776, was thought to reduce fevers and was composed primarily of antimony. The successful use of quinine suggests that she may have had malaria. Compounding Abigail's illness was the fact her housekeeper, Mrs. Brisler, had been taken ill with a lung infection and submitted to three rounds of being bled and blistered, but "lies very ill."[108] Undoubtedly, those heroic measures contributed to the lingering weakness of the patient.

Once ensconced in Philadelphia, Abigail was kept busy unpacking and hosting ceremonial dinner parties, but Mrs. Brisler's health did not allow for much assistance. Though Abigail received many visitors, her fatigue and poor health delayed return visits to her new acquaintances. Moreover, she often had to contend with illnesses among other family members. At the end of November 1790, she wrote Nabby that her son Thomas Adams was ill, "almost helpless with the rheumatism. . . . It seems as sickness follows me wherever I go." Just a month later, Abigail was informed by her daughter that she was suffering from a "violent toothache" and "ague in my face," presumably an inflammation resulting from an infected tooth.[109]

In early 1792, Abigail became dangerously ill with a return of high fever, blinding headaches, and painful rheumatism, symptoms treated by Dr. Rush with "8 pr of Blisters" and three bleedings, and finally doses of quinine, all of which understandably left her weak and thin. During the next decades she would experience repeated episodes of what appears to have been what contemporary medicine would term rheumatoid arthritis, suffering from swollen joints, which sometimes made even walking and writing challenging. For six weeks the normally stoic Abigail was confined to bed with an "Inflamitory Rhumatism . . . my Limbs, it swelled and inflamed them to a high degree, and the distress I suffered in my Head was almost intolerable." These peculiar and very painful symptoms would resurface a number of times for Abigail in the future, and she would sometimes refer to them as her "Feb'ry attacks."[110] Finally on the road to recovery, in late April Abigail returned to the family home for the duration of John's vice presidential term, as he won a second election in 1793. In addition to Abigail's uncertain health, the need to reduce expenses that were draining the couple's limited budget contributed to the decision.[111] In early 1792, northern Braintree became the new town of Quincy, named in honor of Abigail's grandfather. As late as March 10th, John had still been worried about Abigail's health, but once again, in John's absence Abigail capably managed not only the Quincy household but the farm, reflecting her considerable business acumen. John always joined her in Massachusetts during summer congressional recesses, welcoming the opportunity to escape the heat and the rise of summer epidemics in Philadelphia.[112]

Fortunately, Adams was in Quincy during the summer of 1793, for as we have seen, that proved to be the height of the notorious yellow fever epidemic that decimated Philadelphia. John and Abigail were understandably concerned about another outbreak of the disease when he returned to the city at the end of November, but the worst of the plague was over. Moreover, at the beginning of the following year he was able to assure Abigail back in Quincy that "[w]e have frequent Rumours and Allarms about the yellow fever; but when they come to be traced to their Sources they have hitherto proved to be false."[113]

That Abigail was familiar with preventative medical treatment for a number of illnesses, including malaria and other epidemic fevers, is evident from a letter she sent Adams while she was visiting Nabby and her family in New York in the summer of 1795. John and Abigail had traveled together from Quincy as far as New York, but John had gone on to resume his responsibilities in Philadelphia. Abigail reported to her husband that her journey had improved her health. However, to deter illness Abigail avoided "the evening air, and take Bark and drink porter and water as an Antidote to the Ague."[114] Abigail spent most of her time over the next few years in Quincy, and although she was only in her early fifties, good health was only intermittent. To her son Thomas, whom she had not seen in three years, she wrote in late 1796 that she had aged in his absence and that her "frequent indispositions hastens its strides and impair a frail fabric."[115] During the same period John fared much better than his wife. His main health challenges centered on intermittent hand tremors and eye irritations that sometimes interfered with his favored occupations, reading and writing. John rationalized those conditions as an annoying byproduct of aging, and confided to his son John Quincy that sometimes he suffered from "weak Eyes and from a trembling hand."[116]

Health, Medicine, and the American President

On February 8, 1797, at the age of sixty-one, John Adams was elected the second president of the United States, capping a long career of devoted service to the new nation. From Quincy, Abigail sent her heartfelt best wishes and assurances of his worthiness of the office. Philadelphia had never been kind to Abigail's frail health. She begged off from attending the March 4th inauguration there and resisted John's entreaties to join him until October, citing her health and responsibilities in Quincy as well as the poor health of John's mother, Susanna. Over the years Abigail and John exchanged numerous letters about Mrs. Hall's illnesses, which included a severe lung infection, and John often expressed his appreciation to his wife for her "tender care and watchful attention" to his mother.[117] Caring for her infirm mother-in-law appears to have given the normally optimistic Abigail pause about the challenges of aging: "My constant attendance upon her has very much lessened my desire of long life."[118]

Despite Abigail's reluctance to journey to Philadelphia, John still begged his wife to join him so she could tend to him and lend her advice and support as he endured the new stresses of office. As was his habit, he tried to persuade Abigail by bemoaning his poor health, which seems in this instance to have been no more than a minor illness. "I am very unwell—a violent cold and cough," he wrote, "fatigues me, while I have every Thing else to harry me: so that I must entreat you to come on as soon as you can."[119] Abigail, however, solicitously continued to attend John's mother, who died on April 21st.

Abigail finally joined John in Philadelphia in May, having traveled over rain-soaked roads during a two-week stage journey, on which she learned the depressing news that her young niece Mary Smith had succumbed to tuberculosis and that Nabby's family was in dire financial straits due to her husband's failed business schemes. The oppressive heat in Philadelphia in the summer of 1797, which brought fatigue and stomach ailments to the president and his wife and "Cholera Morbis" to Nabby's young son, encouraged them to leave for Quincy in the middle of July for much-needed rest and recuperation. John and Abigail did not return to Philadelphia until November, delayed by reports of yet another yellow fever epidemic in the city, which had caused large numbers to flee until cold weather set in.

The year 1798 was a fateful one with respect to the family's personal health and that of the nation. John had long been interested in medical matters, and his concern for the health of Americans was evidenced as early as 1777, when he expressed satisfaction after the Continental Congress passed legislation that expanded the army's Hospital [Medical] Department, observing, "The expense will be great, but humanity overcame avarice."[120] However, John's most overt foray into public health occurred on July 16, 1798, when he signed into law an act for the care and establishment of hospitals for ill and disabled seamen. Adams had long appreciated that maritime shipping was crucial to American commerce and security. Healthy seamen were paramount to its success, and sick sailors who arrived in American ports taxed local medical services and endangered the health of the local population. Members of Congress from major American ports such as New York and Baltimore initiated the act, which established the Marine Hospital Service and attracted Adams's strong support. To finance the undertaking, sailors' employers (ship owners or captains) withheld a tax of twenty cents per month from their salaries, and the rest of the funding came from the government. In 1799, Adams appointed its first medical officer, Dr. Thomas Welsh, to head the Boston district. This first federal health care program eventually evolved into the modern Public Health Service along with the office of the surgeon general.[121]

Although Adams had never been a sailor, as early as 1769 his interest in the welfare of seamen led to his honorary induction into the Boston Marine Society. Admission to the society was generally limited to men who had served as ship masters, but even then, when John was only in his midthirties, he was known as a shrewd lawyer and a rising political force. The membership fees were even waived to entice him to join. Adams was doubtless impressed with the society's custom that captains

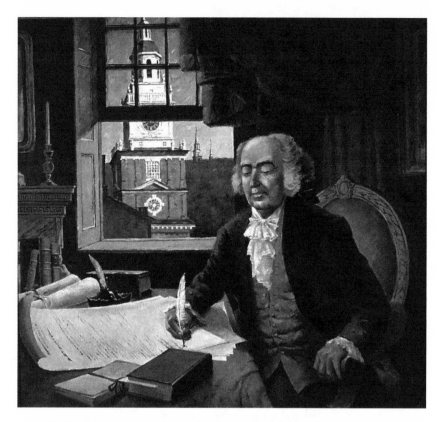

President John Adams Signing the Act for the Relief of Sick and Disabled Seamen, July 16, 1798. Painting by Garnet W. Jex. (Courtesy U.S. National Library of Medicine)

who returned to port safely would deposit some money in a secure box to help others who became needy.[122]

The political stresses endured by her husband and social obligations during her four years as first lady further taxed Abigail's delicate health and affected John as well. When the first couple returned to their remodeled home in Quincy in the hot summer of 1798, Abigail became deathly ill with a recurrence of the severe headaches, fever, insomnia, and rheumatism that had so often troubled her. She was diagnosed with dysentery and diabetes along with the usual vague "bilious intermittent fever," which may have been a recurrence of malaria. So serious was her state that Nabby traveled north from New York to nurse her mother. In a letter to former President Washington in October, a very concerned John lamented that his health was "indifferent" but "Mrs. Adams's is extremely low. Confined to the bed of sickness for two months, her destiny is still very precarious, and mine in consequence of it."[123] Ferling and Braverman go so far as to suggest that John's agitation during the 1798 crisis with France was strongly influenced by a flareup of thyrotoxicosis, which fueled Adams's suspicion of the Federalists and prompted "injudicious" political and diplomatic behavior, ultimately leading to his defeat in the presidential election of 1800.[124]

John remained in Quincy with Abigail through most of her eleven-week illness, both because he was genuinely worried about his wife's state and, probably, to escape the increasingly difficult political environment in Philadelphia. In addition, during that time yellow fever again flared up in many coastal cities, particularly in Philadelphia, where as many as forty thousand people fled to escape contagion. Abigail improved slowly, but after a seven-month absence from the nation's capital, John was finally forced to return without her, arriving in Philadelphia in November. John continued to agonize over conflicts between his public duty and his responsibility to his beloved wife:

> I would resign my office and remain with you, or I would bring you next Winter with me but either of these Plans, the Publick out of the Question, would increase our Difficulties perhaps rather than lessen them. This Climate is a Disease to me, and I greatly fear would be worse to you, in the present State of your Health.[125]

Adams experienced toothaches, but perhaps to cheer Abigail, in late December he informed her that "[y]our solicitude for my Health may subside. I am pretty well." Yet John's underlying hypochondria and pessimism still managed to surface in the very same paragraph. "I am Old, Old, very Old and never shall be very well—certainly while in this Office for the drudgery of it is too much for my Years and Strength," he concluded gloomily.[126] Adams was only sixty-three at the time and would live another twenty-eight active and productive years.

Abigail's many bouts with illness made her appreciate good health keenly. In 1799, she advised her nephew William Shaw to "husband your Health as well as your time, for without Health from experience I tell you,

Life has no enjoyments."[127] In addition to her own physical stresses, Abigail's health was also undoubtedly affected by the difficulties experienced by two of her children, Nabby and Charles. Nabby's husband, the once promising William Smith, had proved irresponsible, and he abandoned his young family for long periods as he pursued flighty economic dealings that ultimately left him bankrupt. Meanwhile, Charles Adams had inexplicably plunged into the depths of depression and alcoholism, causing John to renounce him and Abigail to agonize over the fate of his wife and daughters. Still, yet again Abigail recovered sufficiently to take her place at her husband's side. When George Washington died in late December of 1799, she not only attended a lengthy memorial service in Philadelphia but hosted a reception afterward that was attended by hundreds.

Toward the end of Adams's presidency, in late November 1800, the family situation resulted in tragedy when Charles Adams died at the age of thirty, apparently from complications due to alcoholism and a life of dissipation. Just weeks before his death Abigail had visited her son in New York and found that he was "laid upon a Bed of sickness, destitute of home. A distressing cough, and affection of the liver and a dropsy will soon terminate a Life, which might have been made valuable to himself and others."[128] John would later share his despair with his old friend Thomas Jefferson. In reply to a letter from Jefferson, who apparently was unaware of Charles's death at the time, John mournfully informed him that "[Charles] was once the delight of my Eyes and a darling of my heart, cut off in the flower of his days, amidst very flattering Prospects by causes which have been the greatest grief of my Life."[129] Charles's demise again reminds us that illness and death were a constant factor in the daily lives of people from all walks of life during the era, and the well-to-do and powerful were far from immune.

At the time, alcoholism was not viewed as a disease but rather seen as a vice and character flaw. However, alcoholism was not uncommon in the new nation, which had long exhibited "a hearty drinking tradition."[130] Charles's sad end was indeed a source of deep sorrow and disappointment for his loving but ambitious father. John and Abigail had always been affectionate but demanding parents. Historian Joseph Ellis has speculated that John's repeated lengthy absences from home during his children's formative years may have contributed to the emotional difficulties displayed in differing degrees by all three of his sons.[131]

John and Abigail Adams became the first presidential couple to live in the new capital city of Washington, D.C. When John arrived, half-finished buildings sprouted in the midst of swampy ground and a tree-filled forest, and a population of about five hundred families was augmented by three hundred government members. The future White House, then called the President's House, commanded a beautiful view of the Potomac, but was essentially set in a wilderness. At first it featured only six rooms, and after Abigail joined John in November of 1800, she was forced to entertain dignitaries in modest quarters while her wash hung in the empty East Room. As usual, Abigail rose to the occasion, fulfilling her duties with her customary capability. Within a few weeks she was also called upon to act as nurse to her young granddaughter Susanna Adams, apparently stricken with "the Quincy," diphtheria as we would term it today. One evening Abigail was awakened by the child's hoarse cough and immediately sent for a doctor who dosed her with calomel, placed her feet in warm water, and applied steam from boiling water doused with vinegar.[132] Fortunately, the child recovered despite the dangerous mercury-based medication, but just a week later Abigail lost her son Charles.

John Adams successfully kept America out of war with France, but the rise of bitter partisan politics between the Federalists and Republicans and the notorious Alien and Sedition Acts, which were viewed by many as curtailing the hard-won liberty of Americans, contributed to his unpopularity. Abigail continued to loyally and vehemently defend him against increasing criticism. Adams ran for a second term in 1800 with Aaron Burr, Thomas Jefferson, and Alexander Hamilton as rivals, and was defeated. A tie in the electoral vote between Jefferson and Burr sent the vote to the House of Representatives. In February 1801, on the thirty-sixth ballot, Jefferson was elected president, causing a rift between him and John Adams that lasted for years.

As a fervent Federalist, Abigail never fully overcame her bitterness over what she viewed as a betrayal by Jefferson, formerly a beloved friend. As an equally committed Republican, Jefferson generally favored states' rights and agrarian ideals along with a strong emphasis on individual liberty over Federalist support of a stronger federal government and enlarged commercial interests. Abigail took a keen interest in politics during her husband's term and had supported John's ill-fated sponsorship of the Alien and Sedition Acts. She took her duties as first lady

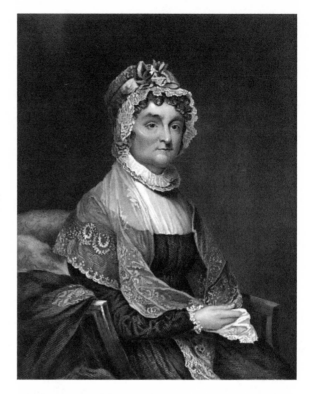

Engraving of Abigail
Adams from an Origi-
nal Painting by Gilbert
Stuart. (Courtesy
Library of Congress)

seriously and carried them out with remarkable good grace under trying personal and public conditions, but John's presidency certainly took
its toll on her health. To her son Thomas Abigail confided that "[a]t my
age and with my body infirmities, I shall be happier at Quincy."[133] Like
Jefferson, Abigail possessed an intuitive understanding of the connection between the mind and the body, which she revealed in a letter to
Catherine Johnson (the mother of her daughter-in-law Louisa Adams):
"I sensibly feel that the Health of the Body depends very much upon
the tranquility of the mind."[134]

Twilight Years and Tragic Illness

After so many years of service to the nation, both John and Abigail looked forward to retirement from public life and their return to
Quincy. The Adams landholdings had grown to about six hundred acres

and featured three separate farms. John appears to have been genuinely happy to shed his political burdens, but Abigail still harbored resentment toward his political foes. Her husband's defeat for a second term as president had left the normally optimistic Abigail despondent about the future of the nation under Republican leadership. Abigail's health had been mixed in Washington. Although she did not suffer much rheumatism, she did experience "Ague and fever," and she believed she would do better permanently at Quincy. Repeated attacks of intermitting fevers over the years sapped her constitution. "I patch up, but it is hard work," she confided to her sister in 1801.[135] Other than the normal disabilities of aging, John's health remained remarkably good during his 25-year retirement. This suggests that the stresses of political life produced many of Adams's ailments. As we will see in the next chapters, Jefferson was also subject to illness when political tensions surfaced.

Back in Quincy, Abigail and John were happy to be surrounded by family and friends and enjoyed the benefits of grandparenthood. Their son Charles's widow and daughters frequently joined the household for long periods, and Abigail virtually raised her granddaughter Susanna. John Quincy Adams continued his work on behalf of the government, but in the company of his cultured, delicate, English-born wife, Louisa Catherine, and their children, he also joined his parents at Peacefield when his schedule permitted. Thomas Adams was also a frequent guest, and when his law practice failed and he could no longer afford to pay his bills, his family augmented his parents' household on a more permanent basis.

Following John Adams's defeat, John Quincy had returned to Massachusetts in 1801 from his diplomatic post in Berlin, accompanied by his wife, Louisa, and their baby son. Like so many women of the era, Louisa had suffered through numerous emotionally and physically draining miscarriages, seven in all, which made the birth of a healthy child even more precious. Louisa gave birth to four living children during her marriage, but only one, future historian Charles Francis Adams, survived to old age. It is interesting to note that before they left Europe, John Quincy and Louisa's first son, named George Washington Adams in honor of America's first president, underwent the safer and more effective Jenner type of smallpox vaccination.[136] During the same time period, as we learned in the introduction, Jefferson would be instrumental in introducing the Jenner method in America.

The feisty Abigail was in her element as the busy matriarch of the household, but she continued to be plagued by multiple often mysterious illnesses. These were diagnosed vaguely as rheumatism coupled with skin rashes and eye infections, which left her with cripplingly painful joints, swellings, and fevers. Most days Abigail was confined to the house or to short journeys in a cushioned carriage. Although she had suffered many painful losses, including the death of her son Charles, Abigail tended to emphasize the positive and was confident that she would be reunited with her loved ones in the afterlife. To her old friend Mercy Warren she wrote in January 1803 that she "had tasted the bitter cup of affliction," and "though not exempt from the infirmities of age . . . enjoy the present with gratitude."[137]

In 1809, Abigail contracted the painful skin condition known as St. Anthony's erysipelas, which left her with a grossly swollen face and inflammation, and she complained to her sister Elizabeth that "[i]t seemed to me as though my blood boiled."[138] For treatment of many of her illnesses, Abigail still sometimes relied on purging, bleeding, and medicinal herbs, but resorted to the use of the opium-based laudanum when necessary to relieve severe pain. However, despite sickness, she retained her uncomplaining manner and wrote optimistically to a granddaughter that while "old age with its infirmities assail me," she was happy that her hearing was still acute, although her memory was not as sharp as it had once been.[139] Remarkably, Abigail could still display her "sunny spirit," as her grandson Charles Francis Adams put it, turning challenges into opportunities. Her lifelong battle with insomnia only grew worse with age and illness, but she chose to look at it as additional time to write letters and accomplish more work at home.[140]

Serious illnesses in the family proved the greatest challenge to Abigail and John's last years together. The year 1811 was a particularly critical one. White-haired and wrinkled at the age of sixty-seven, Abigail considered herself elderly. Indeed, she had already far exceeded the average life expectancy for women at the time, for many died in their twenties and thirties, either through pregnancy and childbirth or from numerous contagious epidemics or untreatable illnesses. One of Abigail's primary concerns was for the health of her son John Quincy Adams, then stationed in Russia as the American minister in St. Petersburg, and that of his wife, Louisa, who was again pregnant. To compound the family's anxiety, Louisa's pregnant sister died in childbirth just as Louisa was approaching the end of her own term. Abigail undoubtedly recalled the many painful experiences Louisa had endured in childbirth. In the hot summer of 1806, for example, Louisa had given birth to a stillborn son in Washington while her husband had gone on ahead to Massachusetts.

Louisa's and John Quincy's younger son, Charles, was with them in Russia, but the two older sons were left behind for schooling in America supervised by John and Abigail. Louisa gave birth to a baby girl named Louisa Catherine in August, and the family was ecstatic, but soon after she received news of her mother's death back in America. Death and illness were a constant in Louisa's life. Tragically, just a little over a year after her birth, the much-beloved baby died in September 1812, a victim of dysentery and high fever, which resulted in convulsions. The doctors could do nothing to treat her effectively. Louisa was heartbroken and recorded in her diary "My child gone to heaven. . . . My heart is buried in my Louisa's grave and my greatest longing is to be laid beside her."[141]

Abigail wrote to console her daughter-in-law, revealing that even many years after the death of her own baby daughter Susanna, she still mourned the loss of the infant. "Forty years has not obliterated from my mind the anguish of my soul upon the occasion," she wrote. Yet in her typical manner, she focused on the blessings of the present: "Let us with gratitude bless our preserver that we have yet so many blessings left to us."[142] Compounding the sadness, in October, Abigail's beloved sister Mary Cranch was seriously ill with tuberculosis, and Mary's husband, Richard, who had generously shared books with Abigail when they were young, was gravely sick after suffering a stroke.

Most distressing was the news from Nabby Adams Smith that she suspected she had a serious breast ailment. But propelled by hope that it was a benign condition, Nabby delayed medical consultation despite increasing pain. On Abigail's insistence, Nabby traveled from upstate New York to Boston with two of her children to consult leading physicians there. After conflicting debate over diagnosis and alternate suggestions for treatment (including the use of hemlock pills), the doctors finally confirmed advanced breast cancer. Their view reflected what Abigail had felt from the first after examining Nabby in person. From his own sickbed in New York, Nabby's husband, William Smith, chimed in with advice to take immediate action.

Physicians at that time understood that some breast tumors were benign, but cancer almost always conferred a death sentence. Once cancer was diagnosed, Nabby decided to consult her father's old friend, Dr. Benjamin Rush, who had published medical articles about the disease. In the absence of modern resources such as chemotherapy and radiation, medical treatment at the time was confined to surgery, and Rush advised speedy and complete removal of the breast, "the remedy of the knife," as he put it. After reviewing Nabby's case, Rush wrote directly to John that time was of the essence for if his daughter were to "wait till it suppurates or even inflames much, it may be too late." Although Rush maintained that "[t]he pain of the operation is much less than her fears represent it be,"[143] this was not the case.

In the end, Nabby courageously endured the painful surgical procedure performed by Dr. John Warren of Boston on October 8th, with only the limited aid of opium in the form of laudanum since the use of ether in operations had not yet been introduced. During Nabby's recuperation, Abigail shuttled between caring for her daughter and her sister's household, where both Mary and Richard Cranch were terminally ill. Richard died within days of Nabby's operation, Mary just a day after her husband. To Abigail's extreme distress, unfortunately Nabby's surgery did prove to be "too late," and another tumor was later found in her other breast, as the cancer metastasized through her entire body. Nabby endured increasing pain and weakness as the disease relentlessly advanced, but she determinedly made the arduous 300-mile journey to spend her last days in the home of her parents. "How she got here is a marvel to me,"[144] Abigail remarked after her first sight of her frail and emaciated dying daughter. Abigail (Nabby) Adams Smith died on August 14, 1813, at the age of forty-nine. To add to the family health tragedies, two of John's and Abigail's infant grandchildren died during the same period— Thomas and Ann Adams's baby daughter Francis of whooping cough and, as we have seen, John Quincy and Louisa's toddler.

Nabby was far from the only woman among the families of America's founders who experienced the terrible ravages of breast cancer. As we learned in the last chapter, Benjamin Franklin's sister was also affected. Eliza Pickney, one of the more visible female supporters of the American Revolution, traveled to Philadelphia in the spring of 1793, hoping to seek expert medical advice and assistance. Although her physician,

Dr. Tate, showed off a number of his "cured" cancer patients to Eliza's daughter, his medicinal potions had little effect on Eliza, who like Nabby suffered great agony before she died just a few weeks later.[145] The death of the Adamses' beloved only living daughter, Nabby, was probably the most heart-wrenching personal tragedy encountered by her grieving parents and undoubtedly contributed to Abigail's physical decline. With Nabby's demise, only two of Abigail's sons remained; four of the six children she had borne had predeceased her. Nabby had fought a long and valiant battle with breast cancer. As her mother later reported to Thomas Jefferson, who sent Abigail a letter of sympathy, "Two years since, she had an operation performed for a cancer in her breast. This she supported, with wonderful fortitude, and we flatterd ourselves that the cure was effectual but it proved otherways. It soon communicated itself through the whole mass of the Blood, and after several sufferings, it terminated her existence."[146] Abigail's frank communication to Jefferson is rather remarkable as at the time breast cancer was a subject that was taboo in society. It reflects not only Abigail's religious faith and stoic attitude toward illness and death but also her advanced views about health and medicine and suggests that she felt that openness on the subject might aid others by disseminating the most up-to-date medical wisdom.

Abigail's letter to Thomas Jefferson also provides us poignant details of Nabby's last days: "Your kind and Friendly Letter found me in great affliction for the loss of my dear and only daughter, Mrs. Smith. She had been with me only three weeks having undertaken a journey from the State of N. York, desirous once more to see her parents, and to close her days under the parental roof." Although Abigail could never bring herself to entirely forgive Jefferson for what she viewed as his political disloyalty, she realized that his own many encounters with the loss of loved ones would allow him to empathize fully with her grief. "You sir, who have been called to separations of a similar kind, can sympathize with your bereaved friend. I have the consolation of knowing that the Life of my dear daughter was pure, her conduct in prosperity and adversity, exemplary, her patience and resignation becoming her religion." The sorrow that John Adams experienced on the loss of his daughter was equally palpable, and in disbelief he lamented in an earlier letter to Jefferson that Nabby had once been "the healthiest and firmest of us all."[147]

Together John and Abigail navigated the path of grief, supporting one another as they had so many times during their long marriage, and religious faith remained a solace, particularly for Abigail. A few years later, Abigail would comment poignantly to Mercy Warren that "if we live to old age string after string is severed from the heart."[148]

After Nabby's death, her daughter, Caroline, moved in with her grandparents, providing great comfort to them. Both Abigail and John were impaired by declining eyesight as they aged, possibly victims to cataracts, but a grandchild or a niece seemed to always be on hand to read to them or help with writing. In his last years John developed an advanced palsy, possibly Parkinson's disease, which he described as "a kind of Paralytic Infection of the Nerves, which makes my hands tremble." Still, John remained remarkably robust, and in 1812, at the age of seventy-six, informed Jefferson that "I walk every fair day, sometimes 3 or 4 miles. Ride now and then but very rarely more than ten or fifteen miles."[149]

Abigail's health was more precarious. In 1815, she was devastated by the loss of her youngest sister, Elizabeth Peabody, with whom she had shared so many joys and sorrows since childhood. In 1816, perhaps prompted by Elizabeth's death, Abigail composed her will, carefully allotting her descendants and many relatives a share in her clothing, jewelry, money, and even property and stock, with a special eye toward the women in the family. Abigail became increasingly frail and was troubled by arthritis and rheumatism. A letter she received from Jefferson in 1816 acknowledged their relative longevity for the time. Mrs. Adams and Jefferson were both then in their early seventies. "You and I, dear Madam, have already more than an ordinary portion of life, and more too of health than the general measure," Jefferson observed. "Your health was, some time ago, not as good as it has been; and I perceive, in the letters communicated, some complaints still . . . I hope it is restored; and that life and health may be continued to you as many years as yourself shall wish."[150]

In the unusually hot summer of 1818, Abigail contracted typhoid, probably through contaminated water, and she developed a high fever, which weakened her further and affected her kidneys. She was visited by Dr. Waterhouse, the physician with whom Jefferson led the battle to introduce the Jenner smallpox vaccination in the United States, and he diagnosed her illness.[151] Although the resilient Abigail Adams had rallied so many times before, this time her illness was probably compounded by a stroke, and she lingered until she died at the old Adams home in Quincy on October 28, 1818, a few weeks short of her seventy-fourth birthday. Her funeral took place three days later, and she was buried beside her daughter Nabby and Mary and Richard Cranch.

Shortly before Abigail's death, John had poured out his sadness to Jefferson, informing his friend that "[t]he dear Partner of my Life for fifty four Years as a Wife and for many more as a Lover, now lyes in extremis, forbidden to speak or be spoken to."[152] After Abigail's death, John continued to praise her for a lifetime of accomplishment and loving support for the entire family. After more than half a century, John had lost his lifelong companion, but took solace from being surrounded by his surviving sons and many grandchildren, and his daughter-in-law Louisa Catherine became one of his strongest sources of support. Though Abigail's elder by nearly a decade, John survived her by eight years. Jefferson, no stranger to the loss of loved ones, counseled Adams that his own "trials have taught me that, for ills so immeasurable, time and silences are the only medicines."[153]

Adams remained in relatively good health. In 1814, he told Jefferson that he was "sometimes afraid that my 'Machine' will not 'surcease motion' soon enough; for I dread nothing so much as 'dying at the top' and thereby becoming a weeping helpless object of compassion for years."[154] John had long feared the effects of dementia, but was certainly mentally acute in the years following Abigail's death. Although he needed the assistance of family members to read letters due to failing eyesight and to write them because of increasing palsy in his hands, he continued to carry on the marvelously sparkling intellectual correspondence with Jefferson, for whom he had developed a remarkable affection. As Adams wrote to Jefferson at the end of 1818, "Sick or Well the friendship is the same of your old Acquaintance." Adams was relieved to hear that Jefferson was recovering from illness, but he confessed, "I envy your Eyes and hands and Horse." Resigned to old age, Adams halfheartedly complained, "Mine are too dim, too tremulous and my head is too dizzy" for deep thinking, the latter patently untrue.[155]

Yet, the following spring the sprightly 83-year-old Adams affirmed that "[t]ho I cannot write I still live and enjoy Life." Adams actually fared better than Jefferson in regard to health and was remarkably vigorous until he neared ninety. At the end of November 1819, having marked yet another birthday, he went so far as to say, "My Health is astonishing to myself. . . . I believe nothing but Distemper will kill me," and he compared himself to the late Benjamin Franklin, who at about the same age enjoyed robust health, a cheerful spirit, and keen intellect.[156]

On the whole, other than a great number of colds, which may have been caused by allergy, and three serious episodes of illness, which may have been related to either malaria, acute stress, or an undiagnosed, untreated thyroid condition, Adams was remarkably free of severe illness during his lifetime, although he tended to grumble about minor sickness and not infrequently predicted his early demise. One writer, who has speculated that Adams ultimately died as a result of heart disease related to hardening of the arteries, has observed that "he was physically one of the healthiest of the American presidents, and when he died at ninety one he had exceeded the life expectancy for men not only in his own time but the present."[157] After a lifetime of devoted service to America, John Adams died peacefully on July 4, 1826, fifty years after the signing of the Declaration of Independence. It is noteworthy that not only had Adams shared the journey to form a new republic and a commitment to the health of the nation's citizens with his revolutionary comrade Thomas Jefferson, but they shared their day of death as well. They were the last living heroes of the struggle for independence.

4

Thomas Jefferson

Advocate for Healthy Living

> [Exercise] is necessary for your health, and health
> is the first of all objects.
> —*Thomas Jefferson to Martha Jefferson, March 28, 1787*

> The state of medicine is worse than that of total
> ignorance.
> —*Thomas Jefferson to William Green Munford, 1799*

In 1766, 23-year-old Thomas Jefferson traveled from Virginia by horse-drawn carriage nearly three hundred miles to Philadelphia to be inoculated for smallpox. Jefferson was at the time a tall, fit, lanky young man in fine health, but he undertook the then-controversial treatment to prevent contracting an acute future case of the devastating disease. Inoculation was illegal in Virginia at the time, as many feared the procedure would spread infection. Jefferson was encouraged to undergo variolation, as the procedure was popularly termed, by his old friend and former classmate at the College of William and Mary, Dr. George Gilmer. Gilmer introduced Jefferson to Dr. John Morgan, who was then advocating inoculation in Philadelphia.[1] Morgan turned Jefferson over to his colleague Dr. William Shippen, as Morgan's practice excluded "surgical" procedures like inoculation.[2] Shippen later served as a surgeon in the American army from 1776 to 1789. Like so many American-trained physicians of the era, Gilmer, Morgan, and Shippen all received their medical degrees from the prestigious University of Edinburgh.

Although Jefferson experienced no ill effects from the smallpox procedure, as we learned, inoculation by live human virus, which produced immunity through a mild case of the disease, could sometimes cause serious illness and was potentially fatal. Like John Adams, Jefferson probably followed the same contemporary prescribed preparation prior to the induction of the human "matter" beneath the skin, which permitted a bland diet but abstention from wine and meat products, followed by the administration of a variety of potions to induce purging to cleanse the system. By undergoing the process, the young Jefferson was demonstrating his familiarity with emerging medical knowledge about infectious diseases and signaling his lifelong progressive commitment to personal and public preventative health. Indeed, his private interest in averting smallpox would evolve into his support of public health initiatives for the nation. Influenced by Enlightenment thought, like Washington, Franklin, Adams, and Madison, Jefferson viewed political, social, economic, and physical health as part of a reciprocal relationship.[3]

Although he is best known for his iconic role in the American Revolution, his authorship of the Declaration of Independence, and his two terms as America's third president, as Jefferson himself famously declared, "Science is my passion, politics my duty."[4] For Jefferson, medicine was perhaps the most important branch of science, and he became one of the first American presidents to make public health policy a significant focus during his tenure in office. A true Renaissance man who possessed a brilliant mind and a wide breath of knowledge in both the arts and the sciences, like his hero Benjamin Franklin, Thomas Jefferson displayed a special interest in health and medicine. Jefferson was never reluctant to question contemporary medical wisdom, nor hesitant to criticize the doctors who practiced it. Although he clearly viewed nature as the best healer and believed in the efficacy of a regimen of healthy living augmented by the use of medicinal herbs and plants, he consulted physicians when he deemed it necessary and approved of the use of medications that proved effective. In other words, his empirical approach to science meant that he always emphasized proven fact over theory.

In many aspects Jefferson's views on health were astute and forward thinking, even revolutionary at times. His Enlightenment outlook on human progress and the belief that science should contribute to the advancement of human welfare and happiness influenced his role as an early leader in the field of American public health. Moreover, Jefferson believed that a free and republican government actually encouraged

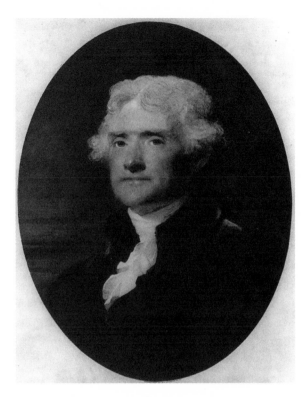

Portrait of Thomas
Jefferson. (Courtesy
Library of Congress)

good health, since he viewed the health of the body and the health of society as intertwined.⁵ In addition to supporting smallpox inoculation by personal example, while president of the United States, Jefferson used his influence to endorse the use of the safer, more effective method of smallpox vaccination introduced by Dr. Edward Jenner in England at the end of the eighteenth century, encouraging its popular use. According to one of his biographers, Jefferson, who regularly read medical litera-ture and closely followed new trends, "was probably as well informed on matters of health, if not even more so, than most physicians of his time."⁶

Jefferson's Family Roots

Future president, statesman, politician, scientist, diplomat, and author Thomas Jefferson was born in Albemarle County, Virginia, on April 13, 1743, to Jane Randolph, the British-born daughter of a distinguished

Virginia family, and Peter Jefferson, a self-made man who trained as a surveyor and became a respected, prosperous tobacco farmer and member of the Virginia House of Burgesses. Peter Jefferson died in the summer of 1757 at the age of fifty, following a two-month unspecified illness when Thomas was only fourteen. The elder Jefferson left his widow, Jane, with eight children, six girls and two boys. Jefferson's baby brother died in 1748 before he reached the age of two months, and two of Jefferson's sisters died as young women. Jane, the eldest child of Peter and Jane Jefferson, and Thomas's favorite sibling, died at the age of twenty-five. His sister Elizabeth, who was probably developmentally disabled, died in her late twenties due to shock and exposure after an earthquake shook the family estate.[7]

The history of the Jefferson family graphically illustrates the fragility of life at the time, particularly in the American South. The life expectancy of men typically did not exceed their fifties and many women died in their thirties, often from complications related to childbirth. Miscarriage and death in infancy and early childhood were common. However, even in an age when mortality was high, Jefferson suffered a disproportionate number of losses of loved ones. He outlived his wife, five of their six children, five of his siblings, and even several grandchildren. Their deaths seem to have left Jefferson with both a heightened sense of family and a predilection to avoid open conflict, perhaps to the detriment of his own health, as it seems to have manifested itself in episodic headaches and stomach distress during stressful periods in his life. Jefferson certainly recognized the abnormally high degree of loss in his life, for while he was living in Paris in 1787 he plaintively wrote Maria Cosway, the object of his affection at the time, "I am born to lose everything I love."[8]

Jefferson's mother lived to age fifty-five, but died suddenly of an apparent stroke in 1776, during a period when Jefferson was a leading member of the Continental Congress and advocating colonial independence from Great Britain. Jefferson reported her demise in a rather matter-of-fact manner to his Uncle William Randolph: "The death of my mother . . . happened . . . after an illness of not more than an hour. We supposed it to have been apoplectic."[9] Jefferson had an apparently ambivalent and distant relationship with his mother, and he may have experienced some degree of guilt when she died. The resultant stress of her death in combination with the complex work that awaited him in

Philadelphia were factors contributing to a vague illness, probably caus-ing one of Jefferson's lifelong intermittent "periodical headaches" as he referred to them, which began to trouble him in his early twenties.

In contrast to most of his blood relations, who died young, Jeffer-son lived to the age of eighty-three, nearly twice the life expectancy of the time. His longevity was undoubtedly due in part to his underlying philosophy of temperate living and perhaps more importantly to his forward-looking ideas on health and preventative medicine, as well as his skepticism about physicians and the medicine they practiced in his day. As we learned in the introduction, most eighteenth-century doctors relied heavily on radical bleeding and purging, treatments that Jeffer-son regarded as scientifically unproven as well as harmful. Nearly forty years younger than Benjamin Franklin, Jefferson was exposed to and influenced by new emerging medical thought from France that rejected heroic medical measures. Jefferson disagreed with Franklin about the efficacy of bleeding but was a great admirer of his fellow patriot, with whom he shared a firm commitment to preventative health and science. Throughout his life, Jefferson ate sparingly and sensibly, emphasized veg-etables in his diet, engaged in regular outdoor exercise, made sure he got adequate sleep, and was a highly controlled man who thrived on order.[10]

Jefferson's father intended that Thomas would receive the advanced formal education he had been denied and provided the means in his will. Dr. Thomas Walker, who attended Peter Jefferson during his last illness, was named Thomas's primary guardian. Walker, a prominent Virginia physician, planter, and politician, undoubtedly served as a dis-tinguished role model for the young Jefferson. Perhaps Jefferson's close association with Dr. Walker encouraged him to undergo smallpox inoc-ulation in 1766. Through inoculation, Jefferson effectively protected himself from the scourge of smallpox during his lifetime.[11]

When he turned twenty-one, Jefferson received control of the family plantation of Shadwell, nearly five thousand acres along with twenty-two slaves. As the eldest son, the precociously bright, handsome, but shy reddish-blond-headed young Jefferson inherited not only considerable property and wealth but also the opportunity to receive a classical edu-cation. At the age of seventeen he began study at the College of William and Mary. Thomas was a brilliant and driven student, attracted to phi-losophy, political thought, and music. It was not uncommon for him to spend fifteen hours a day in study. He was extremely well read, a talented mathematician who used calculus with ease, a fine violinist, and he spoke and read seven languages, including Latin and Greek. Jefferson's developing views on moderation in all life's activities, particularly in diet, were strongly influenced by his admiration of the Greek philosophers Epicurus and Cicero. Following graduation, Jefferson studied law for five years under a beloved mentor, attorney George Wythe, a future signer of the Declaration of Independence. After completing his apprenticeship, at age twenty-four Jefferson was admitted to the bar and became a practicing attorney. Though he found law dull, in the late 1760s and early 1770s he was diligently occupied with his burgeoning business.[12]

Like so many of his educated contemporaries, Jefferson's keen interest in medicine sometimes encouraged him to act as an informal practitioner, as we learned was the case with George Washington. According to family tradition, when a young slave on a neighboring plantation cut his leg badly, Jefferson stepped in and sutured the injury with a needle and thread, probably doing as good a job as a trained surgeon of the time and in a more sanitary manner, as doctors of the period had virtually no understanding of germs and their role in spreading disease. Much later, in his third year of the presidency, Jefferson also personally inoculated neighbors against smallpox during a visit to Monticello. As we learned, Jefferson was generally skeptical about the way medicine was practiced in his era; he believed that the causes and treatment of many diseases were poorly understood because they relied on age-old outdated theories that were not based on true empiric evidence. In particular, he was often disparaging about the medical profession and was once said to have remarked to an acquaintance that "whenever he saw three physicians together, he looked up to discover whether there were not a turkey buzzard hovering overhead."[13]

Although Jefferson became a close friend of many physicians, most notably of Dr. Benjamin Rush, he was extremely critical of the doctor's frequent use of violent bleeding and purging, which, as we have seen, were then the accepted medical wisdom of the era. Jefferson not only disdained bleeding for family members but forbade his plantation overseers from having the medical procedure performed on his slaves.[14] In 1773, he firmly instructed his overseer to "[n]ever bleed a negro."[15] Many years later he informed another overseer that physicians should only be called in sparingly for sick slaves because "in most other cases [other than pleurisy, malaria, and dysentery] they [doctors] oftener do harm than good." Reflecting his belief in the healing powers of nature and limited intervention, he further advised the man in most cases to treat the ill with "a lighter diet and kind attention" and to administer salts since "they are . . . salutary in almost all cases, & hurtful in none."[16]

The Jefferson Family

Although Jefferson involved himself with overseeing a plantation, learning about science and medicine, and nurturing a nascent political career, he made time for several romantic attachments in his teens and early twenties. The young Virginia planter and rising politician, however, did not marry until he was twenty-eight. The personable Jefferson won the heart of an attractive young widow, Martha Wayles Skeleton, whom he married on January 1, 1772, at her family plantation home called "the Forest." The couple shared a love of music, literature, and good conversation and settled into their still-unfinished home of Monticello. In 1771, Jefferson presented his future wife with one of the first pianos imported to America. Through his wife, Martha, within a year and a half of their marriage Jefferson inherited another eleven thousand acres of land and 135 slaves from the estate of her father—and a mound of debt that would plague him throughout his lifetime. Jefferson's financial problems would become extreme in his later years as he struggled to pay for expansions and remodeling at Monticello.

Tragically, illness and death hovered over the Jefferson marriage from the beginning. Martha Jefferson came to the union with her own history of personal tragedy. By the time she was twenty-three, she had already lost her mother, two stepmothers, her first husband, and then her young son—the stepson whom Jefferson looked forward to parenting from Martha's first marriage died soon after they wed. In 1773, Jefferson's brother-in-law and close friend Dabney Carr passed away suddenly, and a few weeks later Martha's father followed. Martha and Thomas's only son died in May 1777 at the age of two weeks, and only three of their five daughters survived their mother.

The death of each of Jefferson's children was a source of deep sadness for Jefferson, and each a tragedy from which he did not recover easily. When his baby son passed away, Jefferson delayed his return to the Continental Congress in Philadelphia for weeks so he could console his wife and begin his own healing process. Baby Jane Randolph, named after Jefferson's mother, died at about eighteen months in 1775, and another daughter, Lucy Elizabeth, at age five months in 1781. Their youngest child, also named Lucy Elizabeth Jefferson, died of whooping cough at the age of only two and half while Jefferson was in France on behalf of the American government. Maria (Polly) died in her midtwenties as a result of complications following childbirth, and only the Jefferson's eldest child, Martha (Patsy), who had been a sickly infant, was still alive when Thomas Jefferson died.[17]

Jefferson's Health and Early Political Career

Although he possessed a strong constitution and was generally in quite good health for the era, during his lifetime Jefferson suffered from several moderate to acute attacks of dysentery (bloody diarrhea), and ultimately that disease was the immediate cause of his death. Jefferson claimed he was able to relieve a severe attack in 1802 through horseback riding, suggesting the psychosomatic origins of his stomach disorder, and he may have actually suffered from colitis. Jefferson also experienced during his lifetime many severe, prolonged "periodic" headaches. At times Jefferson self-medicated these episodes by retreating to a darkened room or by taking lavender or Peruvian bark, which appeared to give him some relief, although it was probably the result of a placebo effect as quinine is used most effectively to treat malaria. Jefferson's recurrent headaches had seemingly psychosomatic origins. Indeed, biographer Fawn Brodie maintains that "they became a reliable indication of when he was most suffering from tension."[18] In 1776, for example, he endured six weeks of pain, while his draft of the Declaration of Independence was under debate, and did not return to his duties at the Continental Congress until May, when revolution appeared imminent.[19]

Like his severe, prolonged "periodic" headaches, most of the bouts with stomach ailments were probably prompted by stress, but some were undoubtedly bacterial in origin. Historian Joseph Ellis maintains that Jefferson's illnesses were often a "typical act of avoidance."[20] His upbringing and innate personality combined to make Jefferson extremely self-controlled and sensitive to criticism and at the same time reluctant to engage in open confrontation and dissension. Balancing these traits certainly may have produced psychosomatic ailments.

Jefferson entered politics as a young man, which no doubt increased the stress in his life. Virginia was the oldest and largest of the thirteen colonies. At the age of twenty-six, in 1768, he was elected to Virginia's governing body, the House of Burgesses, a position he held for six years. In 1774, while a leader of the revolutionary section of that body and the founder of the Committee of Correspondence, Jefferson experienced a violent attack of dysentery en route to a crucial meeting in Williamsburg. Dysentery produced painful intestinal spasms and bloody stools and was a leading cause of illness and death in colonial America. The bacterial infection occurred most often in large cities and generally peaked in summer, spread by flies.

The severity of the illness forced Jefferson to return to Monticello, but always stoic in the face of sickness, he managed to send the draft of his document titled *Summary View of the Rights of British America* to the assembly at the Williamsburg convention. The pamphlet, inspired by the republican ideals of the English philosophers, focused on the outrages perpetrated by the British government on the colonies. We will never know if Jefferson's intestinal distress was bacterial or psychological in origin, but knowing he had been thrust into the revolutionary center and that his writings would have been considered treasonous by the English government certainly may have played a part in his illness. The document proved to be a turning point in Jefferson's political career. His argument highly impressed the delegates, therefore ensuring his election to the Continental Congress in 1775 and foreshadowing his selection as the master draftsman of the Declaration of Independence.[21]

Jefferson remained active in Virginia politics, and it is interesting to note that as early as 1778, when he presented a draft of new laws for the Commonwealth, his keen interest in medical research was evident when he recommended that the bodies of hanged murderers be used for dissection to promote better understanding of anatomy.[22] Jefferson succeeded Patrick Henry as governor of Virginia in 1779 and served a second term from 1780 to 1781. Not only did his time in office coincide with the bleakest period of the American Revolution, but it was a challenging time for Jefferson personally. The death of the Jeffersons' baby daughter

Lucy Elizabeth on April 15, 1781, strengthened Jefferson's desire to end his service as governor and plunged both Jefferson and his wife into depression, a melancholy state that remained with her until her death in 1782.

Jefferson resigned his commission as governor at the end of his second term, partly to be more available to his wife and in response to the criticism he endured while in office after being painted as a coward and criticized for the poor showing of the state militia against the British. Outraged at the slur, he mounted his favorite horse, Caractacus, and took off at great speed in an attempt to dispel his agitated mood. The highly active Jefferson suffered a number of fractured bones and sprains during his lifetime, but usually bounced back quickly due to his underlying good health. Although a superb horseman, in this instance Jefferson broke both his arm and his collar bone after falling from his horse and was unable to resume his normal lifestyle for many weeks, running up a substantial bill from the doctor who attended him. Emotional upheavals often affected Jefferson's health. When Jefferson was later elected to the Continental Congress in 1783, he became chair of the committee to develop federal monetary policies. Stymied by lack of support for his proposals, Jefferson once again experienced a lengthy period of prolonged headaches that probably stemmed from tension.[23]

Over the course of their ten-year marriage, Martha gave birth to six children and suffered several miscarriages. Preoccupied with her growing family, she apparently took little interest in her husband's political career. Frail to begin with, and further weakened by repeated pregnancy and childbirth, she died less than a year and a half after the birth of their youngest child, possibly due to underlying tuberculosis.

Jefferson had often expressed deep anxiety about his wife's ill health and always tried to be at Monticello during at least the last months of Martha's pregnancies. After he completed his draft of the Declaration of Independence in the spring of 1776, Jefferson asked to be released from the Continental Congress to be with Martha during her third pregnancy. In a letter to his friend John Page dated July 30, 1776, Jefferson reported, "Every letter brings me such an account of the state of her health, that it is with great pain that I can stay here."[24] However, his vote was crucial to the Virginia delegation, and Jefferson was required to remain longer than he wished. Sadly, the pregnancy resulted in a miscarriage. In early fall Jefferson apparently decided that his prolonged absence from home made the family situation untenable, and he resigned from Congress on September 2, 1776. Later, as a member of the Virginia assembly, he was frequently absent, most notably after the death of his infant son in 1777. When Martha was recovering from the birth of their daughter Maria in the summer of 1778, Jefferson again missed parts of the fall legislative session to be by her side.[25]

The Death of Martha Jefferson

Although he would be absent from the national political scene for six years, as we have seen, Jefferson did accept state office in 1779. However, despite his duties as governor of Virginia, he remained highly attentive to Martha when her health declined precipitously. By all accounts Jefferson served as a devoted nurse, administering medications and comfort and rarely leaving her side during her last illness. A few weeks after the birth of the second Lucy Elizabeth, Jefferson wrote to his friend future president James Monroe and reported that "Mrs. Jefferson has added another daughter to our family. She has ever since and still continues very dangerously ill."[26]

Jefferson's old friend Dr. Gilmer visited Martha regularly after she gave birth, but it was Jefferson who in reality became her primary medical caregiver. Their daughter Martha Jefferson Randolph later observed,

> As a nurse no female ever had more tenderness or anxiety. . . . For four months that she lingered he [Jefferson] was never out of Calling. When not at her bed side he was writing in a small room which opened immediately at the head of her bed. . . . A moment before the closing scene, he was led from the room in a state of insensibility.[27]

Martha's death sent Jefferson into a deep depression, at first leaving him unable to work or interact with friends or family other than his daughter Martha. To one correspondent he wrote that his grief was "too burdensome to be borne" and left him in a "stupor of mind which . . . rendered me as dead to the world as she was whose loss occasioned it."[28] Although Jefferson was generally of an optimistic, even temperament, he experienced several episodes of intense melancholy, what contemporaries may have termed a "breakdown," in response to the loss of loved ones during his lifetime. After his wife died, he shut himself away with his grief and did not leave his room for three weeks, often keeping his ten-year-old daughter at his side, even when he finally emerged from the house for long rambling horseback rides in the countryside.

Jefferson was only thirty-nine when Martha Wayles Jefferson died on September 6, 1782, and he remained loyal to his deathbed promise that he would never remarry. The oath was witnessed by several of the Monticello female house slaves, including the young Sally Hemings, who may have been John Wayles's illegitimate daughter, making Martha and Sally half-sisters. Despite decades of controversy, many historians now believe that it is unlikely that Jefferson conducted a liaison with Sally Hemings and that there is no verifiable proof that he fathered any of her children. Modern DNA analysis has only established a possible link between Sally's youngest son, Easton, and a member of the Jefferson family, possibly one of Jefferson's nephews or his younger brother Randolph. Certainly Jefferson never publicly acknowledged any of Sally's offspring as his own.[29]

The loss of his wife refocused Jefferson on his political career, which would continue for over a quarter of a century. Just months after her death, he was elected to Congress, but grief took a visible toll on his health. He complained to his friend William Short of "habitual ill health" and reoccurrence of his troubling headaches, which caused him to "avoid reading writing and almost thinking."[30] Despite these ailments, in fact Jefferson continued to work diligently and became known as one of the most productive members of the Congress in Annapolis. Jefferson gradually reestablished ties with old friends like James Madison, with whom he conducted many rich exchanges about politics and philosophy. Jefferson was keenly aware of the mind-body connection. Writing to Madison in early 1784, Jefferson observed that intellectual discourse brought him satisfaction and even provided health benefits. Jefferson maintained that "[a]mong the most valuable [gratifications of life] . . . is rational society. It informs the mind, sweetens the temper, chears our spirits, and promotes health."[31]

James Madison and Jefferson

Because Madison became Jefferson's protégé and Jefferson appears to have regarded the younger man almost as a son, we should pause and provide some background about Madison's legacy of illness. Indeed, Madison's somewhat unusual health experiences also shed light on the state of medicine during the era. Madison was born into a prosperous family of long-time Virginians in Orange County on March 16, 1751. Like Jefferson, Madison was a brilliant, bookish young man and an outstanding student who was attracted to the philosophy of the Enlightenment at an early age. The two first became acquainted in 1779, while Jefferson was serving as governor of Virginia. Jefferson was especially drawn to the work of John Locke, who also influenced Madison's liberal political development and his involvement in guiding the new American nation. Of course, the subject of medical progress and philosophy were intimately intertwined in Enlightenment thought, and like so many gentleman of the elite planter class, such as Washington and Jefferson, Madison became familiar with issues concerning health and disease.

Although America's first three presidents, George Washington, John Adams, and Thomas Jefferson, were robustly built and relatively healthy men for their era, chronic health issues plagued the delicate, weak-voiced James Madison from a young age. Historian Garry Wills described him as a slight, "short frail man," just a shade over five feet tall, and observed that "his sense of discipline and self-restraint stemmed from his concern for his health."[32] Madison, who went on to become known as the respected "Father of the Constitution" and the nation's fourth president, is thought to have suffered from some form of epilepsy, a diagnosis based on inferences in his writings about vaguely described seizures, and he was often troubled by "bilious" stomach upsets and malarial flareups. Certainly Madison often expressed doubts about his potential longevity. When he was only twenty-one, he confided to a college friend that he was unable to formulate firm plans for his future because "my sensations of many months past have intimated to me not to expect a long or healthy life."[33]

As Madison scholar Ralph Ketcham has observed, James Madison exhibited "a hypochondriacal tendency to 'fear the worst.'"[34] "Crossing the sea would be unfriendly to a singular disease of my constitution," Madison wrote in 1785 to Jefferson, his political mentor.[35] The apprehension of serious illness seems to have been a lifetime, if intermittent, preoccupation with Madison, but fortunately increasing political

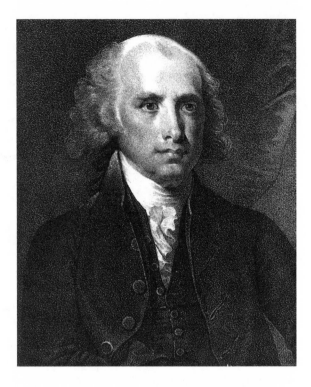

Lithograph of James Madison from a Painting by Gilbert Stuart. (Courtesy Library of Congress)

responsibilities and concerns for his wife, Dolley, often trumped worries about his own health. And like many hypochondriacs, Madison lived to a very ripe age for the era.

Jefferson was sensitive to Madison's tendency to worry about illness. After Jefferson was elected president, Madison joined his cabinet, but expressed concern about moving to Washington. Madison confided that "[m]y health still suffers from several complaints, and I am much afraid that any changes that may take place are not likely to be for the better."[36] Jefferson took Madison's health complaints with a grain of salt, no doubt recalling that, when faced with public responsibility, a refocused Madison often overcame health issues. In his reply to Madison's letter, Jefferson offered an encouraging opinion that emphasized his belief in healthy living: "I think nothing more possible than that a change of climate, even from a better to a worse, and a change in the habits and mode of life, might have a favorable effect on your system."[37]

Biographer Irving Brant has argued that instead of classic epilepsy, Madison suffered from epileptoid hysteria, a psychosomatic condition, and historian Ralph Ketcham has suggested that the underlying problem was a nervous disorder, which, coupled with "an inclination toward hypochondria, strengthen the impression that its cause [ill health] was in part functional."[38] One modern-day physician has speculated that although it is difficult to diagnose a disease retroactively, Madison may have had the petit mal type of epilepsy. Madison's description of episodes in which he was "paralyzed" both mentally and physically for short periods but never experienced convulsions is consistent with this diagnosis. Apparently these types of experiences occurred periodically during Madison's long life, including one witnessed by his wife Dolley when she observed, "I saw you in your chamber unable to move."[39] Given his uncertain health and weak constitution, Madison lived a surprisingly long life, dying at the age of eighty-five, fully mentally alert. But even in old age Madison maintained that he suffered from a "constitutional liability to sudden attacks, somewhat resembling epilepsy and suspending the intellectual functions."[40] Indeed, all of the founders in this study surpassed the common life expectancy, probably aided by their elite status, which gave them access to a relatively high standard of living, their focus on maintaining good health, and their access to the best care available at the time when they were ill.

To return to Jefferson, soon after Martha died, Madison sensed that Jefferson would benefit by an active return to public life and pushed for Jefferson's appointment as American minister plenipotentiary for negotiating peace with England. After several delays Jefferson was deployed to France to move negotiations forward, but after Martha's death Jefferson's children became even more precious to him and their health paramount. After his wife's passing, Jefferson made sure that his three daughters and the children of his sister, Mary Carr, were inoculated for smallpox, once again demonstrating his sophisticated understanding at the time of the danger of contagion and the benefits of inoculation. After the untimely death of his childhood friend and brother-in-law, Dabney Carr, from a "bilious" fever at the age of thirty, the Carr children became Jefferson's wards. According to Jefferson's great-granddaughter Sarah Randolph, Jefferson provided "fatherly affection and guidance" to his sister's six children and "received them into his family as adopted children."[41]

During the smallpox procedure and the subsequent recovery period the Jefferson family members were housed at the home of Jefferson's friend Colonel Archibald Cary, who lived in nearby Chesterfield County. Jefferson served as a medical practitioner, nursing the children through the ordeal and quarantine period. Sarah Randolph later observed that "while engaged as their chief nurse," Jefferson received "notice of his appointment by Congress as the Plenipotentiary to Europe, to be associated with Dr. Franklin and Mr. Adams to negotiate the peace." He had declined the appointment previously because of his promise to his wife Martha Jefferson that he would not become actively involved in public life while she was living. Once the children recovered, four-year-old Maria and the baby Lucy were left in the care of Martha Jefferson's half-sister, Elizabeth Wayles Eppes, and her husband, Francis Eppes. Young Martha was sent to boarding school in Philadelphia. Jefferson stayed in touch with his children through frequent letters during their separations.[42]

American Ambassador to France

In 1784, Jefferson finally set sail from Boston with eleven-year-old Martha for Paris, where he would serve as an American envoy to France. There he would assist John Adams and Benjamin Franklin in their efforts to secure commercial agreements and, ultimately, peace, and the three worked together productively until late in 1785, when Franklin returned to America and Adams was redeployed to London. Martha and her father left on July 5th, and Jefferson would remain in Europe for five years until 1789 amid the first stirrings of the French Revolution. Once in Paris, Jefferson rented a modest house before leasing a finer residence in 1785 on the Champs-Élyseés and placed Martha in a well-run, fashionable convent school. Jefferson would develop into a Francophile and later return to America with dozens of paintings and boxes of books in an effort to import what he considered the most admirable aspects of French culture to his homeland.

The main impetus behind Jefferson's mission to France was to eventually replace the aging Franklin, who was often in pain due to recurrent gout and bladder stones and wanted to return home. Paris at the time was the sophisticated hub of Europe, and diplomats from many countries were stationed there. The city buzzed with the newest cutting-edge trends in art, music, and even medicine. Indeed, Paris, Edinburgh, and Berlin were the medical capitals of the world at the time. Jefferson's position, erudition, and friendship with the popular Benjamin Franklin assured him an entrée into the dazzling Parisian cultural salons, and he led a glittering social life. The elegant Jefferson, who spoke French fluently, loved the first-hand involvement in intellectual cosmopolitan life and exposure to European culture, but often cast a critical eye on the excesses of Parisian luxury and dissipation. He also missed the simpler republican virtues of American agrarianism, and whenever Jefferson could spare the time, he visited the countryside and remained a staunch advocate of fresh air and exercise.

It was Franklin who introduced him to the famous salon of Madame Helvétius. One of the friends Jefferson made there was Pierre-Jean-Georges Cabanis, physician/philosopher, physiologist, and professor of medicine, whose publications would help advance medical theory and practice in both Europe and America in the late eighteenth and early nineteenth centuries. By 1776, the cornerstone for a great medical school had been laid in Paris, and several major hospitals existed in the city by Jefferson's arrival. He admired Cabanis's progressive views on reforming medicine and medical education, and their exchanges undoubtedly contributed to Jefferson's advanced ideas on health and the treatment of illness.[43]

As we learned in chapter 2, during Jefferson's sojourn a new medical treatment introduced by the Austrian physician Dr. Franz Anton Mesmer was capturing the attention of Parisians. Mesmer's theory of "animal magnetism" reflected his belief that all living beings possessed magnetic fluid fields in their bodies and that if those fields were out of sync with the planets, people became ill. Mesmer spent hours at a time waving magnetic rods or wands before his patients, probably "mesmerizing" them with some form of hypnotism, and he claimed to have cured a variety of maladies through this method. Many of Mesmer's patients were probably experiencing common psychosomatic ailments. It is likely that the power of suggestion and belief in the "magical" healing process produced some of the touted cures, a factor Franklin astutely speculated upon after subjecting Mesmer's work to scientific scrutiny.

As was the case with Franklin, Jefferson's rational worldview prompted him to view Mesmer's method with great skepticism and scorn, just as he had reacted toward many of the American medical practices he considered both unscientific and ineffective.[44] When Louis XVI appointed a commission, which included Benjamin Franklin, to investigate Mesmer's claims, Jefferson's initial misgivings were confirmed. In 1784 he wrote a friend, "I send you a pamphlet on the subject of animal magnetism, which has disturbed the nerves of prodigious numbers here. I believe this report will allay the evil."[45]

As much as Jefferson would come to love France, his first encounter with the Paris weather and the "seasoning" for newcomers to the city adversely affected his health, and he was at first troubled by headaches and colds. The adjustment to a new epidemiological environment often presented health challenges to visitors of a new country. Paris winters were notoriously bone-chilling and often led to mysterious and deadly fevers. Jefferson was a frequent and welcome guest at the Adams residence in the Paris suburb of Auteuil, and Abigail Adams played a role in nursing him back to health. In December 1784, she wrote her sister Mary Cranch that "Mr. Jefferson has been sick, and confined to his house for six weeks. He is on the recovery but very weak and feeble."[46]

Jefferson would act as a mentor to both future presidents James Madison and James Monroe of Virginia, and in the spring of 1785 he wrote to Monroe, complaining of illness. "I have had a very bad winter having been confined the greatest part of it," he reported after recovering from a prolonged severe cold that stubbornly held on for several months. "The air is extremely damp, and the waters unwholesome. We have had for three weeks past a warm visit from the Sun (my almighty physician) and I find myself almost reestablished."[47] Jefferson's words reflected his belief in the strong connection between health and locale, the healing powers of nature, and his intuitive understanding that contaminated water bred disease and that sunlight could not only lift moods but sometimes help dispel contagion.

Jefferson frequently expressed his progressive views on healthy living, particularly to family members. Throughout his lifetime he certainly displayed a strong belief in the therapeutic and preventative powers of nature, particularly the benefits of physical activity, a sound diet, and herbal remedies when needed. From his residence in Paris, in 1785 Jefferson wrote a lengthy letter filled with advice to his favorite nephew, Peter Carr. He admonished Carr not to forget his health in the pursuit of education: "Give about two of them [hours] every day to exercise; for health must not be sacrificed to learning. A strong body makes the mind strong."[48] From a young age, Jefferson was a forceful advocate of exercise, which he felt provided both physical and mental benefits, a view that, as we saw, was shared by both Abigail Adams and Franklin.

While Jefferson was in Paris in 1785, he received the tragic news that his young daughter Lucy as well as his niece Lucy Eppes back in Virginia had died of whooping cough months before. In the delayed letter, his brother-in-law wrote rather bluntly:

> I am sorry to inform you that my fears about the welfare of our children, which I mentioned in my last, were too well founded. Yours, as well as our dear little Lucy, have fallen sacrifices to the most horrible of all disorders . . . they both suffered as much pain, indeed more than ever I saw two of their ages experience . . . they were beyond the reach of medicine.[49]

The death of Jefferson's young daughter reminds us of the severity of childhood illnesses of the time and how little medical treatment could be of assistance. Most people, even children, had to endure their pain stoically. Although mild opiates such as laudanum could be obtained relatively easily from a local apothecary, some were reluctant to use it, as many Protestant leaders viewed suffering as a purifying process for the soul.

News of Lucy's death was extremely painful for Jefferson, and it propelled him to send for Maria to join him in France as soon as possible. Abigail Adams's daughter Nabby recorded in her journal that "Mr. J. is a man of great sensibility and parental affection . . . this news has greatly affected him and his daughter."[50] Jefferson had long found Mrs. Adams to be a delightful acquaintance with a sympathetic, nurturing personality, and even though by then she and John Adams were stationed in England, she strongly urged Jefferson to bring Maria to his Paris household. When Maria finally sailed from Virginia to England to join Jefferson in Europe, he turned to Abigail to care for his daughter until she could be brought to Paris. Jefferson's slave, Sally Hemings, then a young teenager, accompanied Maria on the voyage and later attended Jefferson's daughters at the Catholic boarding school in which they were enrolled. It is interesting to note that in the fall of 1787 he paid a local Parisian doctor to inoculate Sally against smallpox, a procedure his immediate family members had all undergone back in Virginia.[51]

Jefferson first met John Adams in 1775 when they both served as delegates to the Continental Congress in Philadelphia, and they had renewed their acquaintance in France. The tall, slender, reticent Jefferson and the short, chubby, garrulous Adams were a stark contrast in personality and appearance, but they shared a deep commitment to the cause of liberty and the welfare of the new American republic. Jefferson and Adams worked closely together in France, and Jefferson came to admire and respect his colleague's skill and work ethic. Moreover, Jefferson and Abigail Adams discovered themselves to be kindred spirits who became friends and confidants in Europe. In France, they visited each other frequently, and the personable but frank Abigail often offered Jefferson her pithy advice. In 1785, John Adams was appointed the first American minister to England, and Abigail and Jefferson continued their friendship through the exchange of friendly letters. Political differences would later drive Jefferson and the Adamses apart, but he and John reconciled in old age (Abigail still remained decidedly distant) and carried out an affectionate, sophisticated level of correspondence that reflected not only their views concerning philosophy, education, political theory, and health but also their facility with the pen. Later John called their long years of correspondence "one of the most agreeable events in my life."[52]

Abigail was happy to watch over the attractive and precocious Maria, for whom she developed a deep and abiding affection, but at the same time urged Jefferson to reunite with his daughter as quickly as possible to restore family stability and her ideal of a close parent/child relationship. Within two weeks, Maria was fetched from London by Jefferson's servant, and although she missed the mother figure Abigail had provided, her affection for her father was rekindled. Maria was enrolled in the same French convent school that Martha attended. Jefferson's two daughters received a superior education for women by the standards of the time, and they were undoubtedly being cultivated to take a place by his side as his political career blossomed. Though Abigail thought boarding away from home an unfortunate separation of the family and a breach of fatherly responsibility, she also understood that it was necessary because of Jefferson's ministerial duties. In addition to social and parental advice, in her usual commonsense style Mrs. Adams also offered a practical remedy for Jefferson's ailments: "I have known very salutary effects produced by the use of British oil upon a spraind joint. I have sent a servant to see if I can procure some. You may rest assured that if it does no good; it will not do any injury."[53]

Jefferson not only skillfully carried out his official governmental duties in Paris but also conducted a romance (perhaps platonic) with the talented and beautiful married artist Maria Cosway. It was during one of their outings that Jefferson seriously injured his wrist, which would cause him lifelong intermittent discomfort. His daughter Martha attributed the fall to an accident that occurred on one of his daily "rambles" of seven miles or so in the countryside when "joined by a friend," but does not specifically refer to Cosway. Yet, in a letter from Cosway to Jefferson, she maintained that she was to blame for the "pains in his wrists." Certainly Cosway was very dear to the infatuated Jefferson, for in October of 1786, as she prepared to leave France, he wrote that "[m]y health is good, except my wrist, which mends slowly, and my mind, which mends not at all, but broods constantly over your departure." Whatever the extent of the affair with Cosway, everyone agrees that the wrist was poorly set by French doctors. Martha noted that the fracture was a complicated one and that Jefferson learned to write with his left hand. When he fell again a few years before his death and this time injured his left hand, he was left unable to write without pain for the rest of his life.[54]

Giving no specific details of the cause of his injury, Jefferson reported the accident to Madison and referred to "[a]n unlucky dislocation of my right wrist."[55] In a letter to Abigail Adams, then in England with her husband John, he revealed the extent of the results of the fall he had taken:

An unfortunate dislocation of my right wrist for three months deprived me of the honor of writing to you. I begin now to use my pen a little, but it is in great pain, and I have no other use of my hand. The swelling has remained obstinately the same for two months past, and the joint, tho I believe well set, does not become more flexible. I am strongly advised to go to some mineral waters at Aix in Provence, and I have it in contemplation.[56]

A few days later Jefferson wrote to Franklin, by then back in Philadelphia after years in Europe on behalf of his country. Jefferson ended his letter by apologizing for its brevity, referring to his "dislocated wrist, not yet re-established."[57] Later, Jefferson visited the hot mineral baths in Aix-en-Provence advised by Abigail Adams, for in 1787 he informed his daughter Martha that he hoped "that the mineral waters of this place might restore strength in my wrist,"[58] but he experienced little improvement.

The connection among exercise, productive activity, and health was a theme that Jefferson often touched upon. During that visit to Aix-en-Provence, Jefferson again wrote Martha, who had remained in Paris, urging her to keep to a busy and productive schedule: "Idleness begets ennui, ennui the hypochondria, and that a diseased body. No laborious person was ever yet hysterical. Exercise and application produce order in our affairs, health of body, cheerfulness of mind, and these make us precious to our friends." Similarly, in a letter to his nephew the same year, he maintained that "an attention to health . . . should take the place of every other object."[59] Jefferson, whose life experiences had graphically taught him the value of good physical health, was himself a constant whirlwind of physical and intellectual energy, and as his writings demonstrate, he also possessed keen psychological insight about mental health.

While the Jeffersons were living in Paris, Martha and Maria both contracted typhoid fever. Jefferson engaged an English physician named Dr. Gem to treat his daughters. Gem shared Jefferson's aversion to aggressive doses of laxatives and bleeding, the common treatment for typhoid at the time. As we have seen, Jefferson understood that radical heroic measures only sapped the energy of patients afflicted with illness and logically could offer little aid to the sick. Instead, he advocated letting the body heal itself through rest augmented by hydration and good nutrition. Gem took a conservative approach, and both young women recovered under a regimen that emphasized nourishing foods and frequent drinks of Madeira wine supplied by Jefferson.[60]

On the basis of Gem's success with Martha and Maria, Jefferson went on to recommend this noninvasive method of treatment for several family members and friends, which according to Jefferson achieved good results. Decades later, in 1821, Jefferson would write about the success of Gem's treatment to Madison, whose family members had contracted typhus. Recalling the illness of his daughters Jefferson wrote, "While I was in Paris, both my daughters were taken with what we formerly called a nervous fever, now a typhus, distinguished very certainly by a thread-like pulse. . . . Dr. Gem, an English physician . . . and certainly the ablest I ever met with, attended them. He never gave them a single dose of physic [medicine]." Instead, Jefferson explained, Gem "forced them to eat . . . some of the farinaceous substances of easy digestion every 2. hours and to drink a glass of Madeira." Moreover, Jefferson asserted that "I have had this fever in my family 3. or 4. times since I have lived at home and have carried between 20. and 30. Patients thro' it without losing a single one, by a rigorous observance of Dr. Gem's plan and principle."[61]

Return to America and Public Life

After five years in Paris, in 1789 Jefferson returned to the United States, just as the French Revolution was igniting. Martha's shocking announcement that she wanted to follow a vocation as a nun was a contributing factor to Jefferson's decision to return quickly to America, where the government was again evolving under the new Constitution. In December of 1789, Jefferson and his daughters arrived at Monticello, where he anticipated a peaceful retirement from public affairs. At least on a symbolic level, Monticello always appeared to be his touchstone, a refuge of comfort, and Jefferson was visibly unhappy when President Washington requested his governmental assistance. However, his return to private life was short-lived, for in 1790 he was appointed America's first secretary of state under Washington. Jefferson was forced to spend most of his time in what was then America's capital of Philadelphia, where he enrolled Maria in a boarding school.

At the same time, Jefferson was pleased with his elder daughter Martha's marriage in 1790 at the age of eighteen to Virginia planter and future politician Thomas Mann Randolph Jr. Martha went on to live a long life, and her twelve children, eleven of whom survived childhood and adolescence, brought Jefferson great joy.[62] In the light of Jefferson's many losses, he was delighted when his daughter Martha had informed him by letter of her first pregnancy soon after her marriage. Jefferson replied that the news had given him "the greatest pleasure of any I have received from you," and admonished her to take special care of her health as she approached childbirth.[63] Jefferson became a doting grandfather and great-grandfather and considered these descendants the "solace of my [old] Age."[64]

Return to public life brought a renewal of headaches, a six-week period of physical discomfort. Jefferson later related that the "severe attach of periodical headache . . . came upon me every day at Sunrise, and never left me till sunset," and was a "paroxysm of the most excruciating pain."[65] A series of chronic but less painful headaches troubled him for months beginning in late 1790 but seemed to only appear in times of stress. In the spring, Jefferson and Madison took a recreational health trip north through New York along the Hudson up to Lake George and Lake Champlain and then through New England. As Jefferson told Washington, one of his goals for the journey was to rid himself of the nagging headaches by "giving more exercise to the body and less to the mind,"[66] suggesting that Jefferson was well aware of the effects of stress on his body.

During Jefferson's tenure as secretary of state, the specter of illness hovered over Philadelphia and demonstrated that epidemics could play havoc even with government plans. Yellow fever and malaria were endemic in the American coastal cities during the summer, as the diseases were spread by mosquitoes in hot weather. As we learned in the introduction, the epidemic of 1793 took thousands of lives, and Dr. Rush's advocacy of bleeding and purging did little to stem the tide of the disease, which declined only with the advent of cold weather and the end of the "plague" of mosquitoes that had descended on the city that summer.

Not only did the yellow fever wreak devastation on humans, but it had political implications as well. At first it exacerbated friction over fiscal matters between the emerging Democratic-Republican and Federalist factions as well as bringing to the fore their divided support of the warring rivals France and Great Britain, with Jefferson and Hamilton the leaders on opposing sides. Soon the debates extended to medical issues, which were also aligned along party lines. Some of the Federalists, led by Alexander Hamilton, claimed the yellow fever was "imported" and had arrived in Philadelphia through French citizens fleeing the French Revolution via Haiti (then St. Domingo). Jeffersonian Republican/Democrats pointed to local domestic conditions as its cause. Not until a century later would Walter Reed identify a particular mosquito as the transmitter of the fever, although an initial group of infected people was needed for transmission.[67]

Jefferson contracted only a few cases of common fevers in his lifetime, wisely retiring to Monticello as often as he could during the dangerous summer months. However, he was in Philadelphia during the height of the 1793 epidemic in the early fall. As always, Jefferson took a deep interest in matters of disease and accurately described the symptoms of the epidemic as beginning "with a pain in the head, sickness in the stomach, with a slight rigor, fever, black vomiting and feces, and death from the 2nd to the 8th day."[68] During the crisis he also kept careful statistics and corresponded with several political colleagues, including Madison, whom he kept updated on the numbers who were afflicted with the disease and those fleeing the city in the hope of outrunning the plague. In early September, Jefferson reported that

[a] malignant fever has been generated in the filth of Water street which gives great alarm. About 70. people had died of it two days ago, and as many more were ill of it. It has now got in to most parts of the city and is considered infectious. . . . Every body who can, is flying from the city, and the panic of the country people is likely to add famine to the disease.[69]

Jefferson was a keen observer and well informed about medical practice. A week later he reported, "The yellow fever increases . . . and it is the opinion of the physicians there is no way of stopping it. . . . [N]o two agree in any one part of their process of cure." Jefferson's pithy summing up of the situation reflected the helplessness of contemporary medicine to deal with the outbreak as well as Jefferson's frequently displayed skepticism about the skills and knowledge of doctors. Jefferson also used the situation to attack his political nemesis Alexander Hamilton as a "timid" coward for claiming to have contracted yellow fever, which Jefferson initially believed to be only a typical "autumnal fever."[70] However, Jefferson later agreed that Hamilton had been a victim of the epidemic and admitted that he himself would have liked to flee Philadelphia as "[t]here is rational danger . . . [but] I do not like to exhibit the appearance of panic."[71]

Another letter written by Jefferson to a member of Congress allows us a first-hand report on the health crisis and how it affected government officials. In September many offices and all the banks shut down, and Jefferson was left with only one clerk. "An infection and mortal fever is broke out in this place," Jefferson reported.

> The deaths under it, the week before last, were about forty; the last week fifty. This week they will probably be about two hundred, and it is increasing. Every one is getting out of the city who can. The President . . . set out for Mount Vernon . . . I shall go in a few days to Virginia. When we shall reassemble again may, perhaps, depend on the course of this malady.[72]

Jefferson stayed in Philadelphia longer than Washington and other cabinet members, leaving in mid-September for Monticello, although still a week earlier than he initially planned. He was accompanied by Maria, propelled by realistic fear of the disease. After a hard frost and the arrival of cold weather in November, Jefferson was able to report with relief to his daughter Martha that "the fever in Philadelphia has almost entirely disappeared."[73] He also informed Madison that "[t]he Physicians say they have no new subjects since the rains. Some old ones are still to recover or die, and it is presumed that will close the tragedy. The inhabitants, refugees, are now flocking back generally."[74]

It is interesting to note that although eighteenth-century medical wisdom generally attributed yellow fever to "malignant" air and lacked any knowledge of its viral origin, Jefferson seems to have understood that lack of sanitation and crowded conditions played at least some role in spreading many diseases. Years later, in 1804, Jefferson would acknowledge to his close friend John Page that he had first considered yellow fever simply an infection brought to America by passengers on incoming ships, but he later came to believe it was endemic and "generated near the water side, in close built cities, under warm climates,"[75] thus arriving at a closer, albeit incomplete, understanding of the origins of the sickness than most physicians of the era. By 1805, after studying local conditions closely, Jefferson concluded to a friend in France that yellow fever was "an endemic, not a contagious disease,"[76] and he was correct in that it was not passed from person to person, although an epidemic did require an infected pool of humans as an initial factor.

With the graphic experience of the 1793 yellow fever epidemic imprinted in his mind, the disease would continue to receive Jefferson's attention after he assumed the presidency. In September 1800, Jefferson wrote a letter to Dr. Rush indicating that the scourge of yellow fever was a threat that he took seriously. After congratulating Rush on "the [current] healthiness of your city [Philadelphia]," he noted that the cities of Norfolk, Baltimore, and Providence were not so lucky and "that we are not clear of our new scourge." Jefferson, the champion of a vision of a bucolic American agrarianism, disliked large urban centers as a potential threat to republican ideals and as hotbeds of disease. Conversely, he viewed airy, open, rural country locations as being most favorable to good health. He was not alone among the founders in his concerns, for as early as the 1750s Franklin had express his own worries about the future of American cities with increasingly dense populations. Although Jefferson sincerely mourned the death of yellow fever victims, he stated that there was for him at least one positive outcome of the epidemic: "The yellow fever will discourage the growth of great cities in our nation, and I view great cities as pestilential to the morals, the health, and the liberties of man."[77] However, even Jefferson realized that urbanization was inevitable, and in an effort to improve public health, he would later offer advice for "building our cities on a more open plan" to avoid the spread of disease through crowded conditions and poor sanitation.[78]

After Jefferson's retirement as secretary of state and what he referred to as the "hated occupation of politics,"[79] at the close of 1793, he returned to Monticello and began a major remodeling project that lasted a decade. Jefferson did not return to active public life until he arrived in Philadelphia in February 1797 as the nation's vice-president elect with John Adams as the Federalist president. To view Jefferson as a politician and statesman is to see only one aspect of his multifaceted life. In addition to all his other many accomplishments, Jefferson was an architect who not only designed his own renowned home at Monticello, but later many of the beautiful classical buildings at the University of Virginia, of which he was a primary founder. At Monticello, he also invented or perfected numerous implements for the estate, such as a more efficient plow, dumbwaiters, and a prototype copy machine. The "polygraph" was used to make copies of his letters, of which he wrote more than eighteen thousand in his lifetime. Jefferson, a gifted Renaissance man, was always engaged in learning. His wide breadth of knowledge, including knowledge of medicine, and his varied accomplishments are astounding.

Time and time again, his beloved plantation would serve as Jefferson's solace from the vicissitudes of personal and public life, even though remodeling Monticello played havoc with his finances. He especially loved his garden, where he grew over ninety plants, including the medicinal herbs he advocated for the prevention of illness as well as healing. Many were those that were used widely for self-medication by early Americans and often also prescribed by physicians and other health practitioners. Jefferson's garden included marjoram, said to be helpful in treating cold symptoms, senna, rhubarb, and tansy, used as mild laxatives, and lavender, sage, mint, and thyme, efficacious in easing headaches, toothaches, and upset stomachs. Jefferson became an expert on the use of medicinal plants, and his library included numerous medical tracts and pharmacopeias, which he consulted to treat his own ailments as well as those of his family and slaves. Jefferson also resorted to patent medicines supplied from an apothecary from time to time and is thought to have occasionally used bark for fevers, mercury and sulphur-based ointments for rashes, and laudanum in his later years to help him sleep and control intestinal disorders.[80]

In late-eighteenth-century Virginia, Jefferson was recognized as the most outstanding scientist in the state during his lifetime.[81] As an enthusiastic student of botany, in his *Notes on Virginia* Jefferson recorded nearly two dozen native medicinal plants, and he also reported on local "Medicinal Springs," some of which were known to "relieve rheumatisms." The *Notes* were primarily composed while Jefferson was confined to his home as a result of a horseback-riding accident in 1782. Jefferson's book also reveals that he had an intuitive and advanced understanding of contagion, and he bemoaned the fact that in many hospitals "the sick, the dying and the dead are crammed together in the same rooms, and often in the same beds."[82]

All was not idyllic during Jefferson's three-year respite from public life, however, as his normally robust health was assaulted by a number of problems. His monetary challenges undoubtedly depressed him, and he would die owing the equivalent of what would be a million dollars today. In severe financial straits and eager to improve his estate, Jefferson commenced a regimen of manual labor that resulted in an injury to his back. In September of 1794, he wrote that he was "in bed under a paroxysm of the rheumatism, which has now kept me for ten days in constant torment, and presents no hope of abatement," and in response to a request from Washington to resume his former post, he firmly replied that "[n]o circumstances . . . will ever more tempt me to engage in anything public."[83] The following month Jefferson was still unable to resume his normal athletic activities, and he wrote Madison that "[t]he day you left me I had a violent attack of the Rheumatism which has confined me ever since. Within these few days I have crept out a little on horseback, but am yet far from being well, or likely to be soon."[84]

The rheumatism passed, probably healed by time, rest, and some herbal remedies sent to him by Dr. Rush. The episode had perhaps given him pause about his usually sound health. The following spring of 1795, he confided to Madison that he would not even consider returning to Washington's cabinet, as "[m]y health is entirely broken down within the last eight months; my age requires that I should place my affairs in a clear state."[85] Just a few months later, during the summer, Maria Jefferson and two of Jefferson's sisters became sick with an undisclosed passing illness and Jefferson was moved to write his daughter despondently that Monticello "has been a mere hospital."[86] Another family tragedy buffeted Jefferson in late August 1795, when Martha Jefferson Randolph's infant baby daughter died within a few days of birth, and Jefferson had the child buried in the family plot at Monticello.

Although Jefferson was only fifty-two at the time, he apparently used his state of health as a convenient excuse since he did eventually return to political affairs and lived to a considerable old age. At the same time, it is clear that Jefferson was in a morose state, alleviated only in part by his Monticello remodeling project. That he felt ill and old during this period is reflected in a letter he wrote in April 1796 to an old friend: "I begin to feel the effects of age. My health has suddenly broken down, with symptoms which give me to believe I shall not have much to encounter of the *tedium vitae*."[87]

However, Jefferson would later recover his optimistic outlook and vigor and resume an active political role as well as the life of a country gentleman surrounded by family. In 1797, Jefferson's old revolutionary comrade John Adams would take office as the second American president, with Jefferson assuming the office of vice president. Because of his many losses, Jefferson's two remaining daughters were especially dear to him, and although he was increasingly involved in politics, their health and happiness were clearly paramount to him. As he wrote in a letter to Maria in the spring of 1797, "I wish to hear that you and your sister continue in health; it is a circumstance on which the happiness of my life depends," Jefferson declared.[88]

Despite his new responsibilities, Jefferson continued to keep his finger on the pulse of his family's health. In April 1797, he wrote his daughter Martha that "I entirely approve of your resolution to have the children inoculated [against smallpox]."[89] In the summer of 1798, at Monticello on a break from his vice-presidential duties, he enjoyed playing babysitter to his granddaughter and wrote Martha that "Ellen appeared feverish the evening you went away; but visiting her a little before I went to bed, I found her quite clear of fever, and was convinced the quickness of pulse which had alarmed me had proceeded from her having been in uncommon spirits and constantly running about."[90]

As Jefferson enjoyed the fruits of his domestic life at Monticello, back in the nation's capital, American political life became more divisive. As we have seen in the previous chapter, during their terms as vice president and president, Jefferson and Adams grew further apart in their political outlooks and ultimately became rivals for the leadership of the nation. For Jefferson the vitality of the new nation depended on strong states' rights and a robust agrarian republic while Adams pushed for a stronger federal position that encouraged urban and commercial growth.

Prior to the presidential election of 1801, Jefferson and Adams had already become bitter enemies with sharply differing views on America's future. In response to the notorious Alien and Sedition Act passed during Adams's term, Jefferson and Madison had written stinging resolutions adopted by Virginia and Kentucky denouncing the legislation as an unacceptable curtailment of freedom of expression, fueling the antagonism between the men. After a prolonged and hotly contested presidential campaign, which pitted the Republican candidate Jefferson against Federalist John Adams, on February 17, 1801, Thomas Jefferson was elected the third president of the United States on the thirty-sixth ballot. He became the first American president to be inaugurated in the new capital of Washington, D.C. As we will see in the next chapter, as president, not only would Jefferson help shape America's political and economic path, but as a leading proponent of scientific and preventative medicine he would also make important contributions to the nation's public health.

5

Thomas Jefferson

The Health of the Nation

I think it important . . . to bring the practice of the [smallpox] inoculation to the level of common capacities; for to give to this discovery the whole of value, we should enable the great mass of the people to practice it on their own families & and without an expense, which they cannot meet.

—*Thomas Jefferson to Dr. John R. Coxe, April 30, 1802*

Having been among the early converts, in this part of the globe, to its [Jenner smallpox vaccination's] efficacy, I took an early part in recommending it to my countrymen. I avail myself of this occasion of rendering you my portion of the tribute of gratitude due to you from the whole human family. Medicine has never before produced any single improvement of such utility. . . . You have erased from the calendar of human afflictions one of its greatest. . . . Future nations will know by history only that the loathsome small-pox has existed and by you has been extirpated.

—*Thomas Jefferson to Dr. Edward Jenner, May 14, 1806*

As president, Thomas Jefferson used his considerable influence to advance American medicine, most notably in his unwavering support of the Jenner method of smallpox vaccination and his insistence that the Lewis and Clark expedition gather information about Indian diseases and treatments as part of its mission. His republican philosophy had long influenced his underlying belief that the health of individuals and the overall health of the nation were interconnected and that a democratic republic was the form of government best suited to physical and mental well-being. Jefferson's most celebrated accomplishment during his first term was the Louisiana Purchase, which doubled the size of the United States. Jefferson's vision of westward expansion was tied to his belief that an abundance of open land was necessary for the vitality of a republic. He especially encouraged settlement of new areas that were not subject to the "unhealthy" factors that characterized America's eastern coastal cities, where epidemics flared in the hot, humid summers. By the early nineteenth century the search for a "salubrious" locale was a significant factor in the decision of where one settled in America. The geography of health became a metaphor that extended beyond the human body and connected to political and economic "health" and the advancement of the nation.[1]

Jefferson often declared that Albemarle County, Virginia, the site of his boyhood home at Shadwell as well as his later plantation at Monticello, was the "healthiest" place in the country. At the first sign of summer heat after he assumed the presidency, Jefferson left the unwholesome environment of Washington for a two-month break at Monticello and informed his secretary of the treasury, Albert Gallatin, "I consider it as a trying experiment for a person from the mountains to pass the two bilious months [when malaria and other fevers were at their height] on the tide-water. I have not done it these forty-two years, and nothing should induce me to do it now."[2]

Jefferson's Medical Outlook

As we saw in the previous chapter, Jefferson's strong views concerning health and his evolving medical philosophy had been profoundly influenced by the French physician Cabanis. Jefferson believed that the practice of medicine should be founded on established fact and decried the theoretical speculation that was common among American physicians at the time. Long after he left France, Jefferson kept abreast of Cabanis's work, which he admired. In 1805 he wrote a French acquaintance that "I am glad to hear that M. Cabanis is engaged in writing on

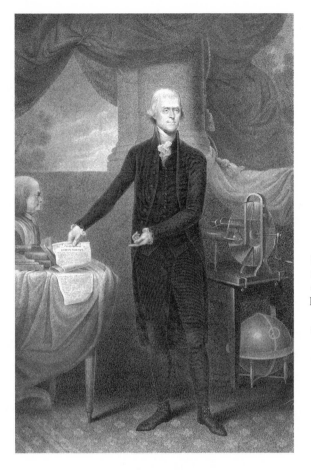

Engraving of Thomas
Jefferson, President of
the United States, c.
1801, from a painting
by Rembrandt Peale.
Jefferson is depicted
holding a copy of the
Declaration of Inde-
pendence, but a world
globe, one of Jefferson's
mechanical inventions,
and a bust of Jefferson's
hero Benjamin Franklin
also appear in the pic-
ture. (Courtesy Library
of Congress)

the reformation of medicine. It needs the hands of a reformer, and cannot be in better hands than his."³

A few years later, within weeks of reading two new works by Cabanis, Jefferson was again moved to criticize doctors who followed
"fanciful theory" and the "adventurous physician who substitutes
presumption for knowledge." Jefferson scoffed at doctors who practiced medicine simply on the basis of theoretical texts or scientifically
unproven treatments, like radical bleeding and purging, that had been
handed down for centuries instead of examining treatment outcomes
on the basis of documented scientific observation. As we will see later
in this chapter, he especially believed in a "hands-on" educational

approach for training doctors, which he would work to implement at the University of Virginia.

In that oft-quoted letter written in 1807 to Dr. Caspar Wistar, a professor of anatomy at the University of Pennsylvania, Jefferson maintained,

> The only sure foundations of medicine are, an intimate knowledge of the human body, and observation on the effects of medicinal substances on that. The anatomical & clinical schools, therefore, are those in which the young physician should be formed. If he enters with innocence that of the theory of medicine, it is scarcely possible that he should come out untainted with error.

In the famous missive, Jefferson, once again, emphasized his faith in the healing power of nature and opined that physicians should only prescribe medicine for the few well-recognized illnesses that had been proven to respond to specific remedies, concluding sardonically that "[t]he patient, treated on the fashionable theory, sometimes gets well in spite of the medicine."[4]

Jefferson as Smallpox Vaccination Advocate

One of the most significant but often overlooked achievements during Jefferson's presidency was his dedicated support of public health, which had its roots in his early work in Virginia as a plantation owner and politician and his deep concern for the physical well-being of all Americans. As was the case with many of his ideas concerning sickness and health, Jefferson was ahead of his time in his grasp of medical subjects, and he speedily embraced the revolutionary scientific advancement of smallpox vaccination over the more risky inoculation procedure. As we learned in the introduction, smallpox continued to be a serious threat throughout the world in the late eighteenth century, and in 1798, Dr. Edward Jenner, a country doctor in England, introduced the more effective procedure of vaccination with cowpox. Inoculation with live human "matter" [virus] had been outlawed in many American colonies because it was generally still believed that its potential dangers outweighed the benefits. Yet, the American medical community remained largely opposed to the introduction of the safer cowpox method as well.

Dr. Benjamin Waterhouse, another American graduate of the University of Edinburgh then living in Boston, where he served as a professor at Harvard Medical School in Cambridge, studied the subject closely. Even in the face of skepticism and outright opposition, Waterhouse became a vocal advocate for vaccination, experimenting first on his own children in 1800.[5] Gradually, variolation gave way to vaccination (the term taken from the Latin word for cow), but as late as the turn of the nineteenth century anti-vaccinationism surfaced in the face of the call for compulsory inoculation during the smallpox epidemic of 1898-1903.[6] Even today, despite scientific proof to the contrary, some parents are still expressing concern about vaccination for their children for a variety of diseases because they worry that the procedure contributes to other conditions, such as autism.

Aware of Jefferson's keen interest in preventative medicine and public welfare, in late 1800 Waterhouse sent him published material about the new method, hoping to win Jefferson as an ally. Vaccination carried the added benefit that those undergoing the procedure could not infect others. Jefferson was eager to try the Jenner method, and he was determined to use his political powers for the sake of the health of the nation. He had already been following updates about vaccination, and he agreed to help Waterhouse encourage physicians in the American South to introduce it by providing them with written information as well as the actual vaccine.

However, the availability of cowpox was limited, and transporting lymph was challenging, particularly in hot climates like that of the South. Waterhouse generally shipped the vaccine using the common combination of glass and threads, but the first several times he sent it to Jefferson the lymph lost its effectiveness before it could be utilized. Jefferson worked with Waterhouse to have samples sent to Reverend Dr. Edward Gantt, the chaplain of Congress in Washington, and ultimately Jefferson used his ingenious mind to design a new container. To increase the chance of preserving its potency, the creative Jefferson advised Waterhouse to send the vaccine in a small phial inserted into a larger one to minimize contact with air and heat.[7] In a letter to Martha, he informed her, "I shall probably be able to carry on some infectious matter with a view of trying whether we can introduce it here [in Virginia]."[8] Eventually threads, glass plates, and lancets were replaced with the more effective method of gathering fresh lymph by arm-to-arm transmission at "vaccine institutes,"[9] but manufacture of the smallpox vaccine as a business did not begin in the United States until the 1870s.[10]

The Jefferson family physician, Dr. William Wardlaw, became the first Virginia doctor to use Jenner's method, but because of Wardlaw's busy schedule, Jefferson and his sons-in-law, Thomas Mann Randolph and John Wayles Eppes, took the project into their own hands and became temporary medical practitioners. Jefferson had been very pleased when his younger daughter, Maria, married Eppes in 1797, and enthused in a letter to Martha that "[s]he could not have been more so to my wishes if I had had the whole earth free to have chosen a partner for her."[11]

For many years Jefferson was especially close to Martha's husband, a charismatic, well-educated, capable Virginian who also rose in politics and served as governor of Virginia. But Thomas Randolph later teetered on the edge of financial disaster and suffered from alcoholism and bouts with mental illness, which pained the family and often made Martha's marriage a troubled one. Still, she appears to have always been a level-headed, cheerful woman who ran her household with great capability. The education and attentive guidance Jefferson had lavished upon her helped shape his older daughter into a charming hostess and cultured conversationalist, and as he aged Jefferson continued to rely on Martha to assist him and provide emotional support.

At Jefferson's insistence, both his daughters visited him twice for extended stays in Washington during his presidency, providing him with the tangible sense of family so essential to his well-being. Martha presented Jefferson with his first grandchild in 1791, and he remained an engaged grandfather to Anne Cary, as the baby was named, and all his other grandchildren. Given Jefferson's emphasis on the healing powers of nature, it is not surprising that late in her pregnancy he sent Martha a medical book that contained advice on the health advantages of breastfeeding for mother and child and cautioned against administering "physic" (medicines) to infants.[12] As the mother of twelve children Martha certainly encountered the prevalent illnesses that were typical at the time in the South. In the winter of 1798, she wrote Jefferson, who was in Philadelphia, that "[p]leurisies, rheumatism and every disorder proceeding from cold have been so frequent that we have scarcely at any one time anyone *well* enough to tend the sick."[13]

When he visited Monticello in the summer of 1801, Jefferson vaccinated his entire household, which included family members and slaves, all of whom experienced minimal negative reactions. In August, Jefferson wrote Madison that "I yesterday performed 6. More inoculations from matter received from Boston and some from England via Boston."[14] In his role of medical practitioner, the new president also kept careful statistics of "his cases." Once he returned to Washington, D.C., he described the undertaking in a letter to Dr. John Coxe of Philadelphia: "In the course of July and August, I inoculated about seventy or eighty of my own family; my sons in law about as many in theirs, and including our neighbors who wished to avail themselves of the opportunity, our whole experiment extended to about two hundred persons."[15]

Jefferson did not stop with his own plantation household, but made a conscious effort to spread the use of vaccination for smallpox across the country. Jefferson was keenly aware of the promise of great public health benefits from the Jenner method and indicated his goal of making it available free of charge to the "masses," who might otherwise not be able to afford the life-saving procedure. In a letter to Waterhouse in July 1801 Jefferson observed, "It will be a great service indeed rendered to human nature to strike off from the catalogue of its evils so great a one as the small pox. I know of no one discovery in medicine equally valuable."[16]

Working in tandem with Waterhouse, Jefferson was able to ensure that the smallpox vaccine was made available throughout the United States by the first years of the nineteenth century. Waterhouse praised Jefferson's efforts, maintaining that they forwarded "the practice of vaccination . . . at least two years."[17] In turn, Jefferson noted that during the Revolutionary War, ten thousand soldiers had died from smallpox and that he considered "not merely the Army, but the whole people of the United States under obligation to him [Waterhouse] for saving an immense number of lives."[18] Later, in 1808, Jefferson would appoint Waterhouse to the Marine Hospital Service, in recognition of his pivotal role in introducing the vaccine to military personnel as well as everyday citizens. As we learned in the introduction, the Marine Hospital Service had been signed into law by President Adams in 1798, while Jefferson served as vice president, and it eventually evolved into the national public health service.

Jefferson did not remark on his own pivotal role in the process, but one early medical historian maintained that "Thomas Jefferson was not

KINE POCK INOCULATION.

Rules to be attended to during the Vaccination.

1. THE diet to be the same as before vaccination.
2. Scratching or rubbing the arm, or shoving up the sleeve should be avoided as much as possible.
3. In case an itching sensation of the vaccinated part should give the patient uneasiness, a little vinegar applied to the part will give immediate relief.
4 No matter to be transferred from the person inoculated to another person. Taking it from another often becomes a snare to individuals, and the source of spurious matter. But even those, who by chance have had the genuine disease in that way, have no certainty of it—and who would wish to have it upon uncertainties ?
5. Women, who do house work, should avoid washing and baking on the 7th and 8th days, the usual time for the symptoms.
6. No danger of washing the hands and face in cold water during the disease.
7. Women may without hesitation receive the Kine Pock in all circumstances without exception, at home or travelling by land or water.
8. No danger of vaccinating children at the period of teething.
9. Labouring men and mechanics need not abstain from their customary employment, provided their indisposition does not require it.
10. Children should never be lifted by the arms,* especially when under the inoculation. The arm should not be bound up, nor confined in tight sleeves.

OBSERVATIONS.

1. It occasions no other disease. On the contrary, it has often been known to improve health ; and to remedy those diseases, under which the patient before laboured.
2. It leaves behind no blemish, but a *blessing ;*—one of the greatest ever bestowed on man ;—*a perfect security against the future infection of the small-pox.*
N. B. Save the scab for examination.   B. WATERHOUSE.

* No prudent person, who is aware of the tenderness of the bone of a young child, would ever lift one by its arms, or lead a child a mile by one arm.

Cambridge, July 3, 1809.

Instructions for Kine [Cow] Pock [Smallpox] Inoculation Issued by Dr. Benjamin Waterhouse, 1809. (Courtesy of the U.S. National Library of Medicine) only a patron and student of vaccination but an active practical disciple of Jenner and the direct introducer of vaccination into Virginia, Pennsylvania and the whole south. . . . Waterhouse and Jefferson were the two men to whom the introduction of vaccination in America was wholly due."[19] Certainly Jefferson developed a high level of medical expertise about vaccination, and Dr. Samuel L. Mitchell, a contemporary observer, related that President Jefferson was able to discuss the Jenner cowpox method "with the intelligence of a physician."[20]

Another example of Jefferson's commitment to preventative medicine and enlarging general medical knowledge occurred when Lewis and Clark began their famous expedition up the Missouri to their ultimate destination of the Pacific Ocean. In preparation for the trip, Jefferson asked Dr. Rush and Dr. Wistar, among others, to help him prepare a group of questions the explorers might research on their journey. The final list was compiled and supplemented by Jefferson and included queries about Indian health practices and the incidence of particular diseases, including bilious fevers and smallpox and their treatment.[21] Jefferson also specifically instructed Captain Meriwether Lewis, his former Virginia neighbor and personal secretary, to "[c]arry with you some matter of the kinepox [cowpox]; inform those of them with whom you may be [American Indians], of its efficacy as a preservative from the smallpox: & instruct & encourage them in the use of it. This may be especially done wherever you winter."[22]

Lewis's mother, Lucy Meriwether Lewis Marks, was a local Virginia medicinal herbalist of some note, two of his brothers became physicians, and as an army officer Lewis was responsible for the health of his men, so he already had some familiarity with medical issues. In addition, Jefferson paid for Lewis to be tutored in botany, zoology, and medicine in Philadelphia in preparation for the expedition. Moreover, Jefferson provided the explorers with a box of contemporary medications, including six hundred of Rush's famous pills, powerful cathartics composed of calomel and jalap, and instructions for medical treatment for a host of common ailments.[23] Constipation, dysentery, and venereal disease proved to be the most common problems for the exploration party, and Rush's potent pills and mercury for syphilis were the medications most frequently employed. Lewis also administered bleeding and bark for malaria, and offered wine, thought to be invigorating, and herb-based tonics and remedies from time to time.[24]

Over the years, Jefferson continued his interest in eradicating smallpox and became quite knowledgeable about the intricacies of vaccination. When Jefferson's daughter Martha wrote that she was worried about a local outbreak of smallpox and begged Jefferson for "matter" for her younger children, who had not yet been vaccinated, he sent her a "scab of vaccine" with detailed instructions on how to use a lancet to perform the procedure on her children.[25] Jefferson's lifelong commitment to the public good stemmed, in part, from his underlying "belief in the intelligence of the common man," as Joseph Ellis has put it.[26] If Americans could be educated about the increased effectiveness and safety of the Jenner vaccine, Jefferson felt most would take advantage of it to protect themselves and their families, ultimately strengthening the vitality of the nation. Over the next years smallpox vaccination gained increasing acceptance over inoculation, and states began to pass laws encouraging the procedure and often provided free services through local boards of health.

The Health of Jefferson and His Family during His Presidency

During his first term as president, in April of 1804 Jefferson suffered the loss of his beloved daughter Maria at the age of twenty-five due to complications following childbirth, graphically demonstrating the high rate of child and maternal mortality at the time and the devastation it frequently wrought on early American families. From childhood Maria had had a long history of serious ailments, and her health had frequently given Jefferson cause for concern. She had apparently inherited her mother's frail constitution, and as an adult was subject to fevers and especially the challenges of pregnancy and childbirth. Less than a year after her marriage, Maria apparently contracted malaria, and Jefferson wrote at the time that he was relieved to hear she was on the mend. His concern was palpable, and he assured her that "I would have gone to you instantly on the receipt of Mr. Eppes's letter, had not that assured me you were well enough to take the bark [quinine]."[27]

When Jefferson received news that Maria had given birth to a daughter in late 1799 he was ecstatic, if understandably worried. "I become daily more anxious to hear from you," he pleaded, "and to know that you continue well, your present state being one which is most interesting to a parent. . . . Take care of yourself, my dear Maria, for my sake, and cherish your affections for me, as my happiness rests solely in you and on that of your sister's and your dear connections."[28] Jefferson's anxiety was not unfounded because the baby died soon after birth. Just a few weeks later he sent his daughter a note of condolence that demonstrated his psychological sensitivity and that his own past experiences had taught him that the passage of grief was indeed an extremely difficult path to navigate. "How deeply I feel it [the death of the baby] in all its bearings. I shall not say—nor attempt consolation when I know that time and silence are the only medicines." Jefferson would offer similar solace to Abigail Adams years later when her adult daughter died of cancer in her forties. Jefferson ended the letter to Maria with assurance of his affection for her, noting, "I have felt perpetual gratitude to Heaven for having given me in you a source of so much pure and unmixed happiness."[29]

Over the next few months Maria received frequent letters from her father expressing his relief at her continuing recovery from a difficult childbirth. Yet, Maria remained sickly after the death of her daughter, worn down by breast infections and back pains related to yet another miscarriage.[30] Her family certainly rejoiced when in September 1801, she gave birth to her son Francis Eppes, her only surviving child. However, Francis was frail from birth and probably suffered from epilepsy, as Martha had noted symptoms, including convulsions and "foaming at the mouth and the drawing back of the head," to her father as early as January 1804, when Francis was only two and a half years old.[31] Certainly there was no effective medical treatment for epilepsy at the time, and to compound matters, it was considered a shameful disease that parents took pains to hide.

The health of his daughters and grandchildren continued to concern Jefferson over the next years. In the summer of 1801, both Martha and Maria were pregnant and moved into Monticello in anticipation of giving birth. Jefferson joined them, arriving from Washington for a much-needed vacation. That year, Jefferson had suffered from severe bouts of diarrhea, which he kept hidden from his family, and "cured" himself through horseback riding. Certainly the strain of his presidential duties and family worries contributed to his stomach ailments. Whether Jefferson experienced much relaxation at Monticello is doubtful, however, as the renovation work at Monticello, coupled with the birth of two new grandchildren, made life frenetic.

Of even more serious concern was a whooping cough epidemic that infected the children of the household in the fall. Two of Martha's daughters, Ellen and Cornelia, became delirious with illness, and Maria watched fearfully over her frail new son, Francis, who also sickened. In a letter to Jefferson, Martha captured the underlying anxiety that pervaded the minds and hearts of parents during the era, for contemporary medicine offered little effective treatment for rampant childhood illnesses. Martha must have recalled that her young sister, Lucy Elizabeth Jefferson, and her first cousin had died as a result of whooping cough many years before and that Maria had been seriously ill with the disease at the same time. Martha's husband, Randolph, appears to have been almost paralyzed with worry, and she poured out her heart to her father: "My God what a moment for a Parent . . . I had to act in the double capacity of nurse to my children and comforter to their Father."[32] Fortunately, all three children recovered.

In early 1802, Jefferson was relieved to hear from Eppes that "Maria was entirely reestablished in her health, and her breast quite well. The little boy too was well and healthy."[33] When Jefferson received word in June that Maria's precarious health was once again uncertain, he expressed his firm agreement with her plan to visit Monticello and then return to her own family home at Eppington, where he believed the healthy air would speed her convalescence. He also took the time to warn her about an outbreak of measles in Martha's family, and instructed her not to visit her sister. Jefferson's considerable medical knowledge made him alert to the fact that measles was "communicable before a person knows they have it." He assured Maria that he would make sure none of the Monticello plantation children would be allowed in the main house during her visit in case they harbored any hidden illness. Moreover, Jefferson advised Maria not to visit any homes during her journey without ascertaining whether measles were present because the illness had assumed near-epidemic proportions. "The disease is now universal throughout the State, and all the States," Jefferson warned.[34]

The severity of measles outbreaks during the era was uneven and affected young adult parents who had not already acquired immunity, as well as children. In 1713, the illness claimed over one hundred lives.[35]

But as Dr. Waterhouse noted in 1783, in some seasons measles outbreaks were very "malignant," at other times "mild." However, he appears to have understood that at times contracting measles weakened a person's immune system, making one more susceptible to other serious diseases like influenza and diphtheria, which together might lead to fatalities.[36]

Both Martha and Maria's husbands were elected to Congress in 1802 and spent time with Jefferson in the President's House in Washington, but his daughters generally remained behind in Virginia with their children. During his presidency, Jefferson commuted back and forth between Monticello and Washington when his schedule permitted. In October 1802, for example, Jefferson reported that his four-day journey was uneventful, but that on arrival he was "much indisposed with a general soreness all over, a ringing in the head, and deafness," which he attributed to traveling in the fog. Jefferson usually made the trips in a one-horse phaeton carriage, and despite his hectic schedule and presidential obligations, he tried to safeguard his health by daily exercise, usually spending two hours on horseback every afternoon.[37]

Jefferson's emphasis on exercising in the fresh air and his underlying strong constitution contributed to his general overall good health. In 1803, he informed a friend that "I retain myself very perfect health, having not had twenty hours of fever in forty-two years past. I have sometimes troublesome headache and some slight rheumatic pains; but now sixty years old nearly, I have had as little to complain of in point of health as most people."[38] He seems to have minimized the troublesome diarrhea that began to affect him after assuming office. Jefferson's biographer Dumas Malone suggests he was close-mouthed about the affliction because he may have felt it was unseemly for others to know such intimate information about the health of a president. He did consult Dr. Rush, however, who over a period of years conservatively suggested changes in diet, rest, and medications such as laudanum and herbal aids such as mint tea. It is unknown whether Jefferson actually availed himself of the medicines, but he did record the prescriptions. If Jefferson disagreed with Rush over the subject of bloodletting, he apparently respected some of his less invasive medical opinions in other areas.[39]

Jefferson's stomach ailments appear to have been intermittent and controllable. However, headaches still continued to plague him, exacerbated no doubt by the stresses of the presidency. In 1808, the last year of his second term, Jefferson wrote from Washington to his granddaughter Cornelia Randolph that he was in the tenth day of his "periodical" headaches and that they were at last moderating and were now "scarcely sensible."[40] The headaches that had troubled him for decades apparently ceased after Jefferson left office, indicating their close connection with tension.

In January of 1804, Jefferson's older sister Mary Bolling died, and he was at the same time worried about the health of Maria, who was pregnant again. When Maria gave birth in early 1804, Jefferson was relieved to hear that his younger daughter was recovering, but the good news was short-lived. When he learned that Maria had contracted a fever, he wrote her that "[n]othing but the impossibility of Congress preceding a single step in my absence presents an insuperable bar [from my joining you]," and advised her husband, John Eppes, to encourage Maria to pursue a diet of good wine and food, which he recommended for curing her illness.[41] Maria was too weak to nurse her baby, and the duty was taken on by her resilient sister, Martha, who was at the time nursing her own baby daughter. Slaves transported Maria by stretcher from the Eppes estate to Monticello so she could die in her own childhood home. In early April, Jefferson rushed to her bedside as soon as he could break away from his duties in Washington and found Maria battling nausea, a low-grade fever, and a raging breast abscess. Jefferson wrote to Madison that she was "[s]o weak as barely able to stand." The following week Maria exhibited "little change. No new imposthume has come on, but she rather weakens," and just two days later Jefferson despondently informed Madison, "I can say nothing favorable of my daughter's situation."[42]

Without the presence of antibiotics, infections and puerperal fevers associated with childbirth were often fatal at the time. Martha attended her sister dutifully, but on April 17, 1804, Maria passed away. Jefferson's diary recorded the event starkly and simply: "This morning between eight and nine o'clock my dear daughter Maria Eppes died."[43] Maria's daughter, named Martha after her grandmother, died a few years later at the age of three.

Jefferson was devastated with grief at the loss of his beloved delicate daughter. Heartbroken, he pessimistically wrote his old friend Governor John Page, "Having lost even the half of all I had, my evening prospects now hang on the slender thread of a single life [Martha]. Perhaps I may be destined to see even this last chord of parental affection broken."[44]

With the death of the fifth of Jefferson's six children, only his eldest child, the lively and intelligent Martha Randolph, survived, although he lived to enjoy many grandchildren and great-grandchildren in his old age. Dolley Madison, who had experienced a similar degree of personal loss, noted Jefferson's daughter's death with great sadness: "This is among the many proofs, my dear sister, of the uncertainly of life! A girl [Maria] so young, so lovely—all the efforts of her Father [Jefferson], doctors and friends availed nothing."[45]

Despite the personal tragedy, Jefferson carried on his presidential duties during a second term in which foreign affairs became a priority as his administration tried to maintain the nation's neutral stance in negotiating with France, England, and Spain. Secretary of State Madison became crucial to Jefferson, but many of their policies had to be developed through correspondence as for several critical months Madison was preoccupied with his wife Dolley's severe knee abscess, which had confined her to bed. When her condition did not improve in Washington, Madison accompanied Dolley to Philadelphia, where the "tumor," as it was referred to, was treated successfully by the aptly named, prominent physician Dr. Phillip Physick. The correspondence between Jefferson and Madison during the summer and fall of 1805 contain many references to her illness interwoven with national issues. Written from Monticello, Jefferson's letter to Madison in July of 1805 expressed his concern that Dolley's illness required the couple to remain in Washington instead of traveling to Montpelier as was their custom. "I sincerely regret that Mrs. Madison's situation confines her and yourself so long at Washington," Jefferson sympathized. Expressing his long-held belief about the efficacy of the Virginia climate that was the site of both their plantations, the president concluded that it was unsafe for both of the Madisons to remain in Washington.[46]

Perhaps to assuage his anxiety about his only remaining offspring, Jefferson brought Martha (then seven months pregnant), her husband, Congressman Randolph, and their six children to join him at the White House for a long stay of many months. Martha safely gave birth to a son in the presidential mansion in the beginning of 1806. The new baby was named James Madison Randolph in honor of the secretary of state, who remained a dear family friend in addition to a political ally. Public health also continued to occupy a significant place on Jefferson's political agenda at the time. In his Fifth Annual Message to Congress on December 3, 1805, he began with a call for effective and judicious uses of quarantine for yellow fever, that "fatal fever which in latter times has visited our shores." Having experienced its ravages first-hand in the epidemic of 1793, Jefferson astutely understood the dangerous nature of yellow fever as well as the fact that it was often confused with other, less serious diseases. As an advocate for medical progress, Jefferson noted that "as we advance in our knowledge of this disease," exact diagnosis would become easier. He exhorted the states, "charged with the care of public health" as he put it, to work with Congress for effective quarantines that would protect the public as well as the nation's commercial interests.[47]

Although Jefferson's overall good health continued, he would experience another bout with severe headaches in the spring of 1807, probably brought on by stress over the increasingly erratic behavior of his son-in-law Thomas Randolph, who had suffered an apparent nervous breakdown. In addition, Jefferson was faced with a host of political challenges, including the unpopular Embargo Act and scandals surrounding Aaron Burr, who had killed Jefferson's political nemesis, Alexander Hamilton, in a duel. Despite popular support, Jefferson announced that he would follow George Washington's path and not seek a third term. Unsurprisingly, Jefferson longed for the end of his presidential term and the day he could retire and return to Monticello, joined by his daughter, Martha, and her family. Certainly Martha painted an idyllic picture of future life at Monticello for Jefferson, surrounded by loving grandchildren and his daughter, who offered the "dear and sacred duty of nursing and cheering your old age."[48]

Jefferson's Retirement

Indeed, when Jefferson returned to Monticello upon his retirement from the presidency and public life in 1809, he looked forward to a peaceful retreat in the Virginia countryside, which also included a second new house called Poplar Forest that he was building some distance from his main plantation. When he left Washington at the age of sixty-six, Jefferson was still fit enough to make the trip to Monticello on horseback, including eight hours in a snowstorm. He wrote America's new president, James Madison, that he felt "no inconvenience from the expedition but fatigue, I have more confidence in my *vis vitae* than I had before entertained."[49]

However, the summer of 1809 proved to be one filled with illness for Jefferson's immediate family, with grandchildren falling sick, the death of a grandchild, and even hardy Martha Randolph succumbing to an infection that confined her to bed. In the fall Jefferson sent his regrets for not having visited the Madisons but explained that he was delayed by the illness of Martha's youngest child.[50] Still, as was their custom, the family served as gracious hosts to many visiting guests, and Jefferson seems to have been left unscathed from the rampant summer sicknesses.[51] However, two years later Jefferson would suffer severe rheumatic pain in his back and legs, making walking difficult. Also, his beloved sister Mary Jefferson Carr, widow of his old friend Dabney Carr, died after several years of a "wasting complaint," but he was comforted by the fact that she passed away "without any increase in pain, or any other than her gradual decay."[52]

Political schisms between the Federalists and Republicans in the 1790s and the rise of political parties had led to the estrangement between Jefferson and John and Abigail Adams. However, in their twilight years, Jefferson and Adams renewed their old friendship, and the rapprochement was brokered by Dr. Rush in 1812. Their resultant correspondence is a dazzling exchange of theological, political, and social ideas as well as a reflection of the state of their health. Jefferson maintained that he and Adams were indeed fortunate to have lived long and relatively healthy lives, although in Jefferson's later years he sometimes suffered from painful rheumatism and arthritis in his joints, which necessitated the use of a cane to aid in walking.

"Of the signers of the Declaration of Independence I see now living not more than half a dozen on your side of the Potomok, and on this side, myself alone," Jefferson observed to Adams.

You and I have been wonderfully spared, and myself with remarkable health, and a considerable activity of body and mind. I am on horseback 3. or 4. hours of every day. . . . I walk little, however, a single mile being too much for me; and I live in the midst of my grandchildren, one of whom has lately promoted me to be a great grandfather. I have heard with pleasure that you also retain good health, and a greater power of exercise in walking than I do.[53]

Certainly Jefferson realized that he and many of his fellow revolutionaries had exceeded the average lifespan of his time. In a later letter written to Abigail Adams in 1816 when Jefferson was seventy-three, he observed, "You and I, dear Madam, have already had more than an ordinary portion of life, and more too of health than the general measure. On this score I owe boundless thankfulness."[54]

Martha Randolph gave birth to twelve children during her childbearing years, at intervals of about one to one and a half years. Jefferson would develop a close relationship and active correspondence with many of them. He obviously endured periods of depression during his lifetime, but for the most part Jefferson remained cheerful, and his grandchildren knew him as a calm and serene man. In 1813, he proudly wrote Abigail Adams, "I have 10 ½ grandchildren, and 2 ¾ great-grand-children; and these fractions will ere long become units. . . . These young scions give us comfortable cares, when we cease to care about ourselves."[55] Acutely conscious of the havoc illness could bring, the following year Jefferson wrote his daughter Maria's only surviving child, his grandson Francis Wayles Eppes, that "[m]y first wish, my dear Francis, is ever to hear that you are in good health, because that is the first of blessings."[56]

Although during his retirement Jefferson continued to keep in touch with Madison, for the most part he steered clear of politics, letting the new president find his own path. In their correspondence Jefferson generally discussed more personal subjects such as health, family, and farm news. He was especially concerned when Madison endured a life-threatening illness in the summer of 1813. Dolley Madison completely curtailed her duties as a hostess to minister to her husband, whose health had been negatively impacted by the stress of a string of unsuccessful military undertakings during the War of 1812 and long hours of work without breaks.

Madison was probably critically ill with an acute attack of "bilious fever," the ubiquitous malaria that was spread by mosquitoes during Washington's hot summers. Those who visited the president during his illness were alarmed by his appearance, and rumors of his impending death rippled through the capital. In early July, Dolley was finally able to report to her cousin that her husband was recovering and that "for the last three weeks his fever has been so slight as to permit him to take bark every hour and with good effect." Madison's doctors had been reluctant to administer the quinine-based bark at first while his fever was still high, and he was bedridden for weeks. Devoted to Madison, Dolley had for three weeks "nursed him night & day—sometimes in despair." When her husband finally recovered, although he remained pale and tired, Dolley could take a breather but admitted, "Now that I see he will get well I feel as if I should die myself, with fatigue."[57]

A letter from Jefferson to Madison in mid-July revealed the generalized worry that had been generated by the president's illness. Jefferson wrote that he hoped Madison was "entirely recovered. If the prayers of millions have been of avail, they have been poured forth with the deepest anxiety."[58] Later in the month Dolley confided to her friend Mrs. Gallatin, the wife of the secretary of the treasury, that "[y]ou can . . . have no idea of its extent and the despair in which I attended his bed for nearly five weeks! Even now I watch over him as I would an infant, so precarious is his convalescence."[59]

Compared to Madison, Jefferson remained resilient. As he aged, Jefferson suffered some sight and hearing loss, and walked with a cane, but like his good friend and fellow healthy older man Benjamin Franklin, he was realistic and even optimistically resigned: "Our machines have now been running for 70 or 80 years," he wrote to Adams in 1814, "and we must expect that worn as they are; here a pivot, there a wheel, now a pinion, next a spring, will be giving way." Two years later he assured Adams that "[m]y temperament is sanguine. I steer my bark [boat] with Hope in the head, leaving Fear astern."[60] Jefferson was proud of his physical endurance and often assured his friends of his "habitual good health." He informed one that "I retain good health, and am rather feeble to walk much, but ride with ease, passing two or three hours a day on horseback," although "[m]y eyes need the aid of glasses by night, and with small print, by day also."[61] It appears that many years earlier Jefferson had taken advantage of Franklin's invention of bifocals. In 1807, he wrote the American artist Charles Willson Peale that "I have adopted Dr. Franklin's plan of half-glasses of different focal distances, with great advantage."[62] In 1816, Jefferson informed still another acquaintance that he had passed the year, which included a "murderous" foul winter season, without "an hour's sickness for a twelvemonth past."[63]

Still, life at Monticello was not without health challenges. In 1815, Martha suffered a miscarriage after a prolonged bout of dysentery. The infectious disease also spread through the slave quarters at Monticello, demonstrating the upheaval an epidemic could cause during the era. A weary Jefferson reported to a relative that

> [w]e have now in our family, both in doors and out, more sickness than I have ever had since I was a housekeeper.... Without doors two or three are taken of a day, so that all the houses of the negroes are mere hospitals requiring great and constant attendance and care; all of an epidemic dysentery now prevailing thro' the neighborhood."[64]

The same year Jefferson's only brother, Randolph Jefferson, passed away at the age of fifty-nine.

In the summer of 1818, Jefferson suffered "[t]he severest attack of rheumatism I have ever experienced," which left him in great discomfort and for weeks unable to walk without pain, only to be followed in the fall by a life-threatening bout with severe constipation.[65] To relieve the rheumatism, Jefferson resorted to the old recommended natural remedy of a trip to the hot mineral waters at Warm Springs, Virginia, informing Martha, "I have tried one to-day the delicious bath and shall do it twice a day hereafter," and his health revived once again.[66]

In his seventies, Jefferson remained both mentally sharp and for the most part remarkably physically fit and was able to ride the ninety miles from Monticello to his second home at Poplar Forest with ease. In early 1819, Jefferson informed Madison that he would soon be traveling to Montpelier on horseback for a meeting since "[m]y health after which you kindly enquire is tolerably established, leaving me indeed in a state of increased debility, yet not so much as to render me unequal to the journey."[67] A year later Jefferson revealed to Madison a more significant decline: "My health is as usual: no pain, but low, weak, able to walk little, and venturing to ride little on account of suspicious symptoms which Dr. Watkins flatters himself will disappear in the spring."[68] Yet as late as 1820, a visitor to Monticello still described Jefferson as being as "straight as a young man."[69]

Jefferson's longevity was undoubtedly tied in part to his lifestyle. Like his hero Franklin, Jefferson adhered to a lifelong consciously healthful moderate diet, with very little consumption of red meat, but one that emphasized vegetables and regular glasses of wine augmented by tea,

coffee, and cider. He also eschewed tobacco. As a devotee of Franklin's recommendation of "early to bed, early to rise," Jefferson generally enjoyed
five to eight hours of sleep a night and rose at dawn. It is probably no coin-
cidence that both revolutionary leaders were progressive in their views on
healthy living, and they lived to an enviably active old age for the era.

As we have seen, because of his own interest in medicine and distrust of the majority of doctors, whose invasive treatments he often felt
hurried many to their deaths, for many illnesses Jefferson relied on the
healing power of nature and medicinal herbs from his own garden at
Monticello, such as thyme for intestinal problems and lavender to aid
headaches. For medical advice he frequently consulted his personal copy
of Thomas's *Modern Practice of Physic*, which had been published in 1817.
When the contents of his library were later catalogued it was found that
Jefferson owned ninety-nine medical texts, eleven books on anatomy,
and seventeen surgical manuals. His wooden medical box, which held
eighteen glass medicine vials, is still on display at Monticello.[70]

In 1819, at the age of seventy-five, Jefferson attributed his good health
to his temperate lifestyle and insisted that he was

> so free of catarrhs [pulmonary afflictions] that I have not had one on an
> average of eight or ten years through life. I ascribe this exemption partly
> to the habit of bathing my feet in cold water every morning for sixty
> years past. A fever of more than twenty-four hours I have not had above
> two or three times in my life . . . except on a late occasion of indisposi-
> tion, I enjoy good health; too feeble, indeed, to walk much, but riding
> without fatigue six or eight miles a day, and sometimes thirty or forty.[71]

Ever the optimist, Jefferson seems to have forgotten that just the previous year he had suffered from life-threatening blood poisoning and
painful boils brought on by the visit to the Blue Ridge mineral springs,
which had left him unable to ride comfortably for weeks. He had visited
Warm Springs both to cure a painful knee as well as to prevent a winter flareup of rheumatism. At first the regimen appeared successful, but
soon complications set in. Several weeks of taking the waters, coupled
with the 100-mile ride home over rough terrain, left him with an infection that produced an abscess, boils, a severe rash, fever, sweats, and
overall "extreme debility." Moreover, the salve of mercury and sulfur he

was prescribed for the rash made him deathly ill, and he did not recover until he ceased applying the ointment. Still his sense of humor was left intact, and he wrote wryly to Adams that he should have known "[t]hat the medicine that makes the sick well, may make the well sick." Jefferson's faith in the therapeutic powers of nature surely must have been shaken by his bad experience. And old age was definitely catching up with him; the next year he informed John Adams that he had "experienced three long and dangerous illnesses within the last 12 months."[72]

Jefferson's family increasingly worried about his health as the years passed. In the fall of 1819, Jefferson's granddaughter, Ellen Randolph Coolidge, wrote her friend Dolley Madison that she was unable to visit her at Montpelier because of a "sudden and violent attack" experienced by her grandfather. His physicians declared him

> entirely out of danger . . . but we cannot expect that at his age his recovery will be a rapid one . . . his complaint was a violent and obstinate cholic lasting about thirty hours . . . a Physician in whom we have great confidence has engaged that if GrandPapa will only stay at home and take care of himself, during this winter, that the warm weather, shall find him restored to the health he enjoyed.

Among other physical problems, Jefferson's old wrist injury continued to be bothersome in his last years, causing painful swelling and stiffening due to rheumatism or arthritis. Knowing how active and strong-willed Jefferson was, it is not surprising that Ellen concluded, "I much fear that he does not know how to take care of himself, to be very attentive to his diet, to use less exercise, and to avoid all fatigue of body or mind, & especially to give up letter-writing, are the points on which the doctor most insists."[73]

Still, Jefferson remained the gracious Virginia gentleman as he aged, although as he neared eighty he confided to John Adams, "I have ever dreaded a doting old age; and my health has been generally so good, and is now so good, that I dread it still. The rapid decline of my strength during the last winter has made me hope some times that I see land [death]."[74] Yet, not only did Jefferson remain mentally acute, but after suffering a broken arm after a fall down the stairs at Monticello, he persisted in riding on his favorite horse, Eagle, despite the necessity of a sling and persistent swelling in his hands and fingers. Jefferson reported the incident to Madison and minimized his accident: "Ten days ago I incured the accident of breaking the small bone of the left fore-arm, and some disturbance of the small bones of the wrist. . . . Dr. Watkins attended promptly, set them well and all is doing well." But weeks later Jefferson was still suffering and reported that "[m]y arm goes on slowly, still in a sling and incapable of any use, and will so continue some time yet."[75] Madison replied in a manner that must have pleased Jefferson with its emphasis on the power of nature over medical treatment: "I was afraid the Docr. was too sanguine in promising so early a cure of the fracture in your arm," wrote Madison. "The milder weather soon to be looked for, will doubtless favor the vis medicatrix which nature employs in repairing the injuries done her."[76]

Over a year later, however, Jefferson's health began a more serious decline. As he wrote to his old French friend the Marquis de Lafayette, dislocated wrists and fingers crippled with arthritis made one of his favorite pastimes, writing, nearly impossible. Jefferson was still able to see the glass half full, however, and continued professing his Enlightenment philosophy, which emphasized faith in progress fueled by advances in science. He noted his infirmities as well as his hopes for the future:

I am again in tolerable health, but extremely debilitated, scarcely able to walk into my garden. The hebetude of age, too, and extinguishment of interest in things around me, are weaning me from them, and dispose me with cheerfulness to resign them to the existing generation, satisfied that the advancement of science will enable them to administer the commonwealth with increased wisdom.[77]

In 1824, Lafayette traveled to Monticello to visit Jefferson, who although weakened by age and suffering from a painful jaw abscess, rushed to welcome him.

Jefferson's Contributions to Medicine and the University of Virginia

One of the crowning achievements of Jefferson's last years, which brought him great personal satisfaction, was the formal opening in 1825 of the University of Virginia, of which he had been principal designer and founder. Jefferson conceived the school buildings with an eye to the physical and mental health of students and the prevention of the spread of infectious diseases among them. To strengthen their bodies, he recommended a daily menu for students that emphasized fruits and vegetables over meat products. More importantly, he employed the principles he had developed in previous studies for the erection of ideal structures for hospitals and prisons, which emphasized fresh air and sanitary surroundings. By 1810, Jefferson had already advised the trustees of the East Tennessee College to design a park-like square, to avoid that academic institution becoming "a large and common den of noise, of filth & fetid air."[78]

As the "father" of the University of Virginia, Jefferson had been involved in the planning of his dream for nearly a decade, and even in old age he played a central role in supervising construction of its campus and the development of its educational program, including the selection of its first professors. "We are determined to receive no one who is not of the first order of science in his line," Jefferson wrote in April 1824, reflecting both his lifelong commitment to high educational standards and the Enlightenment's emphasis on the pursuit of empirical scientific knowledge.[79]

A graduate of the College of William and Mary, Jefferson played a pivotal role in introducing a medical chair there in 1779. Now he played another important part in bringing improved medical education to the state through his establishment of a chair of medicine at the University of Virginia. Back in 1807, Jefferson had written his friend Dr. Caspar Wistar, who was associated with the medical school in Philadelphia, of his plans to send his grandson to that city for medical training in anatomy because the Philadelphia school offered "advantages not to be found elsewhere."[80]

Now Jefferson hoped to bring the best of advanced medical education to Virginia as well. One of Jefferson's most promising academic appointments at the University of Virginia was that of the young, eminent, English-born physician Dr. Robley Dunglison. Dunglison shared Jefferson's affinity for rational scientific inquiry and his antipathy for heroic medical measures such as bloodletting, as well as his underlying belief in preventative medicine and the pivotal role of nature in maintaining and regaining health. As we know, Jefferson had long advocated limited medical intervention and the use of medications with proven value only. Beyond this point, Jefferson maintained, the "judicious, the moral, the humane physician should stop," and Jefferson clearly viewed Dunglison as possessing all three traits. Dunglison received his medical education and training in London, Edinburgh, Paris, and Germany and was appointed at the University of Virginia to a chair of "anatomy, surgery, the history of the progress and theories of medicine, physiology, material medica, and pharmacy." Later, Dr. William Osler, one of the most respected physicians and educators in America in the late nineteenth century, maintained that "Thomas Jefferson did a good work when he imported him from London, as Dunglison had all the wisdom of his day combined with a colossal industry."[81]

It is interesting to note that the goal driving Jefferson's support of medical courses at the University of Virginia in the early years was not only to produce more professionally competent physicians but to provide educated laymen with a good understanding of contemporary medicine. Reflecting his faith in the common man, Jefferson envisioned graduating students who had gained a fundamental medical knowledge that would enable them to make more informed decisions about treatment for themselves and their families and provide them with the tools to lead a healthy lifestyle. Jefferson hoped that medical training at his university would upgrade standards and become a model of scientific medicine for the rest of the country. Classes at the school did not begin until 1825, but Jefferson was closely involved in setting up the medical courses and personally worked with Dunglison to obtain physical specimens of body organs such as a preserved heart, liver, kidney, and uterus so that the future students would have first-hand anatomical exposure through "physiological demonstrations."[82]

Twilight Years

Although Jefferson was notoriously suspicious of doctors, he had great respect for Dunglison, undoubtedly because of the physician's impressive scientific knowledge for the time, high level of medical training, and advocacy of preventative medicine. He became quite fond of the young man, who became his personal physician in his last years, replacing Dr. Thomas Watkins, whom Jefferson had earlier extolled and for whom he felt "indebted to his experience and cautious practice for the restoration of my health."[83] Jefferson notoriously ridiculed those whom he considered medical quacks or incompetent doctors who dispensed medicine without fully understanding their properties, but he appreciated the need for effective, proven treatments and trained, experienced physicians. Jefferson's belief that doctors should emphasize fact over theory and the centrality of clinical evaluation were outlooks apparently shared by Dunglison, who also viewed radical therapy such as bleeding as being inappropriate and ineffective.[84]

Dunglison visited Jefferson numerous times from the spring of 1825 until Jefferson's death in the summer of 1826, and it appears that Jefferson followed his advice and prescriptions meticulously. The first recorded letter concerning Jefferson's health appears in a short, cryptic note from Jefferson to Dunglison in May 1825 when he asked the professor to visit him in the role of physician. "A chronical complaint which has been troublesome for some time has within a few days become too much so to be longer unattended to. I must ask your advice in it therefore as soon as you can come with convenience. It disables me from going out either on horseback or in a carriage."[85] The problem was either an intestinal flareup or, more likely, a urinary tract constriction arising from Jefferson's enlarged prostate. Watkins had already been treating Jefferson for dysuria (painful urination) by prescribing rest, a bland diet, and opium with calomel if the more conservative approach did not bring relief.[86]

It is from Dunglison that we learn of Jefferson's long bout with chronic diarrhea, which the doctor treated conservatively with a bland diet and mild medications, which included laudanum, a derivative of opium, to help soothe Jefferson's intestines and overcome insomnia. Dunglison also realized that Jefferson's nutrition was at risk and advised strong broths and mild but bracing foods. Apparently Dunglison's ministrations brought some relief because in June Jefferson was able to report "Th. J. is going on steadily well. His intervals have proved less than any other symptoms. He will pray a supply of pills by his grandson, either today or tomorrow."[87]

In hindsight it appears that Jefferson may have suffered from colitis or irritable bowel syndrome, exacerbated by tension and, in the end, advancing age. A few weeks later Jefferson happily reported, "I find myself now as well as I have been for several months. . . . All this is from your kind attentions." He requested that Dunglison present him with a bill for his medical services, indicating that Jefferson was accustomed to paying physicians promptly. Dunglison replied that he was gratified to hear of Jefferson's improved health and asserted that the satisfaction he received from being able to aid "one whose existence is so valuable to us all" was sufficient compensation.[88]

Unfortunately, Jefferson had been too optimistic and just a week later he was writing Dunglison again to report, "I find I had been too sanguine in believing that my complaint was wearing off," and again asked for his assistance. For over a week, Dunglison was unable to see his patient at Monticello due to a troublesome medical problem of his own, but he recommended fifty drops of laudanum as a sedative and promised to visit Jefferson the following day. Increasing doses were necessary as time passed to allow Jefferson to rest.[89]

In August, Jefferson confided to a friend only partly in jest that he had "one foot in the grave, and the other uplifted to follow it."[90] From May 17, 1825, until September 20, 1825, Jefferson recorded thirty professional visits from Dunglison, including one notation of a "Bougie," a type of thin catheter similar to the type that Franklin had designed, that Dunglison used to treat the urinary constriction and painful symptoms caused by Jefferson's severely enlarged prostate. The condition caused the former president so much discomfort and inconvenience that at times he was confined to bed. Jefferson's mechanical experience and familiarity with medical treatments enabled him to soon use the mechanical catheter device on his own, although it only afforded him intermittent relief.[91]

By November 1825, Jefferson was philosophical about his health and informed Dunglison that the intestinal problems continued: "I certainly cannot say that I am well, but as much so probably as I ever shall be. . . . I suppose therefore that with care and laudanum I may consider myself in what is to be my habitual state." In the same letter Jefferson also revealed his continuing interest in medical education and told Dunglison he was forwarding information on the "new Medical school approaching nearer to us. I send also the Introductory lecture. It will possess you exactly of the state of Medical instruction in the US."[92]

In Dunglison, Jefferson had found a sympathetic ally who would become a partner in bringing wider attention to his innovative medical ideas concerning public health, particularly for those who could not afford expensive medical treatment. These forward-looking proposals

clearly were evident in a November 1825 draft concerning the introduction of a "Dispensary," or clinic, at the University of Virginia, which had
initially been suggested by Dunglison. Based on the memorandum submitted by Jefferson, the board adopted a resolution that formally connected the dispensary to the medical school. It called for the professor of medicine, at that time Dunglison, to dispense "medical advice,
vaccination, and aid in Surgical cases of ordinary occurrence." All poor
people with the exception of slaves were to receive free treatment, those
who had some means were to pay half a dollar for each visit, and all
smallpox vaccinations were to be offered free of charge. Students in the
medical school were to work alongside the professor of medicine to
gain medical experience and knowledge.[93]

Jefferson's distrust of contemporary medicine, his deeply held underlying belief in natural healing, as well as his regard for Dr. Dunglison
are touchingly revealed in another letter written late in November 1825.
Jefferson remarked sadly that

> the fragment of life remaining to me is likely to be passed in sickness and
> suffering. The young physicians in our neighborhood will probably be
> good ones in time. But time & experience as well as science are necessary
> to make a skillful physician, and Nature is preferable to an unskilled one.
> I had therefore made up my mind to trust to her altogether, until your
> arrival gave me better prospects.[94]

It appears that Dunglison diagnosed Jefferson's recurrent intestinal
disorders as being caused by inflammation and irritation, and in late
December 1825 he instructed Jefferson to "take six grains of Rhubarb
with fifteen of Magnesia," along with a little milk, and to abstain from
vegetables and concentrate instead on eating meat and biscuits. He also
advised him to resume laudanum if his symptoms worsened. Like most
doctors at the time, Dunglison worked with a compilation of information about medications and herbs that he developed over the years
to help treat his patients. When Dunglison later published a medical
textbook in 1843, it carried his accumulated wisdom on a variety of
treatments, and discussed the properties of both rhubarb and magnesia, noting that though they were generally used as cathartics, "gentle"
amounts could have a positive value for intestinal irritation. Moreover,

he asserted that for "inflammation of the lining membrane of the intestinal canal, opium is a most valuable remedy," and laudanum was the easiest form of opium to administer.[95] Dr. Rush had prescribed a laudanum mixture for Jefferson's bouts of diarrhea many years before in 1804, and Jefferson may have prepared the prescription himself, as his account books reveal that he sometimes purchased medicines for home use from an apothecary.[96]

Jefferson's health continued to deteriorate in 1826. Sadly, a few months before his death, Jefferson was yet again to suffer the loss of a beloved family member. His eldest granddaughter, Anne Randolph Bankhead, married to an alcoholic, abusive husband, died at Monticello in February 1826, soon after giving birth to a baby boy. Her death moved the devastated Jefferson to despondently declare, "Heaven seems to be overwhelming us with every form of misfortune."[97]

Dr. Dunglison visited Jefferson frequently during the ex-president's final days and confirmed that at age eighty-two the former president still possessed "his intellectual powers unshaken by age, and the physical man so active that he rode to and from Monticello, and took exercise on foot with all the activity of one twenty or thirty years younger." In May of 1826 Jefferson was optimistic enough to inform James Madison that "[i]n comparison to my sufferings of the last year, my health, although not restored, is greatly better."[98] Apparently Jefferson often shared his lifelong skepticism of doctors with Dunglison, for the doctor also reported that "Mr. Jefferson was considered to have but little faith in physic; and has often told me that he would rather trust to the unaided, or rather, uninterfered with, efforts of nature than to physicians in general." However, Dunglison quoted Jefferson as declaring, "It is not to physic that I object so much, as to physicians."[99]

Although Jefferson may have lost some of his six-foot-three height in his last years, he still stood erect, according to his grandson, Anne's brother Jefferson Randolph, and even in his last days, "his mind was always clear—it never wandered." Randolph recalled that Jefferson's red hair had turned sandy and his skin fragile but that when he died at the age of eighty-four, he still had all his teeth, and his "step was firm and elastic, which he preserved until his death."[100] Similarly, Sally Hemings's son Madison, who claimed that Jefferson was his biological father, observed that he "generally enjoyed excellent health. Till within three weeks of his death he was hale and hearty and at the age of 83 years he walked erect and with a steady tread."[101]

Jefferson exhibited an apparently philosophical reaction to his increasing debilities and, echoing his earlier sentiments to Adams, declared to his grandson, "I am like an old watch, with a pinion worn out here, and a wheel there, until it can go no longer." He managed to keep up his daily horseback rides until three weeks before his death. Throughout his life, time had been a highly valued and precious commodity for Jefferson, and he always rose early to usher in a full day. Randolph noted that during Jefferson's last illness his grandfather maintained that "the sun had not caught him in bed for fifty years."[102]

Indeed, later in the spring of 1826, Jefferson's health began to deteriorate alarmingly. Another visit to a local health springs in June to treat a stubborn rash exacerbated his intestinal problems, and he experienced almost constant severe diarrhea, which sapped his strength. Yet he managed to ride to the University of Virginia one last time in June to oversee work on the Rotunda. Dr. Dunglison had Jefferson's confidence, and Dunglison continued to watch over him. However, by early July it was clear to Jefferson and his family that death was approaching. Jefferson remained cheerful and uncomplaining, as he had during most of his lifetime, concerning himself with the health of his family and minimizing his own illnesses. Still clear-minded, he made final arrangements with the aid of his grandson, before he experienced prolonged periods of unconsciousness.[103]

On July 1, a few days before Jefferson's death, Dunglison wrote Madison that he regrettably had to delay his visit to Montpellier due to "the serious indisposition of Mr. Jefferson." He informed Madison that Jefferson's longstanding intestinal problems had become increasingly serious and due to Jefferson's age, the formerly robust American leader had lost "the power of restoration the existence of which at an earlier period in life render similar affections but trifling moment." Dunglison alluded to Jefferson's imminent demise and sadly concluded that unless there was some miraculous recovery, "My worst apprehensions will soon be realized."[104]

In his diary, Dunglison summarized his evaluation of Jefferson's condition, noting that in his last month Jefferson had become "more impaired, his nutrition fell off." In late June, Jefferson penned his final letter to Dunglison, begging him to stop by Monticello. According to the physician, Jefferson declined an invitation to attend a fiftieth anniversary celebration in Washington marking the Declaration of Independence due to his "indisposition." Dunglison was in attendance on the last day of Jefferson's life when he slipped in and out of consciousness. Aware of his impending death and probably wishing to be as alert as possible, Jefferson instructed his doctor to discontinue the administration of laudanum. His last words to Dunglison on the evening of July 3rd were, "Is it the fourth?" Clearly Jefferson hoped to live long enough to mark the auspicious anniversary.[105]

Jefferson's wish was granted, and he died on the momentous date of July 4, 1826, at the age of eighty-three, surrounded by his family. Even in his weakened state, he was cognizant of the importance of the historic day.[106] Fittingly, his close friend and revolutionary comrade John Adams passed away on the same day in Massachusetts. In a note to her son written just two days after Jefferson's passing, Dolley Madison declared that her husband, who had regarded Jefferson as almost a father, "feels his departure deeply, as no doubt his family must."[107] Not only did Jefferson leave Madison his gold-headed walking stick, but just months before his death, Jefferson revealed to Madison that "[t]o myself you have been a pillar of support through life." He also entreated Madison to "[t]ake care of me when dead."[108] Madison suffered a great personal loss with Jefferson's death and eloquently eulogized his long-time mentor, noting, "He lives and will live in the memory and gratitude of the wise and good as a luminary of science, as a votary of liberty, as a model of patriotism, and as a benefactor of human kind."[109]

All over the United States, citizens were celebrating the half-centennial, and the names of Adams and Jefferson were noted again and again. Jefferson was celebrated for his pivotal role in the founding of the nation, yet few were aware of the central role he had played in advancing medical treatment and education in the United States. Yet, his keen interest in medical knowledge and concern for public health, particularly on behalf of the poor and the "common man," helped lay a usable foundation in America for the later development of progressive medicine. Indeed, the Jeffersonian vision of medicine and politics were intricately intertwined,[110] and Jefferson firmly believed that a liberal political system and an ordered society were necessary ingredients to public as well as individual health.[111] Moreover, like Washington, Franklin,

Adams, and Madison, he recognized the positive and pivotal role government could play in fostering good health on both the national and individual level. Like so many followers of the Enlightenment, particularly Franklin, Jefferson viewed its twin ideals of humanitarianism and progress as being advanced through the platform of preventative medical treatment, including care for those who could not afford it on their own. In Jefferson's view, good health made for active, involved citizens, and Americans who were knowledgeable about medicine could work together toward the prosperity of the nation.

Epilogue

Evolutionary Medicine

Without health we enjoy nothing.
—*Dolley Madison to Anna Cutts, April 8, 1812*

Not only were America's founders political actors on the stage of the eighteenth-century world, but on multiple levels they contributed to advancements in American medicine, illustrating the complex links between politics and health. This was perhaps most visible in the manner in which intellectual leaders like Washington, Franklin, Adams, Jefferson, and Madison used their positions to influence public health and disseminate knowledge about better health practices to their families, communities, and citizens in the nation at large. Their numerous personal encounters with illness and loss made them acutely sensitive to issues surrounding medical practices and disease. Certainly they all believed that the health of the individual and the health of the community were closely intertwined, and that a democratic government and individuals could work together productively to promote the health of all Americans. In other words, they viewed common progress as the best measure of individual progress. As prominent medical historian Charles E. Rosenberg has observed, "There is nothing more fundamental in the history of American health care than the mixture of public and private. . . . It has long been assumed that the state has some role—and an interest—in protecting the health of its citizens generally and of providing at least minimal care for the helpless and indigent."[1]

In the face of terrifying ubiquitous threats of diseases of their era, such as smallpox, cholera, yellow fever, and typhoid, these extraordinarily civic-minded founders often acted not only with personal courage but also with admirable self-sacrifice in order to carry out their political responsibilities and help their neighbors and fellow citizens safeguard their individual and collective health. Franklin's lifelong effort to reduce the incidence of smallpox through education about the benefits of inoculation and his scientific health experiments, Washington's campaign to inoculate his soldiers against smallpox and to provide them with a healthier military camp environment, Adams's concern for isolating potential carriers of disease and caring for maritime sailors through the creation of the Marine Hospital Service, and Jefferson's crusade to make smallpox vaccine more readily available to the American public are just a few examples of their momentous public health activities. Imbued with republican ideas, they all believed that helping to ensure the health of American citizens was not only an admirable humanitarian ideal but a practical way of fostering productivity by increasing the population and growing the economy. Moreover, the government could play a vital role in the process by engaging in health intervention when appropriate.

In 1734, when Franklin reprinted the popular self-help medical manual, *Every Man His Own Doctor*, he was reflecting the medical milieu of the age. Of course, doctors were called in by those who could afford them when deemed necessary, but most farmers, planters, household heads, and their wives were familiar with symptoms of many contemporary diseases and at least basic medical treatment for everyday ills and medical emergencies. As we will see below, not until the late nineteenth century were American physicians able to fully consolidate their elite professional status.

Today Americans almost always consult a doctor for maladies such as bacterial and viral infections, high fevers, and serious diseases such as diabetes and cancer, which our forebears would have at least initially treated themselves.[2] Almost all of America's founders, most notably Franklin, Jefferson, George and Martha Washington, Abigail Adams, and Dolley Madison, were at times medical practitioners themselves, dispensing home remedies and informal medical advice, and in the case of Washington and Jefferson even performing medical procedures, such as inoculation for their families and slaves. Abigail, Martha, and Dolley, often at great personal risk, worked tirelessly to nurse family members and neighbors, setting an example for their entire communities. Certainly medical care at the time was part of everyday "women's work." Some of the founders, especially Jefferson, even took what we would term today a more holistic approach to medicine. His underlying medical belief was based on a philosophy of *vis medicatrix naturae*, that the human body possessed a natural tendency to heal itself—if physicians and the patient would only refrain from derailing that process with invasive heroic measures.

Some of the medical practices followed or suggested by the American founders in this study appear ludicrous to modern ears. As Enlightenment scholar Peter Gay has observed, in the mania to pursue new scientific ideas, outlandish medical theories sprang up in the eighteenth century as emphasis on exclusively theoretical medicine declined. Gay concluded that "[a]ll this stress on experience, on clinical study and experimentation, revolutionized medicine," but even conscientious physicians were often misguided.[3] Today we know that new contradictory scientific research frequently surfaces and that medicine needs to be self-correcting in order to move forward. Recent studies about placebos, for example, indicate that belief about a particular treatment may actually lead to visible improvements in disease symptoms and health through real changes in brain chemicals. Modern research highlights the close interconnection between the mind and the body, a concept that the founders would have accepted as a given.[4] In other words, despite many highly significant advances, much of medicine still exists in a gray zone, where experts often disagree.

Some "incredible" early treatments have even been reintroduced. When Dolley Madison experienced a severe eye inflammation in 1836, one of the remedies proposed was the application of leeches. It is interesting to note that in the beginning of the twenty-first century leeches have been introduced as advanced medical treatment in certain cases to help reestablish circulation in ruptured veins. The medical benefits derived from these parasites are related to powerful anticoagulant chemicals the leeches release, not "bleeding" to regulate hypothetical "humors." In 2004, the American Food and Drug Administration (FDA) approved the use of leeches as medical "devices" or tools and their expanded medicinal possibilities are still being explored. And in 2012, a scientific study concluded that limited phlebotomy (bleeding) had a positive effect on metabolic syndrome (METS) by lowering blood pressure and improving glycemic control.[5] Similarly, the United States Army has begun to offer acupuncture to treat veterans who experience chronic pain. Many patients and their doctors have noted significant reduction in symptoms, but other military physicians have dismissed the procedure as "quackademics" and no better than prescribing sugar pills.[6]

Of course, the American founders worried most often about their own family members, but they were all motivated, to a large degree, by broader goals and were exceptionally public spirited. The revolutionary generation was profoundly influenced by Enlightenment thought and the role of reason and science, including medicine, in promoting well-being and happiness. They imbibed much of their liberalism through the works of John Locke and Scottish philosophers such as David Hume. As avid students of the Enlightenment, they absorbed intellectual ideas about the social contract and human rights that influenced their views about the legitimate role of government, including that in medicine.[7]

All the founders were certainly shrewd and capable politicians, but as we have seen in the previous chapters a fundamental commitment to the public good, including scientific and medical progress, was ingrained in their characters and underlying philosophies. They all shared the conviction that public virtue was an essential ingredient in safeguarding the republic. Indeed, their firm belief in republicanism included an ideal of public virtue that emphasized unselfish devotion to the common good, and they always attempted to incorporate that outlook into their private lives. John Adams may have expressed this idea most clearly when he wrote "Public Virtue is the only Foundation of Republics."[8] It was also evident when in 1777 Adams expressed satisfaction when the Continental Congress passed legislation that expanded the army's Hospital [Medical] Department, observing, "The expense will be great, but humanity overcame avarice."[9] As we have seen, the Washingtons, Franklin, the Adamses, Jefferson, and the Madisons were willing to make extraordinary personal, economic, and political sacrifices to ensure the well-being of the American people. The founders laid the cornerstone for an enduring American legacy that focused on medical progress and appropriate government involvement, and their efforts remain instructive today. Not only did they introduce the revolutionary political notion that ordinary people could govern themselves, but they believed that Americans could and should take an active role in managing their own health.

Unfortunately, the founders' underlying belief in the march of progress led some of them to an almost utopian vision of the future in terms of health. Franklin predicted that as a result of scientific progress, "All Diseases may by sure means be prevented . . . and our Lives lengthened at pleasure even beyond the antediluvian Standard."[10] Also influenced by Enlightenment philosophy, General Washington, at the end of the American Revolution in 1783, issued an optimistic circular letter to state governors about America's future, in which he emphasized that the "foundation of our Empire was not laid in the gloomy age of Ignorance and Superstition" but in an age that reflected "the treasures of knowledge, acquired by the labours of Philosophers, Sages, and legislators."[11] We might safely assume that Washington believed the "treasures of knowledge" would influence medical as well as political progress. Even the conservative Adams expressed optimism in 1787, noting that "[t]he arts and sciences, in general, during the three or four last centuries, have had a regular course of progressive improvement."[12]

Yet, even the European *philosophes* realized that social progress could reflect mixed blessings; growth could be circumscribed and impermanent at times, provoking skepticism.[13] Jefferson's often critical views of contemporary physicians can be viewed in this vein. In old age, Jefferson remained convinced that some areas of medicine still had a good distance to travel: "While surgery is seated in the temple of the exact sciences, medicine has scarcely entered its threshold," he observed.[14]

In 1826, fifty years after the outbreak of the American Revolution and long after he had played a primary role in constructing America's Constitution, Madison would affirm to a friend, "[W]e both have had the happiness of passing through a period glorious to our country, and more than any preceding one, likely to improve the social condition of man."[15] Like the other American founders, Madison believed that social improvement included the promise of a healthier life initiated by the scientific revolution.

It is telling that in his State of the Union Address, when the United States was embroiled in the War of 1812, Madison opened his remarks with a reference to the health of the nation, observing, "On our present meeting it is my first duty to invite your attention to the providential favors which our country has experienced in the unusual degree of health dispensed to its inhabitants," which he tied to the nation's prosperity and the encouraging, supportive backdrop of a democratic republic.[16]

It is noteworthy that the founders were also willing to change their views about disease and medicine when they were confronted with convincing arguments. As we saw in chapter 2, when Franklin and Adams roomed together in 1776 on their way to a meeting in New York, they engaged in an amusing dispute over the efficacy of fresh air. Adams, who considered himself an invalid at the time, was annoyed with Franklin's insistence that the windows be open to allow fresh air to enter their room overnight. Yet, less than a decade later, Adams offered an embryonic theory of germs and speculated in his diary that breathing brought both "salubrious" as well as "noxious Particles" into the lungs and blood. Perhaps due to years of Franklin's influence, by 1783 Adams argued that fresh air and open windows in coaches, dining rooms, and bed chambers helped to dissipate the noxious particles and concluded, "I suspect that the Health of Mankind is much injured by their Inattention to this Subject."[17]

Despite the euphoria after the American Revolution, harsh realities soon confronted the fledgling republic, and for a good part of the nineteenth century both the state of the American government and the state of American medicine were perilously fragile before they emerged stronger after the Civil War. Although one writer has observed that "the late eighteenth century may be looked on as the dawn of modern medicine,"[18] there was certainly a shadow hovering over that dawning for decades in the nineteenth century. Unfortunately, the founders' optimism about the blossoming progress of American medicine did not occur as quickly as they may have hoped, but Thomas Jefferson, for one, would have been pleased that many of his medical theories about radical bleeding and heroic measures were eventually vindicated over time. And in his famous evaluation of eighteenth-century medicine, in 1800 American physician and historian David Ramsay famously observed that, despite setbacks, there had been noticeable improvement and progress during the period.[19] Others have noted that during the era there was some significant decline in maternal and child mortality and smallpox epidemics, as well as more rational medicine based on the principles of pioneer scientist Frances Bacon and greater understanding of the role of good nutrition and clean air in health.[20]

But as medical historian Ronald L. Numbers put it, "Midway through the 19th century American medicine lay in a shambles," and in the decades after 1830, many American citizens were losing their respect for the profession as a whole. Regular doctors who continued to advocate heroic therapies were increasingly challenged and often ridiculed by "irregular" sectarian healers without formal medical degrees who advocated homeopathic and alternative therapies. In response, traditional physicians initiated a reformation, if not a revolution, in medical practice as they successfully consolidated the medical profession and their status through creating a united front, upgrading medical education, and shutting down many institutions that had produced unqualified physicians.[21] Of course, this process was complex. Sectarianism did encourage many regular doctors to distance themselves from therapeutic excesses, but at the same time, it influenced some to "hold on all the tighter to the therapies that represented their own professional tradition," making the transformation challenging.[22]

America's founders may have had public health prominently in their minds, but unfortunately their ideas had little direct impact on the society immediately after them. The Seaman's Act of 1798 and Washington's push for inoculation of the military during the Revolutionary War were significant public health initiatives, but they were limited in their impact on the larger society. Neither program led to any long-range commitment on the part of the federal government. It took a century for the Marine Hospital program to develop into the national United State Public Health Service, and when it did, it was not because of eighteenth-century ideas but because of the push from large-scale immigration, increasing and more widespread epidemics, and the overwhelming need to provide for quarantine of newcomers. As medical historian Margaret Humphreys has so felicitously put it, "Epidemics that visited the republic during the first three or four decades of the nineteenth century caused flickers of reform impulse without creating hearty flames."[23] Not until 1879 did Congress create the National Board of Health.

Today, the state of American medicine reflects remarkable advances in therapeutic effectiveness, a stark contrast to the era of the founders. Then the most popular and effective therapeutic regimens were perhaps the introduction in 1754 of lime juice to fight scurvy, the introduction in 1785 of digitalis (foxglove), which helped treat congestive heart disease, and the use of Peruvian bark for malaria (quinine was not isolated as a specific drug until 1819). Still, it must be acknowledged that even today a "magic bullet" does not exist for all illnesses, and smallpox is the only disease to have been fully conquered. Moreover, third-world countries are still a hotbed of many age-old epidemical diseases. And even in America, treatment of yellow fever in modern times relies only on bed rest, good nursing care, and adequate hydration and fever and pain relievers, although the disease is of course far less common due to improved public health measures.[24] Cancer, malaria, diabetes, and heart disease have yet to be eradicated. Yet in early 2012, one prominent research physician predicted that the future of American medicine would include "a doctor in your pocket," personal electronic monitors that would lead to tailored therapies that could spell the end of many illnesses.[25] At the same time, a recent book written by a prominent physician has taken American hospitals and the doctors who practice there to task for performing unnecessary surgeries and invasive procedures, and causing preventable infections and complications, eerily reminiscent of charges against Dr. Rush and many of his contemporaries.[26]

If the founding mothers and fathers had the opportunity to view American society today, they would probably be both astounded by and pleased with medical progress. In their era modern medicine was in its infancy. Many of the illnesses that were fatal in their age are now preventable or curable. Some of the most serious diseases they encountered, such as stroke, heart disease, and cancer, are still prevalent today, but in many cases they can be treated and successfully controlled, if not cured. But along with the march of progress has come a host of environmentally related health concerns and illnesses connected to our increased standard of living, such as rising rates of diabetes and obesity. While these conditions were certainly not absent during the colonial and early national periods, their rates were nowhere near the epidemic proportions experienced today when technology has provided opportunity for increased sedentary leisure, prolific food and beverage choices, and less physical exercise. As we learned in earlier chapters, most of the American founders were temperate in their eating habits and lifestyles, a model we would perhaps be wise to follow today.

As we stand at the crossroads of American health care with the Obama care debate still ongoing, the experiences of America's founders are instructive. Of course, despite limitations, modern medicine is light years ahead of what it was in the world of America's founders. Nevertheless, a number of their underlying concerns remain. The founders raised questions about responsibility for the sick and indigent and the relationship of individuals and government that continue to command our attention to this day. The founders' commitment to the public good undoubtedly meant that they would have looked with approval on providing the *opportunity* to access good health care for all Americans, particularly to children and the poor, through legislation such as the Federal Affordable Health Care Act. But given their fierce commitment to the principles of individual liberty, they surely would have balked at *requiring* all citizens to purchase health care insurance, as will occur under the new federal mandate. Achieving the delicate balance between social responsibility and individual rights is as challenging an issue for us today as it was for our nation's founders, but the lives of America's founders remind us that it is still a very worthy conversation.

NOTES

Introduction

1. John Duffy, *The Healers: A History of American Medicine* (Urbana: University of Illinois Press, 1976), 50.
2. Peter Gay, *The Enlightenment: An Interpretation*, vol. 2, *The Science of Freedom* (New York: Knopf, 1969), 12-13.
3. Fifth Congress, Chapter 77, July 16, 1798, Statute 605. See also, "Our Public Health Service," *American Journal of Public Health* 29 (September 1939):1044 and John Jensen, "Before the Surgeon General: Marine Hospital in Mid-19th-Century America," *Public Health Reports* 112 (November/December 1997): 525.
4. For a very lucid discussion of the connection between epidemics and commerce specifically in the American South, see Margaret Humphreys, *Yellow Fever and the South* (New Brunswick, NJ: Rutgers University Press, 1992).
5. James Madison, "State of the Union Address" (November 4, 1812), www.globusz. com/ebooks/Madison/00000014.htm , accessed January 27, 2012.
6. Joseph J. Ellis, "Introduction," in Margaret A. Hogan and C. James Taylor, eds., *My Dearest Friend: Letters of Abigail and John Adams* (Cambridge, MA: Belknap Press of Harvard University Press, 2007), vii.
7. Estimates for eighteenth-century mortality rates are based on "imperfect and fragmentary" data, but they do help establish a pattern. Child mortality seems to have been significantly higher in the South than in the North due to a warmer climate and environmental factors that encouraged the spread of deadly diseases in infants. See Michael R. Haines and Richard H. Steckel, eds., *A Population History of North American* (New York: Cambridge University Press, 2000), 4, 161.
8. Abigail Adams to Mary Cranch, September 30, 1785, in Abigail Adams, *The Letters of Mrs. Adams, the Wife of John Adams: With an Introductory Memoir by Her Grandson Charles Francis Adams* (Boston: Wilkins, Carter, 1848), 272.
9. Martha Washington to Fanny Bassett Washington, March 9, 1794, in Joseph E. Fields, ed., *"Worthy Partner": The Papers of Martha Washington* (Westport, CT: Greenwood, 1994), 261.
10. John G. Jackson to Dolley Madison, October 8, 1808, in David D. Mattern and Holly C. Shulman, eds., *The Selected Letters of Dolley Payne Madison* (Charlottesville: University of Virginia Press), 89.
11. See Stanley Finger, *Doctor Franklin's Medicine* (Philadelphia: University of Pennsylvania Press, 2006).
12. See John Duffy's important study, *The Sanitarians: A History of American Public Health* (Urbana: University of Illinois Press, 1990).
13. Duffy, *The Healers*, 18.

14. William Pepper, *The Medical Side of Benjamin Franklin* (Philadelphia: William J. Campbell, 1911), 9.

15. For a comprehensive review of the cause of Washington's death, see Michael L. Cheatham, "The Death of George Washington: An End to the Controversy?" *American Surgeon* 74 (August 2008): 770-74.

16. Oscar Reiss, *Medicine in Colonial America* (Lanham, MD: University Press of America, 2000), 453, estimated that in colonial America, at birth the life expectancy was thirty-two years, but if a child lived past five, his life expectancy increased to forty-seven. Herbert S. Klein, *A Population History of the United States* (New York: Cambridge University Press, 2004), 103, has estimated the life expectancy as higher for those who had survived the very common health crises of infancy, childhood, and adolescence. According to his admittedly "imperfect" data, life expectancy in the period 1750-1789 for men at twenty years of age was sixty-six. His data for women of the same age does not begin until the period 1780-1799, at which point he estimated life expectancy at about sixty-seven years of age. Klein also notes that as late as 1830-1860, life expectancy in Boston, "one of the healthiest urban centers on the Eastern Seaboard," at birth reached only to the uppers thirties. Henry A. Gemery has estimated life expectancy at birth for Harvard graduates in the eighteenth century at just 35-40 years, and for Yale graduates between the years 1701 and 1774 at 49.5. See Henry A. Gremery, "White Population, Colonial United States," in Haines and Steckel, eds., *A Population History of North America*, 163. Michael R. Haines has postulated a life expectancy at birth for both white men and white women as low as 39.5 years as late as 1850. See "The White Population of the United States, 1790-1920," in Haines and Steckel, eds., *A Population History of North America*, 308.

17. Beginning in the 1960s, Thomas McKeown, a professor of social medicine, famously postulated that the decline of tuberculosis mortality in Great Britain was primarily the result of more robust resistance due to a rise in the quality of nutrition and standard of living, rather than medical interventions. See Thomas McKeown, *The Modern Rise of Population* (London: Edward Arnold, 1976) and *The Role of Medicine: Dream, Mirage, or Nemesis* (Princeton, NJ: Princeton University Press, 1979). In "White Population," 175, Gremery has pointed out that the American colonial diet was for the most part high in nutritional levels, even across class lines.

18. Richard Shryock, *Medicine and Society in America, 1660-1860* (New York: New York University Press, 1960), 107.

19. H. Roy Merrens and George D. Terry, "Dying in Paradise: Malaria, Mortality, and the Perceptual Environment in Colonial South Carolina," *Journal of Southern History* 50 (November 1984): 541-42.

20. John Harvey Powell, *Bring Out Your Dead: The Great Plague of Yellow Fever in Philadelphia in 1793* (New York: Arno Press, 1970), 8-12, 219, 232.

21. See Michael McMahon, "Beyond Therapeutics: Technology and the Question of Public Health in Late-Eighteenth-Century Philadelphia," in J. Worth Estes

and Billy G. Smith, eds., *A Melancholy Scene of Devastation: The Public Response to the 1793 Philadelphia Yellow Fever Epidemic* (Canton, MA: Science History Publications, 1997), 97-118.

22. See Powell, *Bring Out Your Dead,* 231-34, for a detailed account of John Todd's experiences and death during the epidemic.

23. Dolley Madison to John Todd, October 1793, in Mattern and Shulman, eds., *Selected Letters of Dolley Madison,* 24-25.

24. Dolley Madison to Eliza Collins Lee, February 10, 1808, in Mattern and Shulman, eds., *Selected Letters of Dolley Madison,* 85.

25. Thomas Jefferson to John Page, August 16, 1804, as cited in William Blanton, *Medicine in Virginia in the Eighteenth Century* (Richmond, VA: Garrett and Massey, 1931), 196, and Thomas Jefferson to Count De Volney, February 8, 1805, in The Thomas Jefferson Papers, Series 1, General Correspondence, 1651-1827, http://hdl.loc.gov/loc.mss/mtj.mtjbib014337.

26. Duffy, *The Sanitarians,* 2, 11, 38-50.

27. Rudolph Marx, *The Health of the Presidents* (New York: Putnam's, 1960), 12, cites the infant mortality rate in London between 1719 and 1809 to have been 41.3 percent and speculates a similar rate in the America.

28. Shryock, *Medicine and Society in America,* 36.

29. Martha Jefferson to Fanny Bassett Washington, July 1789, in Fields, ed., "Worthy Partner," 217.

30. Patricia A. Watson, "The 'Hidden Ones': Women and Healing in Colonial New England," in *Medicine and Healing,* Dublin Seminar for New England Folklore (Boston: Boston University, 1992), 33.

31. In his controversial book, *Bad Medicine: Doctors Doing Harm since Hippocrates* (Oxford: Oxford University Press, 2006), David Wooten argues that until 1865, physicians did their patients more harm than good. He claims that vaguely described psychological and cultural factors were the main obstacles to medical progress, the result of an unholy alliance between elite trained physicians and the lay elite. However, Wooton ignores the positive accomplishments of many dedicated physicians. For example, Jenner's supporters are chastised for not warning about potential risks of smallpox vaccination, but he fails to praise them for significantly reducing smallpox mortality.

32. Eric H. Christianson, "Medicine in New England," in Judith Walzer Leavitt and Ronald L. Numbers, eds., *Sickness and Health in America: Readings in the History of Medicine and Public Health* (Madison: University of Wisconsin Press, 1997), 50-52.

33. Richard H. Shryock, *Medicine in America: Historical Essays* (Baltimore, MD: Johns Hopkins University Press, 1966), 8-9, 239.

34. M. L. Duran-Reynals, *The Fever Bark Tree: The Pageant of Quinine* (New York: Doubleday, 1946), 15.

35. As cited in Peter H. Wood, *Black Majority: Negroes in Colonial South Carolina* (New York: Knopf, 1974), 67.

36. Benjamin Rush, *The Autobiography of Benjamin Rush: His Travels through Life Together with His Commonplace Book for 1789-1813; Edited with Introduction and Notes by George W. Corner* (Princeton, NJ: Princeton University Press, 1948), 182.

37. Wood, *Black Majority*, 73.

38. John Tennett, *Every Man His Own Doctor; or, The Poor Planter's Physician* (Philadelphia: Printed and sold by Benjamin Franklin, 1751).

39. Todd L. Savitt and James Harvey Young, eds., *Disease and Distinctiveness in the American South* (Knoxville: University of Tennessee Press, 1988), 37.

40. William G. Rothstein, *American Physicians in the Nineteenth Century* (Baltimore, MD: Johns Hopkins University Press, 1972), 45-53.

41. See Arthur K. and Elaine Shapiro, *The Powerful Placebo: From Ancient Priest to Modern Physician* (Baltimore, MD: Johns Hopkins University Press, 1997). In *Bad Medicine*, 68, even Wooton acknowledges that in regard to effective modern medicine, a third of patients improve because of positive placebo effects.

42. Samuel X. Radhill, "Thomas Jefferson and the Doctors," *Transactions & Studies of the College of Physicians of Philadelphia*, fourth series, 37 (1969-1970): 107.

43. Charles E. Rosenberg, *The Cholera Years* (Chicago: University of Chicago Press, 1987), 66, 151-52.

44. Ronald L. Numbers, "The Fall and Rise of the American Medical Profession," in Walzer and Numbers, eds., *Sickness and Health in America*, 227.

45. For a concise history of bloodletting in American medicine, see John S. Haller Jr., "Decline of Bloodletting: A Study in 19th-Century Ratiocinations," *Southern Medical Journal* 79 (April 1986): 469-75.

46. Cited in Duffy, *The Healers*, 29.

47. Thomas Jefferson, *The Writings of Thomas Jefferson, Being His Autobiography, Correspondence, Reports, Messages, Addresses, and Other Writings, Official and Private* (Washington, DC: 1853-1854), 4:107, available at University of Denver Libraries, http://o-galenet.galegroup.com.bianca.penlib.du.edu/servlet/Sabin?af =RN&ae=CY105511159&srchtp=a&ste=14.

48. James C. Whorton, *Nature Cures: The History of Alternative Medicine in America* (New York: Oxford University Press, 2002), 6-10.

49. Shryock, *Medicine and Society in America*, 12.

50. Martha Ballard, a successful midwife and contemporary of Adams, Washington, and Madison, noted these accomplishments in her diary. See Laurel Thatcher Ulrich, *A Midwife's Tale: The Life of Martha Ballard, Based on Her Diary, 1785-1812* (New York: Knopf, 1990), 11.

51. Rebecca J. Tannenbaum, "Mary Hale and Ann Edmonds: Gender, Women's Work, and Health in Colonial Massachusetts," in Eric Arnesen, ed., *The Human Tradition in American Labor History* (Wilmington, DE: Scholarly Resources, 2004), 2.

52. J. Worth Estes, "George Washington and the Doctors," *Medical Heritage* 1 (January/February 1985): 46.

53. John P. Kaminski, ed., *Quotable Abigail Adams* (Cambridge, MA: Harvard University Press, 2009), 142.

54. Dorothy Porter and Roy Porter, *Patient's Progress: Doctors and Doctoring in Eighteenth-Century England* (Stanford, CA: Stanford University Press, 1989), 150.

55. For a concise description of the etiology of malaria, see Darrett B. Ruttman and Anita H. Ruttman, "Of Agues and Fevers: Malaria in the Early Chesapeake," *William and Mary Quarterly* 33 (January 1976): 31-60.

56. For a detailed description and analysis of Buchan's work, see "William Buchan's Domestic Medicine," in Charles E. Rosenberg, ed., *Explaining Epidemics and Other Studies in the History of Medicine* (New York: Cambridge University Press, 1992), 33-56.

57. Lamar Riley Murphy, *Enter the Physician: The Transformation of Domestic Medicine, 1760-1860* (Tuscaloosa: University of Alabama Press, 1991), 15.

58. Abigail Adams, diary entry, June 28, 1784, in Lyman Butterfield, ed., *Diary and Autobiography of John Adams*, 4 vols. (Cambridge, MA: Belknap Press of Harvard University Press, 1961), 3:158.

59. See Paul Starr, *Social Transformation of American Medicine* (New York: Basic Books, 1982), 32-35.

60. As cited in Shryock, *Medicine and Society in America*, 12.

61. Reiss, *Medicine in Colonial America*, 59, 63-64, 75.

62. John Duffy, *Epidemics in Colonial America* (Baton Rouge: Louisiana State University Press, 1953), 7.

63. Eric H. Christianson, "Medicine in New England," 48-49.

64. Thomas Jefferson, *The Jefferson-Dunglison Letters*, ed. John M. Dorsey (Charlottesville: University of Virginia Press, 1960), 72.

65. Robert Halsey, *How the President, Thomas Jefferson, and Doctor Benjamin Waterhouse Established Vaccination as a Public Health Procedure* (New York: privately printed, 1936), 6-7.

66. Rush, *Autobiography of Benjamin Rush*, 38.

67. William Rothstein, *American Physicians in the Nineteenth Century*, 34, 41.

68. Whitfield J. Bell Jr., *The Colonial Physician* (New York: Science History Publications, 1975), 8.

69. Rush, *Autobiography of Benjamin Rush*, 98.

70. Richard H. Shryock, "Benjamin Rush from the Perspective of the Twentieth Century," in *Medicine in America: Historical Essays* (Baltimore, MD: Johns Hopkins University Press, 1966), 237.

71. Powell, *Bring Out Your Dead*, vii.

72. Powell, *Bring Out Your Dead*, 40.

73. Ibid. Rush always claimed that his use of bleeding had saved many lives.

74. Benjamin Rush to Julia Rush, September 29, 1793, in L. H. Butterfield, ed., *Letters of Benjamin Rush* (Princeton, NJ: Princeton University Press, 1951), 2: 687.

75. Silvio A. Bedini, *Thomas Jefferson: Statesman of Science* (New York: Macmillan, 1990), 412-313, and Andrew Burstein, *Jefferson's Secrets: Death and Desire at Monticello* (New York: Basic Books, 2005), 32.

76. Rush, *Autobiography of Benjamin Rush*, 84, 106.

77. Gert H. Brieger, ed., *Medical America in the Nineteenth Century: Reading from the Literature* (Baltimore, MD: Johns Hopkins Press, 1972), 90.

78. Paul E. Kopperman, "'Venerate the Lancet': Benjamin Rush's Yellow Fever Therapy in Context," *Bulletin of the History of Medicine* 78 (Fall 2004): 558, 571.

79. David Freeman Hawke, *Benjamin Rush: Revolutionary Gadfly* (Indianapolis: Bobbs-Merrill, 1971), 113, 374.

80. Robert B. Sullivan, "Sanguine Practices: A Historical and Historiographic Reconsideration of Heroic Therapy in the Age of Rush," *Bulletin of the History of Medicine* 68 (Summer 1994): 211-34.

81. Rush, *Autobiography of Benjamin Rush*, 234.

82. Thomas Jefferson to Dr. Thomas Cooper, October 7, 1814, in Dorsey, ed., *The Jefferson-Dunglison Letters*, 105.

83. David Ramsey, "A Review of the Improvement, Progress, and State of Medicine in the Eighteenth Century, Delivered January 1, 1800," *Transactions of the American Philosophical Society* 55 (1965): 211.

84. Cited in Marx, *Health of the Presidents*, 48.

85. Thomas Jefferson to John Adams, May 27, 1813, in Lester J. Cappon, ed., *The Adams-Jefferson Letters* (New York: Simon & Schuster, 1971), 323.

86. John Adams to Thomas Jefferson, June 11, 1813, in Cappon, ed., *Adams-Jefferson Letters*, 328.

87. Shryock, *Medicine and Society*, 52, 64.

88. Elizabeth Smith Shaw Peabody to Abigail Adams, October 6, 1797, in Adams Papers, http://rotunda.upress.virginia.edu/founders/FOEA-03-01-02-1551.

89. For a lucid explanation of the technical aspects of smallpox and a fine study of its high visibility during the American Revolution, see Elizabeth A. Fenn, *Pox Americana: The Great Smallpox Epidemic of 1775-82* (New York: Hill and Wang, 2001).

90. John T. Barrett, "The Inoculation Controversy in Puritan New England," *Bulletin of the History of Medicine* 12 (1942): 169.

91. Adams, *Letters of Mrs. Adams, the Wife of John Adams*, xxiii.

92. Shryock, *Medicine and Society in America*, 56-57.

93. Cotton Mather, *A Letter about the Good Management under the Distemper of the Measles, etc.* (Boston: 1739).

94. Duffy, *Epidemics in Colonial America*, 29. For a popular account of Boston's 1721 smallpox epidemic, see Ola Elizabeth Winslow, *A Destroying Angel: The Conquest of Smallpox in Colonial Boston* (Boston: Houghton Mifflin, 1974).

95. Benjamin Franklin and William Heberden, *Some Account of the Success of Inoculation for Small-Pox in England and America* (London: William Strahan, 1759).

96. Fenn, *Pox Americana*, 3, 9.

97. James Madison to Thomas Jefferson, April 14, 1794, in James Morton Smith, ed., *The Republic of Letters: The Correspondence between Thomas Jefferson and James Madison, 1776-1826* (New York: Norton, 1995), 2:840.

98. Twelfth Congress, Chapter XXXVII, Statute II, February 27, 1813.

99. See Fiammetta Rocco, *The Miraculous Fever-Tree: Malaria and the Quest for a Cure That Changed the World* (New York: HarperCollins, 2003).

100. For a recent overview of malaria see Sonia Shah, *The Fever: How Malaria Has Ruled Humankind for 500,000 Years* (New York: Farrar, Straus, Giroux, 2010).

Chapter 1

1. Joseph J. Ellis, *His Excellency George Washington* (New York: Knopf, 2004), xiv.

2. Wyndham B. Blanton, "Washington's Medical Knowledge and Its Sources," *Annals of Medical History* 5 (1933): 54.

3. George Washington to Marquis de Lafayette, December 8, 1784, in W. W. Abbot, ed., *The Papers of George Washington: Colonial Series* (Charlottesville: University Press of Virginia, 1998-1999), 2:145-46.

4. J. Worth Estes, "George Washington and the Doctors," *Medical Heritage* 1 (January/February, 1985): 46.

5. Staff of the Mayo Clinic, "The Medical History of George Washington (1732-1799)," *Proceedings of the Mayo Clinic*, February 18, 1942, 107.

6. Harlow Giles Unger, *The Unexpected George Washington* (New York: Wiley, 2006), 12-18.

7. George Washington to Ann Fairfax Washington, c. September–November 1749, in Abbot, ed., *Papers of George Washington: Colonial Series*, 1:38.

8. Herbert S. Klein, *A Population History of the United States* (New York: Cambridge University Press, 2004), 53-57.

9. Rudolph Marx, *The Health of the Presidents* (New York: Putnam's, 1960), 19.

10. Staff of the Mayo Clinic, "The Medical History of George Washington," 92.

11. J. Worth Estes, "George Washington and the Doctors," 48.

12. George Washington to Lawrence Washington, May 4, 1749, in Abbot, ed., *Papers of George Washington: Colonial Series*, 1:38.

13. Oscar Reiss, *Medicine in Colonial America* (Lanham, MD: University Press of America, 2000), 176.

14. George Washington, *The Diaries of George Washington*, ed. Donald Jackson and Dorothy Twohig (Charlottesville: University Press of Virginia, 1976), 1:73, 82-83.

15. For an excellent account of smallpox and its pivotal effect on the American Continental Army, see Elizabeth A. Fenn, *Pox Americana: The Great Smallpox Epidemic of 1775-82* (New York: Hill and Wang, 2001).

16. George Washington to William Fauntleroy, May 20, 1752, in Abbot, ed., *Papers of George Washington: Colonial Series*, 1:49.

17. George Washington to James Innes, July 2, 1755, in Abbot, ed., *Papers of George Washington: The Colonial Series*, 1:319, 331.

18. George Washington to Mary Ball Washington, July 18, 1755, and George Washington to John Augustine Washington, July 18, 1755, in Abbot, ed., *Papers of George Washington: The Colonial Series*, 1:333-37, 343.

19. George Washington to Warner Lewis, August 14, 1755, in Saxe Commins, ed., *Basic Writings of George Washington* (New York: Random House, 1948), 41.

20. Robert Stewart to Robert Dinwiddie, October 24, 1757, in Abbot, ed., *Papers of George Washington: Colonial Series*, 5:63.

21. James Craik to George Washington, November 25, 1757, in Abbot, ed., *Papers of George Washington: Colonial Series*, 5:64.

22. Ludwig M. Deppisch, *The White House Physician: From Washington to George W. Bush* (Jefferson, NC: McFarland, 2007), 8-9.

23. Ellis, *His Excellency George Washington*, 38.

24. Ron Chernow, *Washington: A Life* (New York: Penguin, 2010), xviii.

25. For a study of Washington's often overlooked political aspirations and agenda see John Ferling, *The Ascent of George Washington: The Hidden Political Genius of an American Icon* (New York: Bloomsbury, 2009). Chernow also views Washington as a shrewd politician.

26. Estes, "George Washington and the Doctors," 47.

27. Patricia Brady, *Martha Washington: An American Life* (New York: Viking, 2005), 46.

28. Martha Washington to Anna Maria Dandridge Bassett, April 6, 1762, in Joseph E. Fields, ed., *"Worthy Partner": The Papers of Martha Washington* (Westport, CT: Greenwood Press, 1994), 147.

29. Lillian B. Miller, ed., *The Selected Papers of Charles Willson Peale and His Family* (New Haven, CT: Yale University Press, 1988), 2:695.

30. Martha Washington to Fanny Bassett Washington, February 25, 1788, in Fields, ed., *"Worthy Partner,"* 206.

31. Martha Washington to Mrs. Burwell Bassett, June 1, 1760, in Fields, ed., *"Worthy Partner,"* 129.

32. Martha Washington to Anna Maria Dandridge Bassett, April 18, 1761, in Fields, ed., *"Worthy Partner,"* 134.

33. Rebecca J. Tannenbaum, *The Healer's Calling: Women and Medicine in New England* (Ithaca, NY: Cornell University Press, 2002), 24.

34. Bill from Dr. James Carter, November 28, 1757, in Fields, ed., *"Worthy Partner,"* 15-16.

35. Tannenbaum, *The Healer's Calling*, 29.

36. Brady, *Martha Washington: An American Life*, 49-50

37. Martha Washington to John Hanbury, August 20, 1757, in Fields, ed., *"Worthy Partner,"* 6.

38. For an interesting account of domestic medicine in the early South, see Kay K. Moss, *Southern Folk Medicine, 1750-1820* (Columbia: University of South Carolina Press, 1999).

39. Patricia Brady Smith, *Nelly Custis Lewis's Housekeeping Book* (New Orleans: Historic New Orleans Collection, 1982), 127.

40. Martha Washington to Fanny Bassett Washington, June 15, 1794, in Fields, ed., *"Worthy Partner,"* 268.

41. Martha Washington to Mrs. Margaret Green, September 29, 1760, in Fields, ed., *"Worthy Partner,"* 131.

42. Washington, *The Diaries of George Washington*, 2:122-23, 128, 202.

43. Washington, *The Diaries of George Washington*, April 14, 1769, 2:141.

44. Washington, *The Diaries of George Washington,* 2:257.
45. John Johnson to Martha Washington, 21 March, 1772, in Fields, ed., *"Worthy Partner,"* 150.
46. George Washington to Burwell Bassett, June 20, 1773, in Commins, ed., *Basic Writings of George Washington,* 93.
47. George Washington to Reverend Jonathan Boucher, July 9, 1771, in Commins, ed., *Basic Writings of George Washington,* 87.
48. Washington, *Diaries of George Washington,* 11:47, 168.
49. Benson John Lossing, *Martha Washington* (New York: J.C. Buttre, 1861), 19; and Brady, *Martha Washington,* 139-40, 147.
50. Abbot, ed., *Papers of George Washington,* 7:2, 7.
51. As cited in Todd D. Savitt, *Medicine and Slavery: The Diseases and Health Care of Blacks in Antebellum Virginia* (Urbana: University of Illinois Press, 1978), 150, 162.
52. Staff of the Mayo Clinic, "The Medical History of George Washington," 93.
53. Estes, "George Washington and the Doctors," 51.
54. Invoice of Goods from Robert Cary Esqr. & Company for George Washington, July 1759, in Fields, ed., *"Worthy Partner,"* 86-91.
55. David R. Curfman, "The Medical History of the Father Our Country: General George Washington," www.founderspatriots.org/articles/gw_medical_history.htm.
56. Blanton, "Washington's Medical Knowledge and Its Sources," 54.
57. For a study of later popular resistance to enforced smallpox vaccination campaigns, see Michael Willrich, *Pox: An American History* (New York: Penguin, 2011).
58. Blanton, "Washington's Medical Knowledge and Its Sources," 57.
59. Martha Washington to Mrs. Margaret Green, June 26, 1761, in Fields, ed., *"Worthy Partner,"* 135.
60. George Washington to Andrew Burnaby, July 27, 1761, in Abbot, ed., *Papers of George Washington,* 7:59.
61. George Washington to Charles Green, August 26, 1761, in Abbot, ed., *Papers of George Washington,* 7:68.
62. George Washington to Richard Washington, October 20, 1761, in Abbot, ed., *Papers of George Washington,* 7:80.
63. Fields, ed., *"Worthy Partner,"* xxiii.
64. Carol Berkin, *Revolutionary Mothers: Women in the Struggle for America's Independence* (New York: Knopf, 2005), 43.
65. Fields, ed., *"Worthy Partner,"* xxiii.
66. George Washington, General Orders, July 4, 1775, in Commins, ed., *Basic Writings of George Washington,* 122-23.
67. George Washington to the President of Congress, July 20, 1775, in Commins, ed., *Basic Writings of George Washington,* 141.
68. Fenn, *Pox Americana,* 47-48, 50.
69. Fenn, *Pox Americana,* 78.
70. George Washington to John Augustine Washington, May 31, 1776, in Commins, ed., *Basic Writings of George Washington.*

71. John Parke Custis to Martha Washington, June 9, 1776, in Fields, ed., "*Worthy Partner,*" 168.

72. Oscar Reiss, *Medicine and the American Revolution: How Diseases and Their Treatments Affected the Colonial Army* (Jefferson, NC: McFarland, 1998), 228.

73. George Washington to William Shippen, January 6, 1777, in *Writings of George Washington*, 6:473-74.

74. John Adams to Abigail Adams, April 13, 1777, in L. H. Butterfield, ed., *Adams Family Correspondence* (Cambridge, MA; Harvard University Press, 1963-), 2:209.

75. As cited in Fenn, *Pox Americana*, 93-94.

76. Report of the Commissioners to Benjamin Franklin, 1777, in Leonard W. Larabee et al., eds., *The Papers of Benjamin Franklin* (New Haven, CT: Yale University Press, 1959-), 24:15.

77. Fenn, *Pox America*, 134, 260.

78. Sonia Shah, *The Fever: How Malaria Has Ruled Humankind for 500,000 Years* (New York: Farrar, Straus, Giroux, 2010), 90.

79. Reiss, *Medicine and the American Revolution*, 10-16.

80. George Washington, General Orders, July 14, 1775, in Commins, ed., *Basic Writings of George Washington*, 138.

81. Stanhope Bayne-Jones, *The Evolution of Preventative Medicine in the United States Army, 1607-1939* (Washington, DC: Office of the Surgeon General, 1969), 11.

82. Reiss, *Medicine and the American Revolution*, 17-20, 55-60.

83. George Washington to Marquis de Lafayette, December 8, 1784, in Abbot, ed., *Papers of George Washington*, 2:145-46.

84. Reiss, *Medicine and the American Revolution*, 230-31.

85. Chernow, *Washington: A Life*, 438-39.

86. Curfman, "The Medical History of the Father of Our Country," and Reiss, *Medicine and the American Revolution*, 231.

87. Reiss, *Medicine and the American Revolution*, 230.

88. Brady, *Martha Washington: An American Life*, 148-50.

89. Martha Washington to Fanny Bassett Washington, February 18, 1793, in Fields, ed., "*Worthy Partner,*" 244.

90. Martha Washington to Elizabeth Powell, January 18, 1788, in Fields, ed., "*Worthy Partner,*" 201.

91. For an overview on tuberculosis treatment in America, see Jeanne Abrams, "On the Road Again: Consumptives Traveling for Health in the American West, 1840-1925," *Great Plains Quarterly* 30 (Fall 2010): 271-85.

92. Martha Washington to Hannah Stockton Boudinot, January 15, 1784, in Fields, ed., "*Worthy Partner,*" 193.

93. The Staff of the Mayo Clinic, "The Medical History of George Washington," 110.

94. Diary Entry for January 10, 1787, in Dorothy Twohig, ed., *George Washington's Diaries: An Abridgement* (Charlottesville: University of Virginia Press, 1999), 313.

95. Alexander Donald to Thomas Jefferson, October 1787, in Abbot, ed., *Papers of George Washington: Confederation Series*, 5:425.

96. See Chernow, *Washington: A Life.*
97. George Washington to James Craik, September 8, 1789, in Abbot, ed., *Papers of George Washington: Presidential Series*, 4:1.
98. Benjamin Franklin to Cadwallader Colden, November 28, 1745, in Leonard W. Larabee et al., eds., *The Papers of Benjamin Franklin* (New Haven, CT: Yale University Press, 1959-), 3:49.
99. Deppisch, *The White House Physician*, 7, 9, 14-15.
100. James Madison to Thomas Jefferson, June 30, 1789, in James Morton Smith, ed., *The Republic of Letters: The Correspondence between Thomas Jefferson and James Madison* (New York: Norton, 1995), 1:622.
101. George Washington to James McHenry, July 3, 1789, in Abbot, ed., *Papers of George Washington: Presidential Series*, 3:112.
102. Thomas Jefferson to James Madison, July 24, 1791, in Smith, ed., *Republic of Letters*, 2:701.
103. George Washington to Benjamin Franklin, September 23, 1789, in Commins, ed., *Basic Writings of George Washington*, 565, 662.
104. Martha Washington to Mercy Otis Warren, December 26, 1789, in Fields, ed., *"Worthy Partner,"* 224.
105. Martha Washington to Fanny Bassett Washington, June 5, 1791, in Fields, ed., *"Worthy Partner,"* 232.
106. Martha Washington to Mr. Whitelock, April 14, 1794, in Fields, ed., *"Worthy Partner,"* 265.
107. Washington, *Diary of George Washington*, April 4, 1790, 6:56.
108. May 9, 1790, in Abbot, ed., *Papers of George Washington: Presidential Series*, 5:393.
109. George Washington to David Stuart, June 15, 1790, in Abbot, ed., *Papers of George Washington: Presidential Series*, 5:527.
110. Deppisch, *The White House Physician*, 15-16.
111. Stephen Decatur, *Private Affairs of President Washington* (Boston: Houghton Mifflin, 1933), 133.
112. Cited in James Thomas Flexner, *Washington: The Indispensable Man* (Boston: Little, Brown, 1974), 232.
113. David McCullough, *John Adams* (New York: Simon & Schuster, 2001), 423.
114. Silvio A. Bedini, *Thomas Jefferson: Statesman of Science* (New York: Macmillan, 1990), 203.
115. Martha Washington to Mercy Otis Warren, June 12, 1790, in Fields, ed., *"Worthy Partner,"* 226.
116. Cited in Chernow, *George Washington: A Life*, 581, 677.
117. Cited in Flexner, *Washington*, 288.
118. Ibid., 300.
119. Martha Washington to Fanny Bassett Washington, August 4, 1793, and Martha Washington to Elizabeth Schuler Hamilton, September 1793, in Fields, ed., *"Worthy Partner,"* 250, 253.

120. As quoted in John Harvey Powell, *Bring Out Your Dead: The Great Plague of Yellow Fever in Philadelphia in 1793* (New York: Arno, 1970), 113-16.

121. Ibid., 116-17, 277-79, 282.

122. George Washington to James Madison, October 14, 1793, in John C. Fitzpatrick, ed., *The Writings of George Washington* (Washington, DC: Government Printing Office, 1931-44), 33:125.

123. Powell, *Bring Out Your Dead*, 292-93.

124. Martha Washington to Fanny Bassett Washington, January 14, 1794, and Martha Washington to Fanny Bassett Washington, February 10, 1794, in Fields, ed., "*Worthy Partner,*" 254, 256.

125. Martha Washington to Fanny Bassett Washington, March 2, 1794, in Fields, ed., "*Worthy Partner,*" 259.

126. Martha Washington to Fanny Bassett Washington, August 3, 1794, in Fields, ed., "*Worthy Partner,*" 272.

127. Martha Washington to Fanny Bassett Washington, March 9, 1794, and Martha Washington to Fanny Bassett Washington, March 16, 1794, in Fields, ed., "*Worthy Partner,*" 261, 262.

128. Martha Washington to Fanny Bassett Washington, August 3, 1794, in Fields, ed., "*Worthy Partner,*" 272.

129. Martha Washington to Fanny Bassett Washington, September 15, 1794, and Martha Washington to Fanny Bassett Washington, September 29, 1794, in Fields, ed., "*Worthy Partner,*" 274, 276.

130. Martha Washington to Fanny Bassett Washington, June 30, 1794, and Martha Washington to Fanny Bassett Washington, July 14, 1794, in Fields, ed., "*Worthy Partner,*" 270, 271.

131. Martha Washington to Tobias Lear, March 30, 1796, in Fields, ed., "*Worthy Partner,*" 291.

132. Martha Washington to Elizabeth Dandridge Henley, November 22, 1797, and Martha Washington to T. C. Radcliffe, August 18, 1799, in Fields, ed., "*Worthy Partner,*" 308, 321.

133. Martha Washington to Mary Stillson Lear, November 11, 1800, in Fields, ed., "*Worthy Partner,*" 394.

134. "Tobias Lear's Journal Account of George Washington's Last Illness and Death," in T. J. Crankel, ed., *The Papers of George Washington*. Digital Edition. University of Virginia Press, Rotunda, 2007. Available at: http://rotunda.upress. virginia.edu. Accessed August 13, 2010.

135. White McKenzie Wallenborn, "George Washington's Terminal Illness: A Modern Medical Analysis of the Last Illness and Death of George Washington,"1999, *The Papers of George Washington*, available at http://gwpapers.virginia.edu/ articles/wallenborn.html.Accessed August 13, 2010.

136. "Tobias Lear's Account of the Death of George Washington."

137. William Pepper, *The Medical Side of Benjamin Franklin* (1910; reprint New York: Argosy-Antiquarian, 1970), 23.

138. For a detailed description of Washington's final illness and treatment, see Michael L. Cheatham, "The Death of George Washington: An End to the Controversy?" *American Surgeon* 74 (August 2008): 770-75.

139. Benjamin Rush, *The Autobiography of Benjamin Rush* (Princeton, NJ: Princeton University Press, 1948), 249.

140. Abigail Adams to Mary Cranch, December 22, 1799, in Stewart Mitchell, ed., *New Letters of Abigail Adams* (Boston: Houghton Mifflin, 1947), 222.

Chapter 2

1. Benjamin Franklin to Joseph Huey, June 6, 1753, in Leonard W. Larabee, ed., *The Papers of Benjamin Franklin* (New Haven, CT: Yale University Press, 1961), 4:504-6.

2. Whitefield J. Bell Jr., "Medicine in Boston and Philadelphia: Comparisons and Contrasts, 1750-1820," in *Medicine in Massachusetts, 1620 -1820* (Boston: Colonial Society of Massachusetts, 1980), 164.

3. John Duffy, *The Sanitarians: A History of American Public Health* (Urbana: University of Illinois Press, 1990), 159.

4. Benjamin Franklin to Abiah Franklin, 1750, in Larabee, ed., *Papers of Benjamin Franklin*, 3:475.

5. Joyce E. Chaplin, *The First Scientific American: Benjamin Franklin and the Pursuit of Genius* (New York: Basic Books, 2006).

6. Stanley Finger, *Doctor Franklin's Medicine* (Philadelphia: University of Pennsylvania Press, 2006), 9.

7. Walter Isaacson, *Benjamin Franklin: An American Life* (New York: Simon & Schuster, 2003), 3, 102.

8. Benjamin Franklin, *Autobiography and Other Writings*, edited with an introduction and notes by Russel B. Nye (Boston: Houghton Mifflin, 1958), 20.

9. William Pepper, *The Medical Side of Benjamin Franklin* (1910; reprint New York: Argosy-Antiquarian, 1970), 3, 6.

10. Benjamin Franklin, *Autobiography*, 20.

11. Benjamin Franklin, *Autobiography,* 47.

12. John Duffy, *The Healers: A History of American Medicine* (Urbana: University of Illinois Press, 1979), 12.

13. Donald R. Hopkins, *Princes and Peasants: Smallpox in History* (Chicago: University of Chicago Press, 1983).

14. Judith Walzer Leavitt, "'Be Safe. Be Sure': New York City's Experience with Epidemic Smallpox," in Judith Walzer Leavitt and Ronald L. Numbers, eds., *Sickness and Health in America: Readings in the History of Medicine and Public Health* (Madison: University of Wisconsin Press, 1997), 409-12.

15. Benjamin Franklin to Jane Mecom, June 19, 1731, in Nathan G. Goodman, ed., *A Benjamin Franklin Reader* (New York: Crowell, 1945), 541.

16. Benjamin Franklin, *Autobiography*, 93.

17. H. W. Brands, *The First American* (New York: Doubleday, 2000), 456.

18. Whitfield J. Bell, "Benjamin Franklin and the Practice of Medicine," in *The Colonial Physician* (New York: Science History Publications, 1975), 121.

19. Benjamin Franklin and William Heberden, *Some Account of the Success of Inoculation for the Small-Pox in England and America* (London: William Strahan, 1749), 4.

20. Elizabeth A. Fenn, *Pox Americana: The Great Smallpox Epidemic of 1775-82* (New York: Hill and Wang, 2001), 41, 83.

21. David Freeman Hawke, *Benjamin Rush: Revolutionary Gadfly* (Indianapolis: Bobbs-Merrill, 1971), 83.

22. See Robert Hunter, "Benjamin Franklin and the Rise of Free Treatment of the Poor by the Medical Profession of Philadelphia," *Bulletin of the History of Medicine* 31 (1957): 137-46.

23. Benjamin Franklin, *Autobiography*, 110.

24. Benjamin Franklin to Cadwallader Evans, May 5, 1767, in Pepper, *The Medical Side of Benjamin Franklin*, 45.

25. Benjamin Franklin, "Appeal for the Hospital," *Pennsylvania Gazette*, August 15, 1751.

26. Benjamin Franklin, *Some Account of the Pennsylvania Hospital* (Philadelphia: Printed by Benjamin Franklin, 1754).

27. Benjamin Franklin to Josiah and Abiah Franklin, September 6, 1744, in Larabee, ed., *Papers of Benjamin Franklin*, 2:413.

28. Benjamin Franklin to Deborah Franklin, March 21, 1756, in Larabee, ed., *Papers of Benjamin Franklin*, 6:425.

29. Benjamin Franklin to Abiah Franklin, October 16, 1747, in Larabee, ed., *Papers of Benjamin Franklin*, 3:179.

30. Benjamin Franklin to Richard Jackson, June 1, 1764, in Larabee, ed., *Papers of Benjamin Franklin*, 11:216.

31. Benjamin Franklin to Benjamin Rush, July 14, 1773, in William B. Wilcox, ed., *Papers of Benjamin Franklin* (New Haven, CT: Yale University Press, 1959-), 20:315.

32. See Barbara B. Olberg, ed., *The Papers of Benjamin Franklin* (New Haven, CT: Yale University Press, 2000), 35:283-85.

33. Benjamin Franklin to Jane Mecom, June 19, 1731, in Goodman, ed., *A Benjamin Franklin Reader*, 541.

34. Benjamin Franklin to Cadwallader Colden, April 23, 1752, in Larabee, ed., *Papers of Benjamin Franklin*, 4:301.

35. John Duffy, *The Sanitarians: A History of Public Health* (Urbana: University of Illinois Press, 1990), 21-22.

36. Benjamin Franklin to Cadwallader Colden, November 28, 1745, in Larabee, ed., *Papers of Benjamin Franklin*, 3:46-49.

37. Benjamin Franklin, *Poor Richard: The Almanacks for the Years 1733-1758 by Richard Sanders* (New York: Heritage Press, 1964).

38. *Pennsylvania Gazette*, May 14, 1730.

39. Benjamin Franklin, "Introduction to John Pringle's Account of Gaol Fever," *Pennsylvania Gazette*, September 4, 1755.

40. Benjamin Franklin, *Autobiography*, 89.

41. Thomas A. Horrocks, *Popular Print and Popular Medicine: Almanacs and Health Advice in Early America* (Amherst: University of Massachusetts Press, 2008), 7, 11.

42. Benjamin Franklin, Afterword to John Tennent, *Every Man His Own Doctor; or, The Poor Planter's Physician*, 4th ed. (Philadelphia: Printed and sold by B. Franklin, 1736).

43. Benjamin Franklin, *Poor Richard: The Almanacks for the Years 1733-1758*.

44. Benjamin Franklin to Barbeau Duboung, 1773? in Goodman, ed., *A Benjamin Franklin Reader*, 532.

45. Benjamin Franklin to Samuel Johnson, September 13, 1750, in Larabee, ed., *Papers of Benjamin Franklin*, 4:63.

46. Benjamin Franklin, *Poor Richard Improved* (Philadelphia: Printed and sold by B. Franklin and D. Hall, 1749).

47. Benjamin Franklin to Samuel Johnson, September 13, 1750, in Larabee, ed., *Papers of Benjamin Franklin*, 4:63.

48. L. H. Butterfield et al., eds., *Diary and Autobiography of John Adams* (Cambridge, MA: Harvard University Press, 1961), 3:418.

49. Benjamin Franklin to Jean-Baptiste LeRoy, June 22, 1773, in Wilcox, ed., *Papers of Benjamin Franklin*, 20:241-42.

50. Benjamin Franklin to Jaques Barbeu Dubourg, July 28, 1768, in Nathan, ed., *A Benjamin Franklin Reader*, 545.

51. Bell, "Benjamin Franklin and the Practice of Medicine," 122-23.

52. Ibid., 124.

53. Ibid., 125-26.

54. Edward J. Huth, "Benjamin Franklin's Place in the History of Medicine," James Lind Library, www.jameslindlibrary.org, 3.

55. See Sherry Ann Beaudreau and Stanley Finger, "Franklin and the Revolutionary Body," in Jack Lynch, ed., *Critical Insights: Benjamin Franklin* (Pasadena, CA: Salem Press, 2010), 95-114.

56. "Using Electricity, Magnets for Mental Illness," *Wall Street Journal*, January 11, 2011, D3; and "Wiring the Brain, Literally, to Treat Stubborn Disorders," *Wall Street Journal*, January 17, 2012, D1.

57. Benjamin Franklin to John Franklin, December 8, 1752, in Goodman, ed., *A Benjamin Franklin Reader*, 542-43.

58. Benjamin Franklin to George Whately, May 23, 1785, in Goodman, ed., *A Benjamin Franklin Reader*, 553.

59. Benjamin Franklin to Jane Mecom, July 17, 1771, in Goodman, ed., *A Benjamin Franklin Reader*, 546-57.

60. Benjamin Franklin, "Proposals Relating to the Education of Youth in Pennsylvania," 1749, *Papers of Benjamin Franklin* (New Haven, CT: Yale University Press, 1961), 3:402.

61. Benjamin Franklin to William Franklin, August 19, 1772, in Goodman, ed., *A Benjamin Franklin Reader*, 548.

62. Gordon S. Woods, *The Americanization of Benjamin Franklin* (New York: Penguin, 2004), 12-13.

63. J. A. Leo Lemay, "The Life of Benjamin Franklin," in Page Talbott, ed., *Benjamin Franklin: In Search of a Better World*, (New Haven, CT: Yale University Press, 2005), 51.

64. Claude-Anne Lopez, *Mon Cher Papa* (New Haven, CT: Yale University Press, 1990), 1, 20-24.

65. Franklin's Description of his Ailments, October 1, 1777 through February 28, 1778, *The Papers of Benjamin Franklin* (New Haven, CT: Yale University Press, 1986), 25:77-80.

66. Benjamin Franklin to Jane Mecom, April 22, 1779, in Goodman, ed., *A Benjamin Franklin Reader*, 654.

67. Franklin's Journal of His Health, October 4, 1778[-January 16, 1780] , *The Papers of Benjamin Franklin*, 27:496-99.

68. John Fothergill to Benjamin Franklin, October 25, 1780, in Barbara B. Oberg, ed., *The Papers of Benjamin Franklin* (New Haven, CT: Yale University Press, 1959–), 35:458-61.

69. Benjamin Franklin, *The Writings of Benjamin Franklin; Collected and Ed. with a Life and Introduction, by Albert Henry Smyth* (New York: Macmillan, 1905), 113-14.

70. Benjamin Franklin to Vicq d' Azyr, July 20[-24], 1781, in Oberg, ed., *Papers of Benjamin Franklin*, 35:293-94.

71. Benjamin Franklin to Thomas Bond, February 5, 1772, in Pepper, *The Medical Side of Benjamin Franklin*, 55.

72. Pepper, *The Medical Side of Benjamin Franklin*, 6.

73. Benjamin Franklin to *La Sabliere de la Condamine*, March 19, 1784, in Goodman, ed., *A Benjamin Franklin Reader*, 552.

74. Benjamin Franklin, et al., "Report of Dr. Benjamin Franklin, and Other Commissioners," reprinted in Maurice M. Tinterow, *Foundations of Hypnotism* (Springfield, IL: Charles C. Thomas, 1970).

75. Benjamin Franklin to the Speaker and Committee of Correspondence of the Pennsylvania Assembly, August 22, 1766, 383, and Benjamin Franklin to Stephen Crane, February 6, 1772, in Larabee, ed., *Papers of Benjamin Franklin*, 13:383 and 19:67.

76. Benjamin Franklin to Deborah Franklin, November 22, 1757, in Larabee, ed., *Papers of Benjamin Franklin*, 7:272-74.

77. Benjamin Franklin to Deborah Franklin, July 4, 1771, in William B. Wilcox, ed., *Papers of Benjamin Franklin* (New Haven, CT: Yale University Press, 1959–), 18:161.

78. Benjamin Franklin to John Fothergill, [1757?], in Larabee, ed., *Papers of Benjamin Franklin*, 7:173.

79. Benjamin Franklin to John Fothergill, [October 1757?], and Benjamin Franklin to Deborah Franklin, February 21, 1760, and March 18, 1760, in Larabee, ed., *Papers of Benjamin Franklin*, 7:271 and 9:25, 35-36.

80. Benjamin Franklin to Deborah Franklin, May 11, 1765, in Larabee, ed., *Papers of Benjamin Franklin*, 12:127.

81. Benjamin Franklin to Deborah Franklin, February 13, 1768, in Wilcox, ed., *Papers of Benjamin Franklin*, 15:45-46.

82. Benjamin Franklin to Deborah Franklin, October 5, 1768, in Wilcox, ed., *Papers of Benjamin Franklin*, 15:223.

83. Benjamin Franklin to Deborah Franklin, June 10, 1770, in Wilcox, ed., *Papers of Benjamin Franklin*, 17:166-67.

84. Benjamin Franklin to Deborah Franklin, August 22, 1772, in Wilcox, ed., *Papers of Benjamin Franklin*, 19:274-75.

85. Benjamin Franklin, "Dialogue between Franklin and the Gout," October 22, 1780, in Goodman, ed., *A Benjamin Franklin Reader*, 731-37.

86. Benjamin Franklin to Alexander Small, July 22, 1780, in Goodman, ed., *A Benjamin Franklin Reader*, 551.

87. Benjamin Franklin to John Temple, July 15, 1781, in Oberg, ed., *Papers of Benjamin Franklin*, 35:270.

88. Benjamin Franklin to George Whatley, May 23, 1785, www.franklinpapers.org.

89. John Adams to Benjamin Franklin, October 22, 1781, in Oberg, ed., *Papers of Benjamin Franklin*, 35:630.

90. Margaret A. Hogan and C. James Taylor, eds., *My Dearest Friend: Letters of Abigail and John Adams* (Cambridge, MA: Belknap Press of Harvard University Press, 2007), 265.

91. Butterfield et al., eds., *Diary and Autobiography of John Adams*, 3:26, 38.

92. Abigail Adams to Mary Cranch, December 9, 1784, in *Abigail Adams: Letters of Mrs. Adams, the Wife of John Adams; With an Introductory Memoir by Her Grandson, Charles Francis Adams* (Boston: Wilkins, Carter, 1848), 216.

93. Benjamin Franklin to Mary Stevenson Hewson, September 7, 1783, www.franklinpapers.org.

94. Benjamin Franklin to Comte De Vergennes, December 6, 1783, in Pepper, *The Medical Side of Benjamin Franklin*, 98.

95. Andrea-Holger Maehle, *Drugs on Trial: Experimental Pharmacology and Therapeutic Innovation in the Eighteenth Century* (Atlanta, GA: Rodopi-B.V., 1999), 55, 104-7.

96. Benjamin Franklin to John Jay, January 6, 1784, in Goodman, ed., *A Benjamin Franklin Reader*, 26-27.

97. Quoted in Claude-Anne Lopez, *Mon Cher Papa*, 9.

98. Thomas Jefferson to John Adams, November 23, 1819, in Lester J. Cappon, ed., *The Adams-Jefferson Letters* (New York: Simon & Schuster, 1959), 548.

99. Silvio A. Bedini, *Thomas Jefferson: Statesman of Science* (New York: Macmillan, 1990), 126.

100. Benjamin Franklin, "Case History of Stone with Medical Opinions," July 18, 22, 1785, www.franklinpapers.org.

101. Benjamin Franklin to Jan Ingenhousz, August 28, 1785, www.franklinpapers.org.

102. Benjamin Franklin, Diary, 1785, www.franklinpapers.org.

103. Benjamin Franklin, "The Art of Procuring Pleasant Dreams," 1786, in Goodman, ed., *A Benjamin Franklin Reader*, 556-58.

104. Benjamin Rush's diary entries for August 1786 and November 1786, quoted in Benjamin Franklin, *The Writings of Benjamin Franklin*, 116-17.
105. Benjamin Franklin to Benjamin Vaughan, July 31, 1786, in Goodman, ed., *A Benjamin Franklin Reader*, 554-56.
106. Benjamin Franklin to Jonathan Shipley, February 24, 1786, in Goodman, ed., *A Benjamin Franklin Reader*, 30.
107. Benjamin Franklin to Louis-Guillaume le Veillard, April 15, 1787, quoted in Isaacson, *Benjamin Franklin*, 439-40.
108. Isaacson, *Benjamin Franklin*, 446.
109. Benjamin Franklin to Marianne-Marie-Jeanne-Francoise Camasse, July 13, 1787, www.franklinpapers.org.
110. Bell, "Benjamin Franklin and the Practice of Medicine," 129.
111. Benjamin Franklin to Louis-Guillaume le Veillard, September 5, 1789, in Goodman, ed., *A Benjamin Franklin Reader*, 34.
112. Benjamin Franklin to Benjamin Vaughn, November, 1789, in Goodman, ed., *A Benjamin Franklin Reader*, 34.
113. George Washington to Benjamin Franklin, September 23, 1789, in Saxe Commins, *Basic Writings of George Washington* (New York: Random House, 1948), 564-65.
114. Benjamin Franklin to Catherine Ray Greene, March 2, 1789, www.franklinpapers.org.
115. Benjamin Franklin to Elizabeth Partridge, November 25, 1788, www.franklinpapers.org.
116. Thomas Jefferson to Madame d' Houdetot, April 2, 1790, in Julian P. Boyd, ed., *The Papers of Thomas Jefferson* (Princeton, NJ: Princeton University Press, 1943-), 16:292.
117. Sarah Randolph, *The Domestic Life of Thomas Jefferson* (New York: Ungar, 1958), 173.
118. Ibid., 179.
119. Benjamin Rush, *The Autobiography of Benjamin Rush* (Princeton, NJ: Princeton University Press, 1948), 182.
120. L. H. Butterfield, et al., eds., *Diary and Autobiography of John Adams* (Cambridge, MA: Harvard University Press, 1961), 3:419.
121. Stanley Finger and Ian S. Hegeman, "Benjamin Franklin's Risk Factors for Gout and Stones: From Genes and Diet to Possible Lead Poisoning," *Proceedings of the American Philosophical Society* 152 (June 2008): 189-207.
122. *The Pennsylvania Gazette*, April 21, 1790.
123. Ibid.
124. Bell, "Benjamin Franklin and the Practice of Medicine," 119.
125. I. Bernard Cohen, *Science and the Founding Fathers* (New York: Norton, 1995), 136.
126. Finger, *Dr. Franklin's Medicine*, 3.

Chapter 3

1. Woody Holton, *Abigail Adams* (New York: Free Press, 2009), 4, 7. John P. Kaminski, ed., *The Quotable Abigail Adams* (Cambridge, MA: Belknap Press of Harvard University Press, 2009), introduction, provides a very helpful, concise summary of the life of Abigail Adams.

2. John Duffy, *Epidemics in Colonial America* (Baton Rouge: Louisiana State University Press, 1953), 125.

3. For an insightful description of the role of wives in colonial New England, see Laurel Thatcher Ulrich, *Good Wives: Image and Reality in the Lives of Women in Northern New England, 1650-1970* (New York: Knopf, 1982).

4. Charles Francis Adams, the grandson of John and Abigail Adams, provided invaluable information about Abigail and John's early life in his memoir. See Abigail Adams, *Letters of Mrs. Adams, the Wife of John Adams: With an Introductory Memoir by Her Grandson, Charles Francis Adams* (Boston: Wilkins, Carter, 1848).

5. Joseph J. Ellis, *First Family: Abigail and John* (New York: Knopf, 2010), 12.

6. Abigail Smith to John Adams, April 8, 1764, in L. H. Butterfield, Marc Friedlander, Mary-Jo Kline, eds., *The Book of Abigail and John: Selected Letters of the Adams Family, 1762-1784* (Cambridge, MA: Harvard University Press, 1975), 25.

7. Abigail Smith to John Adams, April 7, 1764, and John Adams to Abigail Smith, April 7, 1764, in Margaret A. Hogan and C. James Taylor, eds., *My Dearest Friend: Letters of Abigail and John Adams* (Cambridge, MA: Belknap Press of Harvard University Press, 2007), 8, 9.

8. L. H. Butterfield, ed., *Diary and Autobiography of John Adams,* 4 vols. (Cambridge, MA: Belknap Press of Harvard University Press, 1961), 3:276.

9. Ibid., 280.

10. John Duffy, *The Healers: A History of American Medicine* (Urbana: University of Illinois Press, 1979), 38.

11. Catherine Drinker Bower, *John Adams and the American Revolution* (New York: Grosset & Dunlap, 1950), 621-22.

12. Letter from John Adams to Abigail Smith, 13 April 1764, *Adams Family Papers: An Electric Archive.* Massachusetts Historical Society, http://www.masshist.org./digitaladams.

13. Ibid.

14. John Adams to Abigail Smith, April 30, 1764, in L. H. Butterfield, ed., *Adams Family Correspondence* (Cambridge, MA: Harvard University Press, 1963-), 1:41.

15. Butterfield, ed., *Diary and Autobiography of John Adams,* 257.

16. Rudolph Marx, *The Health of the Presidents* (New York: Putnam's, 1960), 30.

17. Meribeth Meixner Reed, "Describing the Life Cycle of U.S. Marine Hospital #17, Port Townsend, Washington, 1855-1933," *Military Medicine* 170 (April 2005): 260.

18. I. Bernard Cohen, *Science and the Founding Fathers* (New York: Norton, 1995), 196.

19. Adams, *The Letters of Mrs. Adams,* xxx.

20. Butterfield, ed., *Diary and Autobiography of John Adams,* 2:37, 3:296.

21. John Adams to Isaac Smith, April 11, 1771, in Butterfield, ed., *Adams Family Correspondence,* 1:75.

22. For a detailed analysis of Adams's possible thyroid condition, see John Ferling and Lewis E. Braverman, "John Adams's Health Reconsidered," *William and Mary Quarterly* 55 (January 1998): 83-104.

23. Kaminski, ed., *The Quotable Abigail Adams*, introduction.
24. Cited in Drew R. McCoy, *The Elusive Republic: Political Economy in Jeffersonian America* (Chapel Hill: University of North Carolina Press, 1980), 69.
25. For an interesting perspective on the marriage partnership of John and Abigail Adams, see a review by Gordon S. Wood, "Pursuit of Happiness," *New Republic Online*, April 8, 2004.
26. Abigail Adams to John Adams, October 21, 1775, in Butterfield, ed., *Adams Family Correspondence*, 1:308.
27. For a fine analysis of Abigail Adams's literary talents, see Edith B. Gelles, *Abigail Adams: A Writing Life* (New York: Routledge, 2002).
28. Benjamin Rush, *The Autobiography of Benjamin Rush* (Princeton, NJ: Princeton University Press, 1948), 144.
29. Henry Colman, A *Sketch of the Character of John Adams: Delivered in the Church in Barton Square, Salem, 9th June, 1826, the Lord's Day, after His Interment* (Salem, MA: 1826), 17.
30. Abigail Adams to John Adams, October 22, 1775, in Hogan and Taylor, eds., *My Dearest Friend*, 86.
31. Paul C. Nagel, *The Adams Women: Abigail and Louisa Adams, Their Sisters and Daughters* (New York: Oxford University Press, 1987), 19.
32. Paul Starr, *The Social Transformation of American Medicine* (New York: Basic Books, 1982), 32, 48.
33. Rebecca J. Tannenbaum, "'What Is Best to Be Done for These Fevers': Elizabeth Davenport's Medical Practice in New Haven Colony," *New England Quarterly* 70 (June 1997): 278.
34. Joan R. Gundersen, *To Be Useful to the World: Women in Revolutionary America, 1740-1790* (New York: Twayne, 1996), 55.
35. Laurel Thatcher Ulrich, "Martha Moore Ballard and the Medical Challenge to Midwifery," in Judith Walzer Leavitt and Ronald L. Numbers, eds., *Sickness and Health in America: Readings in the History of Medicine and Public Health* (Madison: University Press of Wisconsin, 1997), 72.
36. Ulrich, *Good Wives*, 134.
37. Gundersen, *To Be Useful to the World*, 56-57.
38. Lauren Thatcher Ulrich, *A Midwife's Tale: The Life of Martha Ballard, Based on Her Diary, 1785-1812* (New York: Knopf, 1990), 173-74.
39. See Judith Walzer Leavitt, "Science Enters the Birthing Room: Obstetrics in American since the Eighteenth Century," *Journal of American History* 70 (September 1983): 281-304.
40. John Adams to Abigail Adams, May 12, 1774, in Butterfield et al., eds., *The Book of Abigail and John*, 54-55.
41. Abigail Adams to John Adams, September 14, 1774, in Hogan and Taylor, eds., *My Dearest Friend*, 43.
42. Abigail Adams to John Adams, June 16, 1775, in Hogan and Taylor, eds., *My Dearest Friend*, 60-61.

43. John Adams to Abigail Adams, July 7, 1775, in Hogan and Taylor, eds., *My Dearest Friend*, 71.
44. As cited in Ferling and Braverman, "John Adams's Health Reconsidered," 87-88.
45. Ferling and Braverman, "John Adams's Health Reconsidered," 88, 89. According to the authors, "today patients suffering from many of the symptoms experienced by Adams would be evaluated for hyperthyroidism" (91).
46. Abigail Adams to John Adams, September 8, 1775, in Butterfield, ed., *Adams Family Correspondence*, 1:276.
47. Ibid.
48. Abigail Adams to John Adams, September 16, 1775, in Butterfield, ed., *Adams Family Correspondence*,1:278-79.
49. Abigail Adams to John Adams, September 10, 1775, in Hogan and Taylor, eds., *My Dearest Friend*, 75.
50. Abigail Adams to Mary Cranch, April 21, 1790, in Stewart Mitchell, ed., *New Letters of Abigail Adams, 1788-1801* (Boston: Houghton Mifflin, 1947), 45.
51. Nagel, *The Adams Women*, 59.
52. Abigail Adams to John Adams, October 1, 1775, in Hogan and Taylor, eds., *My Dearest Friend*, 77.
53. Abigail Adams to John Adams, October 1775, in *Letters of Mrs. Adams*, xxxvii.
54. John Adams to Abigail Adams, October 13, 1775, in Hogan and Taylor, eds., *My Dearest Friend*, 81.
55. Abigail Adams to John Adams, November 27, 1775, in Hogan and Taylor, eds., *My Dearest Friend*, 88-89.
56. Joseph J. Ellis, *American Sphinx: The Character of Thomas Jefferson* (New York: Knopf, 1997), 37.
57. Letter from Abigail Adams to John Adams, 31 March–5 April 1776 (electronic edition), *Adams Family Papers*.
58. Letter from Abigail Adams to John Adams, 21 April 1776 and 7-9 May 1776 (electronic edition), *Adams Family Papers*.
59. Letters from Abigail Adams to John Adams, 2-10 March 1776 (electronic edition), *Adams Family Papers*.
60. John Adams to Abigail Adams, June 26, 1776, in Butterfield et al., eds., *Book of Abigail and John*, 137-38.
61. John Adams to Colonel Hitchcock, October 1, 1776, in Butterfield, ed., *Diary and Autobiography of John Adams*, 442.
62. Abigail Adams to John Adams, July 13, 1776, in Hogan and Taylor, eds., *My Dearest Friend*, 128.
63. Abigail Adams to John Adams, July 14, 1776, in Hogan and Taylor, eds., *My Dearest Friend*, 130.
64. John Adams to Abigail Adams, July 27, 1776, in Butterfield, ed., *Adams Family Correspondence*, 2:63.
65. John Adams to James Warren, July 25, 1776, as cited in David G. McCullough, *John Adams* (New York: Simon & Schuster, 2001), 144.

66. Abigail Adams to John Adams, July 21, 1776, in Hogan and Taylor, eds., *My Dearest Friend*, 132.
67. Abigail Adams to John Adams, August 1, 1776, Butterfield, ed., *Adams Family Correspondence*, 2:72.
68. Joyce D. Goodfriend, "New York City in 1772: The Journal of Solomon Drowne, Junior," *New York History* 82 (Winter 2001): 43, 51.
69. Abigail Adams to John Adams, August 14, 1776, in Hogan and Taylor, eds., *My Dearest Friend*, 139.
70. Ibid., 141.
71. Abigail Adams to John Adams, September 7, 1776, in Hogan and Taylor, eds., *My Dearest Friend*, 150-51.
72. Abigail Adams to John Adams, July 9, 1777, in Hogan and Taylor, eds., *My Dearest Friend*, 186.
73. John Adams to Abigail Adams, July 10, 1777, in Hogan and Taylor, eds., *My Dearest Friend*, 188.
74. Abigail Adams to John Adams, July 16, 1777, Butterfield, ed., *Adams Family Correspondence*, 2:282.
75. John Adams to Abigail Adams, July 28, 1777, in Hogan and Taylor, eds., *My Dearest Friend*, 190.
76. Abigail Adams to John Adams, August 5, 1777, in Butterfield, ed., *Adams Family Correspondence*, 2:301.
77. John Adams to Abigail Adams, September 30, 1777, in Butterfield, ed., *Adams Family Correspondence*, 2:350.
78. Abigail Adams to Thomas Jefferson, May 20, 1804, in Lester J. Cappon, ed., *The Adams-Jefferson Papers* (New York: Simon & Schuster, 1971), 169.
79. John Adams to Abigail Adams, December 2, 1781, in Hogan and Taylor, eds., *My Dearest Friend*, 252.
80. Ferling and Braverman, "John Adams's Health Reconsidered," 93, 99.
81. John Adams to Abigail Adams, October 9, 1781, in Butterfield et al., eds., *The Book of Abigail and John*, 298.
82. Cited in David McCullough, *John Adams*, 265-66.
83. Benjamin Franklin to John Adams, October 5, 1781, and Benjamin Franklin to John Adams, October 12[-16], 1781, in Barbara B. Oberg, ed., *The Papers of Benjamin Franklin* (New Haven, CT: Yale University Press, 2000), 35:565, 583.
84. John Adams to Benjamin Franklin, October 22, 1781, in Oberg, ed., *Papers of Benjamin Franklin*, 35:630, 632.
85. John Adams to Abigail Adams, October 14, 1783, in Richard Alay Ryerson et al., eds., *Adams Family Correspondence* (Cambridge, MA: Harvard University Press, 1963–), 5:255.
86. Abigail Adams to John Adams, October 19, 1783, in Ryerson et al., eds., *Adams Family Correspondence*, 5:257.
87. Abigail Adams to John Adams, May 25, 1784, in Ryerson, et al., eds., *Adams Family Correspondence*, 5:292.

88. "Abigail Adams' Diary of Her Voyage," in Butterfield, ed., *Diary and Autobiography of John Adams*, 155.
89. Abigail Adams to Mary Cranch, July 6, 1784, and Abigail Adams to Mary Cranch, July 20, 1784, in *Letters of Mrs. Adams*, 157-58, 168.
90. Abigail Adams to Mercy Warren, September 5, 1784, in *Letters of Mrs. Adams*, 200-206, and Abigail Adams to Mary Cranch, December 9, 1784, 213, 214.
91. Abigail Adams to Mary Cranch, May 8, 1785, in *Letters of Mrs. Adams*, 248.
92. Abigail Adams to Elizabeth Shaw, December 14, 1784, in Kaminski, ed. *The Quotable Abigail Adams, 143* and Abigail Adams to Mary Smith Cranch, April 24, 1786, in Margaret A. Hogan et al., eds., *Adams Family Correspondence*, vols. 7-9 (Cambridge, MA: Harvard University Press, 1963-), 7:147.
93. Abigail Adams to Elizabeth Smith Shaw, December 14, 1784, in Ryerson, ed., *Adams Family Correspondence*, 6:29.
94. Abigail Adams to Elizabeth Shaw, December 14, 1784, and Abigail Adams to John Quincy Adams, January 17, 1787, in Kaminski, ed., *The Quotable Abigail Adams*, 139.
95. Abigail Adams to John Adams, December 30, 1786, in Hogan et al., eds., *Adams Family Correspondence*, 7:414.
96. Abigail Adams to John Quincy Adams, November 28, 1786, in Kaminski, ed., *The Quotable Abigail Adams*, 139.
97. Abigail Adams to John Quincy Adams, October 12, 1787, *Letters of Mrs. Adams*, 341.
98. Kaminski, ed., *The Quotable Abigail Adams*, 142.
99. Abigail Adams to John Quincy Adams, January 17, 1787, in Kaminski, ed., *The Quotable Abigail Adams*, 137.
100. Abigail Adams to Mary Cranch, July 9, 1798, in Mitchell, ed., *New Letters of Abigail Adams*, 201.
101. Abigail Adams to Thomas Boylston Adams, January 2, 1801, and Abigail Adams to Susanna B. Adams, May 5, 1817, in Kaminski, ed., *The Quotable Abigail Adams*, 138.
102. John Adams to Abigail Adams, June 6, 1789 (electronic edition), *Adams Family Papers*.
103. Abigail Adams to John Adams, October 20, 1789, and John Adams to Abigail Adams, November , 1789, in Hogan and Taylor, eds., *My Dearest Friend*, 330-31.
104. Abigail Adams to Mary Cranch, March 15, 1790, in Mitchell, ed., *New Letters of Abigail Adams*, 41.
105. Abigail Adams to Mary Cranch, April 28, 1790, in Mitchell, ed., *New Letters of Abigail Adams*, 46.
106. Abigail Adams to Mary Cranch, May 30, 1790, in Mitchell, ed., *New Letters of Abigail Adams*, 49.
107. Abigail Adams to Mary Cranch, June 9, 1790, in Mitchell, ed., *New Letters of Abigail Adams*, 50.
108. Abigail Adams to Mary Cranch, October 25, 1790, in Mitchell, ed., *New Letters of Abigail Adams*, 63.

109. Abigail Adams to Nabby Smith, November 28, 1790, and December 26, 1790, *Letters of Mrs. Adams*, 350.

110. Abigail Adams to Mary Cranch, March 20, 1792, and Abigail Adams to Mary Cranch, February 21, 1798, in Mitchell, ed., *New Letters of Abigail Adams*, 78, 134.

111. Holton, *Abigail Adams*, 284-85.

112. John Adams to Abigail Adams Smith, March 10, 1792, in Hogan et al., eds., *Adams Family Correspondence*, 9:268.

113. John Adams to Abigail Adams, January 22, 1794, in Hogan and Taylor, eds., *My Dearest Friend*, 351.

114. Abigail Adams to John Adams, June 10, 1795, in Hogan and Taylor, eds., *My Dearest Friend*, 187.

115. Abigail Adams to Thomas B. Adams, November 8, 1796, in *Letters of Mrs. Adams*, 373.

116. John Adams to John Quincy Adams, April 26, 1795, cited in Ellis, *First Family*, 157.

117. John Adams to Abigail Adams, February 17, 1794, in Hogan and Taylor, eds., *My Dearest Friend*, 360.

118. Abigail Adams to John Adams, February 26, 1794, cited in Ellis, *First Family*, 158.

119. John Adams to Abigail Adams, March 27, 1797, in Hogan and Taylor, eds., *My Dearest Friend*, 443.

120. John Adams to Abigail Adams, April 11, 1777, in John Adams, *Letters of John Adams Addressed to His Wife*, vol. 1 (Boston: Little, Brown, 1841), 209.

121. Reed, "Describing the Life Cycle of U.S. Marine Hospital #17," 260.

122. "Boston Marine Society History," www.bostonmarinesociety.org.

123. John Adams to George Washington, October 9, 1798, as quoted in Edith B. Gelles, *Abigail and John: Portrait of a Marriage* (New York: Morrow, 2009), 254.

124. John Ferling and Lewis E. Braverman, "John Adams's Health Reconsidered," 103.

125. John Adams to Abigail Adams, November 19, 1798, in Hogan and Taylor, eds., *My Dearest Friend*, 375.

126. John Adams to Abigail Adams, December 25, 1798 (electronic edition), *Adams Family Papers*.

127. Abigail Adams to William Smith Shaw, January 3, 1799, in Kaminski, ed., *The Quotable Abigail Adams*, 140.

128. Abigail Adams, November 10, 1800, in Mitchell, ed., *New Letters of Abigail Adams*, 255.

129. John Adams to Thomas Jefferson, March 24, 1801, in Cappon, ed., *Adams-Jefferson Letters*, 264.

130. For a lively discussion of the subject, see W. J. Rorabaugh, *The Alcoholic Republic: An American Tradition* (New York: Oxford University Press, 1979).

131. Ellis, *First Family*, 43.

132. Abigail Adams to Mary Cranch, December 1, 1800, in Mitchell, ed., *New Letters of Abigail Adams*, 260.

133. Abigail Adams to Thomas B. Adams, November 13, 1800, in *Letters of Mrs. Adams*, 380.

134. Abigail Adams to Catherine Johnson, January 19, 1800, in Kaminski, ed., *The Quotable Abigail Adams*, 141.

135. Abigail Adams to Mary Cranch, January 15, 1801, in Mitchell, ed., *Letters of Abigail Adams*, 262.

136. Woody Holton, *Abigail Adams*, 336-37.

137. Abigail Adams to Mercy Warren, January 16, 1803, in *Letters of Mrs. Adams*, 387-89.

138. Abigail Adams to Elizabeth Shaw, June 5, 1809, in *Letters of Mrs. Adams*, 401.

139. Abigail Adams to Caroline DeWindt, in Caroline DeWindt, ed., *Journal and Correspondence of Miss Adams: Daughter of John Adams* (New York: Wiley & Putnam, 1841), 220.

140. Nagel, *The Adams Women*, 153.

141. Diary Entry of October 25, 1812, in DeWindt, ed., *Journal of Louisa Adams*.

142. Abigail Adams to Louisa Adams, January 20, 1813, in DeWindt, ed., *Journal of Louisa Adams*.

143. Benjamin Rush to John Adams, September 20, 1811, in Lyman H. Butterfield, ed., *The Rush Letters* (Princeton, NJ: Princeton University Press, 1951), 2:1104.

144. Nagel, *The Adams Women*, 145.

145. Cokie Roberts, *Founding Mothers: The Women Who Raised Our Nation* (New York: Morrow, 2004), 265-66.

146. Abigail Adams to Thomas Jefferson, September 20, 1813, in Cappon, ed., *Adams-Jefferson Letters*, 377.

147. Abigail Adams to Thomas Jefferson, September 20, 1813, and John Adams to Thomas Jefferson, August 16, 1813, in Cappon, ed., *Adams-Jefferson Letters*, 377, 366.

148. Abigail Adams to Mercy Warren, May 4, 1814, in *Letters of Mrs. Adams*, 417.

149. John Adams to Thomas Jefferson, January 1812, in Cappon, ed., *Adams-Jefferson Letters*, 2:296.

150. Thomas Jefferson to Abigail Adams, 1816, in Cappon, ed., *Adams-Jefferson Letters*, 2:504.

151. Nagel, *The Adams Women*, 156.

152. John Adams to Thomas Jefferson, October 20, 1818, in Cappon, ed., *Adams-Jefferson Letters*, 2:529.

153. Jefferson to Adams, November 13, 1818, in Cappon, ed., *Adams-Jefferson Letters*, 2:529.

154. John Adams to Thomas Jefferson, July 16, 1814, in Cappon, ed., *Adams-Jefferson Letters*, 2:430, 435.

155. John Adams to Thomas Jefferson, December 8, 1818, and John Adams to Thomas Jefferson, December 30, 1818, in Cappon, ed., *Adams-Jefferson Letters*, 2:530, 531.

156. John Adams to Thomas Jefferson, May 21, 1819, and John Adams to Thomas Jefferson, November 23, 1819, in Cappon, ed., *Adams-Jefferson Correspondence*, 2:540, 547-48.

157. Marx, *Health of the Presidents*, 39.

Chapter 4

1. George Gilmer to John Morgan, May 11, 1766, in Julian P. Boyd, et al., eds., *The Papers of Thomas Jefferson* (Princeton, NJ: Princeton University Press, 1950-), 1:18.

2. Oscar Reiss, *Medicine and the American Revolution: How Diseases and Their Treatments Affected the Colonial Army* (Jefferson, NC: McFarland, 1998), 56.

3. For an early salient analysis of Jeffersonian views about political, social, and health issues, see George Rosen, "Political Order and Human Health in Jeffersonian Thought," *Bulletin of the History of Medicine* 26 (1952): 32-44.

4. Quoted in Silvio A. Bedini, *Thomas Jefferson: Statesman of Science* (New York: Macmillan, 1990), 1.

5. Rosen, "Political Order and Human Health in Jeffersonian Thought," 34-35.

6. Bedini, *Thomas Jefferson*, 314.

7. Rudolph Marx, *The Health of the Presidents* (New York: Putnam's, 1960), 47.

8. Thomas Jefferson to Maria Cosway, July 1, 1787, in Boyd et al., eds., *Papers of Thomas Jefferson*, 11:520.

9. Thomas Jefferson to William Randolph, June 1776, in Boyd et al., eds., *Papers of Thomas Jefferson*, 1:408-10.

10. Norm Ledgin, *Diagnosing Jefferson* (Arlington, TX: Future Horizons, 2000), has attempted to specifically tie some of Jefferson's personality traits to a highly functional case of Asberger's, a forms of autism, and portrays Jefferson as a troubled genius. However, practicing psychological analysis on a person deceased for over two centuries is fraught with difficulties, and Ledgin's examples are often far-fetched.

11. Robert Halsey, *How the President, Thomas Jefferson, and Doctor Benjamin Waterhouse Established Vaccination as a Public Health Procedure* (New York: New York Academy of Medicine, 1936), 2-3.

12. Henry S. Randall, *The Life of Thomas Jefferson* (New York: Derby and Jackson, 1858), 1:20-28.

13. Marx, *Health of the Presidents*, 48-49.

14. Samuel X. Radbill, "Thomas Jefferson and the Doctors," *Transactions & Studies of the College of Physicians* 37 (1969-70): 107.

15. Entry for May 22, 1773, in Edwin M. Betts, ed., *Thomas Jefferson's Garden Book* (Philadelphia: American Philosophical Society, 1944), 41.

16. Thomas Jefferson to Jeremiah A. Goodman, December 1811, in Betts, ed., *Thomas Jefferson's Garden Book*, 467.

17. Randall, *Life of Thomas Jefferson*, 1:133.

18. Fawn M. Brodie, *Thomas Jefferson: An Intimate History* (New York: Norton, 1974), 115.

19. Bedini, *Thomas Jefferson: Statesman of Science*, 70.

20. Joseph J. Ellis, *American Sphinx: The Character of Thomas Jefferson* (New York: Knopf, 1997), 29.

21. Marx, *Health of the Presidents*, 50-51.

22. Radbill, "Thomas Jefferson and the Doctors," 109.

23. Marx, *Health of the Presidents*, 53.

24. Thomas Jefferson to John Page, July 30, 1776, in Boyd et al., eds., *Papers of Thomas Jefferson*, 1:483.
25. Brodie, *Thomas Jefferson: An Intimate History*, 131-32.
26. Thomas Jefferson to James Monroe, May 20, 1782, in Boyd et al., eds., *Papers of Thomas Jefferson*, 6:186.
27. Randall, *Life of Thomas Jefferson*, 1:371, 382.
28. Thomas Jefferson to the Marquis de Chastellux, November 26, 1782, in Boyd et al., eds., *Papers of Thomas Jefferson*, 6:203-4.
29. In *Thomas Jefferson: An Intimate History* (1974), Fawn Brodie postulated an affair between Jefferson and Hemings. Later, in *Thomas Jefferson and Sally Hemings: An American Controversy* (Charlottesville: University of Virginia Press, 1997), Annette Gordon-Reed argued that Jefferson *could* have fathered Sally's children. However, a study conducted by a group of prestigious scholars in 2001 but just recently published offers highly persuasive arguments to the contrary. See Robert F. Turner, ed., *The Jefferson-Hemings Controversy: Report of the Scholars Commission* (Durham, NC: Carolina Academic Press, 2011).
30. Thomas Jefferson to William Short, March 1, 1784, in Boyd et al., eds., *Papers of Thomas Jefferson*, 6:570.
31. Thomas Jefferson to James Madison, February 17, 1784, in James Morton Smith, ed., *The Republic of Letters: The Correspondence between Thomas Jefferson and James Madison* (New York: Norton, 1995), 1:297.
32. Garry Wills, *James Madison* (New York: Holt, 2002), 13-15.
33. William T. Hutchinson, ed., *The Papers of James Madison* (Chicago: University of Chicago Press, 1962-), 1:75.
34. Ralph Ketcham, "James Madison," in Henry F. Graff, ed., *The Presidents: A Reference History* (New York: Scribner's/Gale, 2002), 58.
35. James Madison to Thomas Jefferson, 1785, in Boyd et al., eds., *Papers of James Madison*, 8:270.
36. James Madison to Thomas Jefferson, January 10, 1801, in Smith, ed., *Republic of Letters*, 1159.
37. Thomas Jefferson to James Madison, February 12, 1801, in Smith, ed., *Republic of Letters*, 1160.
38. See Irving Brant, *The Fourth President: The Life of James Madison* (New York: Bobbs-Merrill, 1970) and Ralph Ketcham, *James Madison* (Charlottesville: University Press of Virginia, 1990), 52-53.
39. John R. Bumgarner, *Health of the Presidents* (Jefferson, NC: MacFarland, 1994), 27.
40. Ketcham, *James Madison*, 51.
41. Sarah Randolph, *The Domestic Life of Thomas Jefferson* (New York: Ungar, 1958), 47.
42. Ibid., 67-69.
43. Radbill, "Thomas Jefferson and the Doctors," 108, and Courtney R. Hall, "Jefferson on the Medical Theory and Practice of His Day," *Bulletin of the History of Medicine* 31 (1957): 236-38.

44. Marx, *Health of the Presidents*, 55.
45. Thomas Jefferson to Charles Thompson, November 11, 1784, cited in E. J. Huth, "Benjamin Franklin's Place in the History of Medicine," James Lind Library (www.jameslindlibrary.org), 2006, 4.
46. Abigail Adams to Mary Cranch, December 9, 1784, in *Abigail Adams: Letters of Mrs. Adams, the Wife of John Adams; With an Introductory Memoir by Her Grandson, Charles Francis Adams* (Boston: Wilkins, Carter, 1848), 216.
47. Thomas Jefferson to James Monroe, March 18, 1785, in Boyd et al., eds., *Papers of Thomas Jefferson*, 8:43.
48. Thomas Jefferson to Peter Carr, August 19, 1785, in Adrienne Koch and William Peden, eds., *The Life and Selected Writings of Thomas Jefferson* (New York: Modern Library, 1944), 375.
49. Randolph, *Domestic Life of Thomas Jefferson*, 101-2.
50. Brodie, *Thomas Jefferson: An Intimate History*, 190.
51. Ibid., 233. For the reference to Hemings's smallpox inoculation, see James A. Bear and Lucia C. Stanton, eds., *Jefferson's Memorandum Books: Accounts, with Legal Records and Miscellany, 1767-1826* (Princeton, NJ: Princeton University Press, 1997), 2:1502.
52. John Adams to Thomas Jefferson, March 1, 1787, in Lester J. Cappon, ed., *The Adams-Jefferson Letters* (New York: Simon & Schuster, 1959), 177.
53. Abigail Adams to Thomas Jefferson, January 29th, 1787, in Cappon, ed., *Adams-Jefferson Letters*, 168.
54. Randolph, *Domestic Life of Thomas Jefferson*, 74, 86, 89.
55. Thomas Jefferson to James Madison, December 16, 1786, in Smith, ed., *Republic of Letters*, 1:457.
56. Thomas Jefferson to Abigail Adams, December 21, 1786, in Cappon, ed., *Adams-Jefferson Letters*, 159.
57. Thomas Jefferson to Benjamin Franklin, December 23, 1786, www.franklinpapers.org.
58. Thomas Jefferson to Martha Jefferson, in Edwin M. Betts and James A. Bear, eds., *The Family Letters of Thomas Jefferson* (Columbia: University of Missouri Press, 1966), 34.
59. Thomas Jefferson to Martha Jefferson, March 28, 1787, and Thomas Jefferson to Thomas Mann Randolph Jr., 1787, in Koch and Peden, eds., *The Life and Selected Writings of Thomas Jefferson*, 417, 394.
60. Marx, *Health of the Presidents*, 49.
61. Thomas Jefferson to James Madison, January 13, 1821, in Smith, ed., *Republic of Letters*, 3:1828.
62. Marx, *Health of the Presidents*, 51.
63. Randolph, *Domestic Life of Thomas Jefferson*, 192.
64. Thomas Jefferson to John Adams, January 23, 1812, in Cappon, ed., *The Adams-Jefferson Letters*, 247.
65. Thomas Jefferson to Thomas Cooper, October 27, 1808, in Andrew A. Lipscomb and Albert E. Bergh, eds., *The Writings of Thomas Jefferson* (Washington, DC: Thomas Jefferson Memorial Association, 1903), 12:292.

66. Thomas Jefferson to George Washington, May 15, 1791, in Boyd et al., eds., *Papers of Thomas Jefferson*, 20:417.

67. For an illuminating discussion of the political strife related to the yellow fever epidemic of 1893, see Martin Pernick, "Politics, Parties, and Pestilence: Epidemic Yellow Fever in Philadelphia and the Rise of the First Party System," *William and Mary Quarterly* 29 (October 1972): 559-86.

68. Thomas Jefferson to Thomas Mann Randolph Jr., September 2, 1793, in John Catazariti, ed., *The Papers of Thomas Jefferson* (Princeton, NJ: Princeton University Press), 27:21.

69. Thomas Jefferson to James Madison, September 1, 2, 1793, in Smith, ed., *Republic of Letters*, 2:814.

70. Thomas Jefferson to James Madison, September 8, 1793, in Paul Leicester Ford, ed., *The Writings of Thomas Jefferson* (New York: Putnam's, 1895), 6:419.

71. Thomas Jefferson to James Madison, September 8, 1793, in Smith, ed., *Republic of Letters*, 2:818-19.

72. Thomas Jefferson to Mr. Morris, September 11, 1793, in Randolph, *Domestic Life of Thomas Jefferson*, 219.

73. Thomas Jefferson to Martha Randolph Jefferson, November 10, 1793, in Betts and Bear, *The Family Letters of Thomas Jefferson*, 125.

74. Thomas Jefferson to James Madison, November 9, 1793, in Smith, ed., *Republic of Letters*, 2:829.

75. Thomas Jefferson to James Madison, 1793, and Thomas Jefferson to John Page, 1804, quoted in Wyndham B. Blanton, *Medicine in Virginia in the Eighteenth Century* (Richmond, VA: Garrett & Massey, 1931), 193, 196.

76. Thomas Jefferson to Comte de Volney, February 8, 1805, in Lipscomb and Berg, eds., *Writings of Thomas Jefferson*, 11:65.

77. Thomas Jefferson to Dr. Benjamin Rush, September 23, 1800, in Lipscomb and Berg, eds., *Writings of Thomas Jefferson*, 10:173.

78. Thomas Jefferson to Comte de Volney, February 8, 1805, in Lipscomb and Berg, eds., *Writings of Thomas Jefferson*, 11:66.

79. Cited in Smith, ed., *Republic of Letters*, 881.

80. For a detailed description of Jefferson's knowledge of botanical medications, see John M. Holmes, *Thomas Jefferson Treats Himself* (Fort Valley, VA: Loft Press, 1997), 39, 105. Holmes's chapter "A Garden Pharmacy" is particularly informative.

81. Blanton, *Medicine in Virginia in the Eighteenth Century*, 62.

82. Thomas Jefferson, *Notes on Virginia*, in Koch and Peden, eds., *Life and Selected Writings of Thomas Jefferson*, 233.

83. Thomas Jefferson to Edmund Randolph, September 7, 1794, in Randolph, *Domestic Life of Thomas Jefferson*, 231.

84. Thomas Jefferson to James Madison, October 30, 1794, in Smith, ed., *Republic of Letters*, 2:858.

85. Thomas Jefferson to James Madison, April 27, 1795, in Smith, ed., *Republic of Letters*, 877.

86. Thomas Jefferson to Martha Jefferson Randolph, July 31, 1795, in Betts and Bear, eds., *Family Letters of Thomas Jefferson*, 219.
87. Thomas Jefferson to Philip Mazzei, April 24, 1796, in Lipscomb and Berg, eds., *Writings of Thomas Jefferson*, 9:336.
88. Thomas Jefferson to Maria Jefferson, May 25, 1797, in Randolph, *Domestic Life of Thomas Jefferson*, 244.
89. Thomas Jefferson to Martha Jefferson Randolph, April 9, 1797, in Betts and Bear, eds., *Family Letters of Thomas Jefferson*, 143.
90. Thomas Jefferson to Martha Jefferson Randolph, August 15, 1798, in Randolph, *Domestic Life of Thomas Jefferson*, 251.

Chapter 5

1. For an important study on health and migration see Conevery Bolton Valencius, *The Health of the Country: How American Settlers Understood Themselves and Their Land* (New York: Basic Books, 2002).
2. Thomas Jefferson to Albert Gallatin, September 18, 1801, cited in James Morton Smith, ed., *The Republic of Letters: The Correspondence between Thomas Jefferson and James Madison* (New York: Norton, 1995), 2:1172.
3. Thomas Jefferson to Count Volney, February 8, 1805, quoted in Courtney R. Hall, "Jefferson on the Medical Theory and Practice of His Day," *Bulletin of the History of Medicine* 31 (1957): 238.
4. Thomas Jefferson to Dr. Caspar Wistar, June 21, 1807, in Merrill D. Peterson, ed., *Thomas Jefferson: Writings* (New York: Library of America, 1984), 1181-85.
5. Robert Hurtin Halsey, *How the President, Thomas Jefferson, and Doctor Benjamin Waterhouse Established Vaccination as a Public Health Procedure* (New York: privately printed, 1936), 11-12.
6. For a fine detailed study of that smallpox epidemic, see Michael Willrich, *Pox: An American History* (New York: Penguin, 2011).
7. Andrea Rusnock, "Catching Cowpox: The Early Spread of Smallpox Vaccination," *Bulletin of the History of Medicine* 83 (2009): 26.
8. Thomas Jefferson to Martha Jefferson Randolph, July 16, 1801, in Edwin M. Betts and James A. Bear, eds., *The Family Letters of Thomas Jefferson* (Columbia: University of Missouri Press, 1966), 207.
9. Rusnock, "Catching Cowpox," 85.
10. Willrich, *Pox: An American History*, 180.
11. Thomas Jefferson to Martha Jefferson Randolph, June 8, 1797, in Sarah Randolph, *The Domestic Life of Thomas Jefferson: Compiled from Family Letters and Reminiscences of His Great-Granddaughter* (New York: Ungar, 1878; reprint 1958), 245.
12. Elizabeth Langhorne, *Monticello: A Family Story* (Chapel Hill, NC: Algonquin, 1987), 62-63.
13. Martha Jefferson Randolph to Thomas Jefferson, January 22, 1798, in Betts and Bear, eds., *Jefferson Family Letters*, 153.

14. Thomas Jefferson to James Madison, August 14, 1801, in Smith, ed., *Republic of Letters*, 2:1187.

15. Thomas Jefferson to Dr. John Coxe, November 5, 1801, in Henry A. Martin, "Jefferson as a Vaccinator," *North Carolina Medical Journal* (January 1881): 32.

16. Halsey, *How the President, Thomas Jefferson, and Doctor Benjamin Waterhouse Established Vaccination as a Public Health Procedure*, 31.

17. Benjamin Waterhouse to Thomas Jefferson, September 2, 1801, in Halsey, *How the President, Thomas Jefferson*, 38.

18. Samuel X. Radbill, "Thomas Jefferson and the Doctors," *Transactions & Studies of the College of Physicians* 37 (1969-70): 111-12.

19. Martin, "Jefferson as a Vaccinator,"33.

20. Henry Martin, *Thomas Jefferson: Scientist* (New York: Henry Schuman), 1952, 7.

21. For a highly detailed study on the medical aspects of the undertaking, see Drake W. Will, "The Medical and Surgical Practice of the Lewis and Clark Expedition," *Journal of the History of Medicine and Applied Sciences* 14 (July 1959): 273-97.

22. Thomas Jefferson to Meriwether Lewis, June 20, 1803, "Instructions to Captain Lewis," in Peterson, ed., *Thomas Jefferson: Writings*, 1130.

23. Halsey, *How the President, Thomas Jefferson*, 6. See also, Volney Steele, *Bleed, Blister, and Purge: A History of Medicine on the American Frontier* (Missoula, MT: Mountain Press, 2005), 47-48.

24. Will, "The Medical and Surgical Practice of the Lewis and Clark Expedition," 282, 288, 290.

25. Martha Jefferson Randolph to Thomas Jefferson, November 24, 1808, and Thomas Jefferson to Martha Jefferson Randolph, November 29, 1808, in Betts and Bear, eds., *Jefferson Family Letters*, 361, 366.

26. Joseph J. Ellis, *American Sphinx: The Character of Thomas Jefferson* (New York: Knopf, 1997), xii.

27. Thomas Jefferson to Maria Jefferson Eppes, July 13, 1798, in Randolph, *Domestic Life of Thomas Jefferson*, 250.

28. Thomas Jefferson to Maria Jefferson Eppes, January 17, 1800, in Randolph, *Domestic Life of Thomas Jefferson*, 259.

29. Thomas Jefferson to Maria Jefferson Eppes, February 12, 1800, in Randolph, *Domestic Life of Thomas Jefferson*, 263.

30. Fawn Brodie, *Thomas Jefferson: An Intimate History* (New York: Norton), 328 and footnote 18, 537.

31. Martha Jefferson Randolph to Thomas Jefferson, January, 14, 1804, in Betts and Bear, eds., *Family Letters of Thomas Jefferson*, 252.

32. Martha Jefferson Randolph to Thomas Jefferson, November 27, 1801, in Betts and Bear, eds., *Family Letters of Thomas Jefferson*, 213.

33. Thomas Jefferson to Martha Jefferson Randolph, January 17, 1802, in Betts and Bear, eds., *Family Letters of Thomas Jefferson*, 216.

34. Thomas Jefferson to Maria Jefferson Eppes, July 2, 1802, in Randolph, *Domestic Life of Thomas Jefferson*, 285-86.

35. Eric H. Christianson, "Medicine in New England," in Judith Walzer Leavitt and Ronald L. Numbers, *Sickness and Health in America: Readings in the History of Medicine and Public Health* (Madison: University of Wisconsin Press, 1978), 54.

36. Ernest Caulfield, "Early Measles Epidemics in America," *Yale Journal of Biology and Medicine* 15 (1942): 545-46.

37. Thomas Jefferson to Maria Jefferson Eppes, October 7, 1802, in Randolph, *Domestic Life of Thomas Jefferson*, 288-89.

38. Randolph, *Domestic Life of Thomas Jefferson*, 292.

39. Dumas Malone, *Jefferson the President: First Term, 1801-1805* (Boston: Little, Brown, 1970), 185-88.

40. Thomas Jefferson to Cornelia Randolph, April 3, 1808, in Randolph, *Domestic Life of Thomas Jefferson*, 316.

41. Thomas Jefferson to Maria Jefferson Eppes, March 3, 1804, and Thomas Jefferson to John Eppes, March 15, 1804, in Randolph, *Domestic Life of Thomas Jefferson*, 297-98.

42. Thomas Jefferson to James Madison, April 9, 1804, April 13, 1804, April 15, 1804, in Smith, ed., *The Republic of Letters*, 2:1304, 1307, 1309.

43. *Thomas Jefferson's Memorandum Book*, April 17, 1804, cited in Langhorne, *Monticello*, 130.

44. Thomas Jefferson to Governor John Page, June 25, 1804, cited in Cappon, ed., *The Adams-Jefferson Letters*, 265.

45. Dolley Madison to Anna Cutts, April 26, 1804, in David B. Mattern and Holly C. Shulman, eds., *The Selected Letters of Dolley Payne Madison* (Charlottesville: University of Virginia Press, 2003), 53.

46. Thomas Jefferson to James Madison, July 25, 1805, in Smith, ed., *The Republic of Letters*, 3:1373.

47. Thomas Jefferson's Fifth Annual Message to Congress, December 3, 1805.Yale Law School Avalon Project, http://avalon.yale.edu/19th_century/jeffmes5.asp.

48. Martha Jefferson Randolph to Thomas Jefferson, March 20, 1807, in Betts and Bear, eds., *Family Letters of Thomas Jefferson*, 303.

49. Thomas Jefferson to James Madison, March 15, 1809, in Randolph, *Domestic Life of Thomas Jefferson*, 327.

50. Thomas Jefferson to James Madison, September 12, 1809, in Smith, ed., *The Republic of Letters*, 3:1602

51. Merrill D. Peterson, ed., *Visitors to Monticello* (Charlotte: University of Virginia, 1989), 46, 51.

52. Thomas Jefferson to Randolph Jefferson, September 6, 1811, in Bernard Mayo, ed., *Thomas Jefferson and His Unknown Brother* (Charlottesville: University of Virginia, 1981), 26.

53. Thomas Jefferson to John Adams, January 21, 1812, in Lester J. Cappon, ed., *The Adams-Jefferson Letters* (New York: Simon & Schuster, 1959), 292.

54. Thomas Jefferson to Abigail Adams, August 22, 1813, and Thomas Jefferson to Abigail Adams, Winter 1816, in Cappon, ed., *Adams-Jefferson Letters*, 366, 504.

55. Thomas Jefferson to Abigail Adams, August 22, 1813, in Cappon, ed., *Adams-Jefferson Letters*, 367.

56. Thomas Jefferson to Francis Wayles Eppes, September 9, 1814, in Betts and Bear, eds., *Family Letters of Thomas Jefferson*, 407.

57. Dolley Payne Madison to Edward Coles, July 2, 1813, in Mattern and Shulman, eds., *Selected Letters of Dolley Madison*, 177.

58. Thomas Jefferson to James Madison, July 13, 1813, in Smith, ed., *Republic of Letters*, 1725.

59. Quoted in Ethel Stephen Arnett, *Mrs. James Madison, The Incomparable Dolley* (Greensboro, NC: Piedmont Press, 1972), 214.

60. Thomas Jefferson to John Adams, July 5, 1814, and Thomas Jefferson to John Adams, April 8, 1816, in Cappon, ed., *Adams-Jefferson Letters*, 2:430, 466.

61. Thomas Jefferson to Caesar A. Rodney, March 16, 1815, and Thomas Jefferson, Spring 1816, in Randolph, *Domestic Life of Thomas Jefferson*, 360, 361.

62. As quoted in Stanley Finger, *Doctor Franklin's Medicine* (Philadelphia: University of Pennsylvania Press, 2006), 264.

63. Thomas Jefferson to Mrs. Trist, April 28, 1816, in Randolph, *Domestic Life of Thomas Jefferson*, 363.

64. Thomas Jefferson to Mrs. M. B. Jefferson, August 2, 1815, in Edwin M. Betts, ed., *Thomas Jefferson's Farm Book* (Princeton, NJ: Princeton University Press, 1953), 39.

65. Thomas Jefferson to Wilson Cary Nicholas, August 11, 1819, cited in Alan Pell Crawford, *Twilight at Monticello: The Final Years of Thomas Jefferson* (New York: Random House, 2008), 176,181.

66. Thomas Jefferson to Martha Jefferson Randolph, August 7, 1818, in Betts and Bear, eds., *Family Letters of Thomas Jefferson*, 424.

67. Thomas Jefferson to James Madison, February 19, 1819, in Smith, ed., *Republic of Letters*, 3:1807.

68. Thomas Jefferson to James Madison, February 16, 1820, in Smith, ed., *Republic of Letters*, 3:1822.

69. Cited in Ralph Ketcham, *The Madisons at Montpelier* (Charlottesville: University of Virginia Press, 2009), 114.

70. Norman G. Schneeberg, "The Medical History of Thomas Jefferson (1743-1826)," *Journal of Medical Biography* 16 (2008): 118.

71. Thomas Jefferson to Doctor Vine Utley, March 21, 1819, in Randolph, *Domestic Life of Thomas Jefferson*, 371.

72. Thomas Jefferson to John Adams, November 7, 1819, and Jefferson to John Adams, October 7, 1818, in Cappon, ed., *Adams-Jefferson Letters*, 546, 527.

73. Ellen Wayles Randolph Coolidge to Dolley Madison, October 15, 1819, in Mattern and Shulman, eds., *Selected Letters of Dolley Payne Madison*, 236-37.

74. Thomas Jefferson to John Adams, June 1, 1822, in Cappon, ed., *Adams-Jefferson Letters*, 578.

75. Thomas Jefferson to James Madison, November 22, 1822, and January 6, 1823, in Smith, ed., *Republic of Letters*, 3:1841, 1853.

76. James Madison to Thomas Jefferson, January 15, 1823, in Smith, ed., *Republic of Letters*, 3:1855.

77. Thomas Jefferson to Lafayette, November 4, 1823, in Randolph, *Domestic Life of Thomas Jefferson*, 384.

78. Quoted in Martin Clagett, *Scientific Jefferson Revealed* (Charlottesville: University Press of Virginia, 2009), 53. For a detailed exploration of Jefferson's understanding of the spread of infectious diseases in relation to architectural design, see chapter 4, "Social Architecture and Public Health."

79. Thomas Jefferson to Richard Rush, April 26, 1824, in John M. Dorsey, ed., *The Jefferson-Dunglison Letters* (Charlottesville: University of Virginia Press, 1960), 13.

80. Edwin M. Betts, ed., *Thomas Jefferson's Garden Book* (Philadelphia: American Philosophical Society, 1944), 349.

81. Dorsey, ed., *Jefferson-Dunglison Letters*, 72, 85, 101.

82. Dorsey, ed., *Jefferson-Dunglison Letters*, 14-16, and Jefferson to Dr. Greenhow, March 8, 1825, 17 and April 14, 1825, 21-23.

83. Thomas Jefferson to James Madison, January 28, 1821, in Smith, ed., *Republic of Letters*, 3:1829.

84. Oscar A. Thorup, "Jefferson's Admonition," *Mayo Medical Ventures for Mayo Foundation for Medical Education and Research* 47 (1972): 199-201.

85. Thomas Jefferson to Dr. Dunglison, May 17, 1825, in Dorsey, ed., *Jefferson-Dunglison Letters*, 13.

86. Thomas Watkins to Thomas Jefferson, May 11, 1825, *Thomas Jefferson Papers*, Library of Congress.

87. Thomas Jefferson to Dr. Dunglison, June 16, 1825, in Dorsey, ed., *Jefferson-Dunglison Letters*, 30.

88. Thomas Jefferson to Dr. Dunglison, July 2, 1825, and Dr. Dunglison to Thomas Jefferson, July 2, 1825, in Dorsey, ed., *Jefferson-Dunglison Letters*, 34-35.

89. Thomas Jefferson to Dr. Dunglison, July 8, 1825, and Dr. Dunglison to Thomas Jefferson, July 18, 1825, in Dorsey, ed., *Jefferson-Dunglison Letters*, 36-37.

90. Thomas Jefferson to Fanny Wright, August 7, 1825, in Paul Leicester Ford, ed., *The Works of Thomas Jefferson* (New York: Putnam's, 1904-05), 10:344.

91. Dorsey, ed., *Jefferson-Dunglison Letters*, 38-39.

92. Thomas Jefferson to Dr. Dunglison, November 17, 1825, in Dorsey, ed., *Jefferson-Dunglison Letters*, 41-42.

93. Dorsey, ed., *Jefferson-Dunglison Letters*, 47-48.

94. Thomas Jefferson to Dr. Dunglison, November 26, 1825, in Dorsey, ed., *Jefferson-Dunglison Letters*, 44-45.

95. Dr. Dunglison to Thomas Jefferson, December 21, 1825, in Dorsey, ed., *Jefferson-Dunglison Letters*, 48-51.

96. John M. Holmes, *Thomas Jefferson Treats Himself* (Fort Valley, VA: Loft Press, 1997), 61-63.

97. Thomas Jefferson to Thomas Jefferson Randolph, February 11, 1826, in Randolph, *Domestic Life of Thomas Jefferson*, 416.

98. Thomas Jefferson to James Madison, May 1826, in Smith, ed., *Republic of Letters*, 3: 1970.

99. "Dr. Dunglison's Memoranda," in Henry S. Randall, *The Life of Thomas Jefferson* (New York: Derby and Jackson, 1858), 3:547-49.

100. Jefferson Randolph to Henry S. Randall, in Randall, *Life of Thomas Jefferson*, 3:543.

101. "Reminiscences of Madison Hemings," in Brodie, *Thomas Jefferson: An Intimate History*, 474.

102. Jefferson Randolph to Henry S. Randall, in Randall, *Life of Thomas Jefferson*, 3:544.

103. Ibid.

104. Dr. Dunglison to James Madison, July 1, 1826, in Dorsey, ed., *Jefferson-Dunglison Letters*, 66-67.

105. Dorsey, ed., *Jefferson-Dunglison Letters*, 68-69.

106. Randolph, *Domestic Life of Thomas Jefferson*, 423-25.

107. Dolley Madison to John Payne Todd, July 6, 1826, in Mattern and Shulman, eds., *Selected Letters of Dolley Payne Madison*, 264.

108. Thomas Jefferson to James Madison, February 17, 1826, in Smith, ed., *Republic of Letters*, 3:1967.

109. James Madison to Nicholas Trist, July 6, 1826, in Gaillard Hunt, ed., *The Writings of James Madison* (New York: Putnam's, 1910), 9:248.

110. See Andrew Burstein, *Jefferson's Secrets: Death and Desire at Monticello* (New York: Basic Books, 2005).

111. George Rosen, "Political Order and Human Health in Jeffersonian Thought," *Bulletin of the History of Medicine* 26 (1952): 258.

Epilogue

1. Charles E. Rosenberg, *Our Present Complaint: American Medicine, Then and Now* (Baltimore, MD: Johns Hopkins University Press, 2007), 186, 189.

2. Lamar Riley Murphy, *Enter the Physician: The Transformation of Domestic Medicine, 1760-1860* (Tuscaloosa: University of Alabama Press, 1991), xiii.

3. Peter Gay, *The Enlightenment: An Interpretation*, vol. 2, *The Science of Freedom* (New York: Knopf, 1969), 19, 23.

4. Shirley S. Wang, "Why Placebos Work Wonders," *Wall Street Journal*, January 3, 2012, D1–D2.

5. Khosrow S. Houschyar, et al., "Effects of Phlebotomy-Induced Reduction of Body Iron Stores on Metabolic Syndrome," *BMC Medicine* (2012), http://www.biomedcentral.com/1741-7015/10/54.

6. "Military Pokes Holes in Acupuncture Skeptics," *Morning Edition*, National Public Radio, February 16, 2012.

7. Douglass Adair, "'That Politics May Be Reduced to a Science': David Hume, James Madison, and the Tenth Federalist," *Huntington Library Quarterly* 20 (August 1957): 343-60.

8. Cited in Drew R. McCoy, *The Elusive Republic: Political Economy in Jeffersonian America* (Chapel Hill: University of North Carolina Press, 1980), 69.

9. John Adams to Abigail Adams, April 11, 1777, in John Adams, *Letters of John Adams Addressed to His Wife*, (Boston: Little, Brown, 1841), 1:209.

10. Nathan G. Goodman, ed., *A Benjamin Franklin Reader* (New York: Crowell, 1945), 360.

11. Jared Sparks, ed., *The Writings of George Washington: Being His Correspondence, Addresses, and Messages, and Other Papers, Official and Private* (Boston: Little, Brown, 1885), 8:441.

12. Cited in Peter Gay, *The Enlightenment*, 98.

13. Peter Gay, *The Enlightenment* 101-7, 362-68.

14. Thomas Jefferson to Dr. John Crawford, January 2, 1812, in Andrew A. Liscomb and Albert E. Bergh, eds., *The Writings of Thomas Jefferson*, (Washington, DC: Thomas Jefferson Memorial Foundation, 1904), 13:117-19.

15. James Madison to Richard Peters, September 8, 1826, cited in Ralph Ketcham, *The Madisons at Montpelier* (New York: Norton, 2009), 131.

16. James Madison, "State of the Union Address," November 4, 1812, www.globusz. com/ebooks/Madison/00000014.htm , accessed January 27, 2012.

17. May 21, 1783, in L. H. Butterfield, *Diary and Autobiography of John Adams* (Cambridge, MA: Belknap Press of Harvard University Press, 1961), 3:123.

18. Kay K. Moss, *Southern Folk Remedies, 1750-1820* (Columbia: University of South Carolina Press, 1999), 219.

19. Ramsay, David, "A Review of the Improvement, Progress, and State of Medicine in the Eighteenth Century," delivered January 1, 1800, *Transactions of the American Philosophical Society* 55 (1965): 96-217.

20. Peter Gay, *The Enlightenment*, 23.

21. Ronald L. Numbers, "The Fall and Rise of the American Medical Profession," in Judith Walzer Leavitt and Ronald L. Numbers, eds., *Sickness and Health in America* (Madison: University of Wisconsin Press, 1978), 225, 226–28, 231-32.

22. John Harley Warner, "Medical Sectarianism, Therapeutic Conflict, and the Shaping of Orthodox Professional Identity in Antebellum American Medicine," in J. Worth Estes and Billy G. Smith, eds., *A Melancholy Scene of Devastation: The Public Response to the 1793 Philadelphia Yellow Fever Epidemic* (Canton, MA: Science History Publications, 1997), 234.

23. Margaret Humphreys, "Appendix II: Yellow Fever since 1793; History and Historiography," in Estes and Smith, eds., *A Melancholy Scene of Devastation*, 184.

24. Estes, "Introduction: The Yellow Fever Syndrome and Its Treatment in Philadelphia, 1793," in Estes and Smith, eds., *A Melancholy Scene of Devastation*, 7.

25. David B. Agus, "A Doctor in Your Pocket," *Wall Street Journal*, January 14-15, 2012, C3.

26. Marty Makary, *Unaccountable: What Hospitals Won't Tell You and How Transparency Can Revolutionize Health Care* (New York: Bloomsbury), 2012.

BIBLIOGRAPHY

Primary Sources

Abbot, W. W., ed., et al. *The Papers of George Washington* (Charlottesville: University Press of Virginia, 1983-1998).

Adams, Abigail. *The Letters of Mrs. Adams, the Wife of John Adams: With an Introductory Memoir by Her Grandson Charles Francis Adams*. 4th ed. (Boston: Wilkins, Carter, 1848).

Adams, John. *Letters of John Adams Addressed to His Wife*. Charles Francis Adams, ed. 2 vols. (Boston: Little and Brown, 1841).

Adams Family. *Adams Family Papers: An Electronic Archive*. Massachusetts Historical Society. http:///www.masshist.org/digitaladams.

Bear, James A., and Lucia C. Stanton, eds. *Jefferson's Memorandum Books: Accounts, with Legal Records and Miscellany, 1767-1826*. 2 vols. (Princeton, NJ: Princeton University Press, 1997).

Betts, Edwin Morris, ed. *Thomas Jefferson's Farm Book* (Princeton, NJ: Princeton University Press, 1953).

Betts, Edwin Morris, ed. *Thomas Jefferson's Garden Book, 1766-1824* (Philadelphia: American Philosophical Society, 1944).

Betts, Edwin Morris, and James Adam Bear Jr., eds. *The Family Letters of Thomas Jefferson* (Columbia: University of Missouri Press, 1966).

Boyd, Julian P., et al., eds. *The Papers of Thomas Jefferson*. 34 vols. to date. (Princeton, NJ: Princeton University Press, 1950-).

Butterfield, Lyman H., ed. *Diary and Autobiography of John Adams*. 4 vols. (Cambridge, MA: Harvard University Press, 1961).

Butterfield, L. H., ed. *The Letters of Benjamin Rush* (Princeton, NJ: Princeton University Press, 1951).

Butterfield, Lyman H., et al., eds. *Adams Family Correspondence*. 9 vols. (Cambridge, MA: Harvard University Press, 1963-).

Butterfield, Lyman H., Marc Friedlander, and Mary-Jo Kine, eds. *The Book of Abigail and John: Selected Letters of the Adams Family, 1762-1784* (Cambridge, MA: Harvard University Press, 1975).

Cappon, Lester J., ed. *The Adams-Jefferson Letters* (New York: Simon & Schuster, 1971).

Cohen, Ellen R., et al., eds. *The Papers of Benjamin Franklin* (New Haven, CT: Yale University Press, 1959-), vols. 36-39.

Colman, Henry. *A Sketch of the Character of John Adams: Delivered in the Church in Barton Square, Salem, 9th June, 1826, the Lord's Day, after His Interment* (Salem, MA, 1826).

Commins, Saxe, ed. *Basic Writings of George Washington* (New York: Random House, 1948).

DeWindt, Caroline, ed. *Journal and Correspondence of Miss Adams, Daughter of John Adams* (New York: Wiley & Putnam, 1841).

Fields, Joseph E., compiler. *"Worthy Partner": The Papers of Martha Washington* (Westport, CT: Greenwood, 1994).

Fitzpatrick, John C. *The Writings of George Washington from the Original Manuscript Sources, 1748-1799*. 39 vols. (Washington, DC: Government Printing Office, 1931-1944).

Ford, Paul Leicester, ed. *The Works of Thomas Jefferson* (New York: Putnam's, 1904-1905).

Franklin, Benjamin. "Afterword" to *John Tennent, Every Man His Own Doctor; or, The Poor Planter's Physician*. 4th ed. (Philadelphia: Printed and Sold by B. Franklin, 1736).

Franklin, Benjamin. *Autobiography and Other Writings*. Edited with an introduction and notes by Russell B. Nye (Boston: Houghton Mifflin, 1958).

Franklin, Benjamin. *Some Account of the Pennsylvania Hospital, from Its First Rise, to the Beginning of the Fifth Month, Called, May, 1754* (Baltimore, MD: Johns Hopkins University Press, 1954).

Franklin, Benjamin. *The Almanacs for the Years 1733-1758 by Richard Sanders* (New York: Heritage, 1964).

Franklin, Benjamin. *The Papers of Benjamin Franklin*. American Philosophical Society and Yale University. www.franklinpapers.org.

Franklin, Benjamin. *The Writings of Benjamin Franklin; Collected and Ed. with a Life and Introduction, by Albert Henry Smyth* (New York: Macmillan, 1905).

Franklin, Benjamin, and William Heberden. *Some Account of the Success of Inoculation for Small-Pox in England and America* (London: William Strahan, 1759).

Goodman, Nathan G., ed. *A Benjamin Franklin Reader* (New York: Crowell, 1945).

Hogan, Margaret A., et al., eds. *Adams Family Correspondence*, vols. 7-9 (Cambridge, MA: Harvard University Press, 1963–).

Hogan, Margaret A., and C. James Taylor, eds. *Dearest Friend: Letters of Abigail and John Adams* (Cambridge, MA: Harvard University Press, 2007).

Hunt, Gaillard, ed. *The Writings of James Madison* (New York: Putnam's, 1900-1910).

Hutchinson, William T., ed. *The Papers of James Madison* (Chicago: University of Chicago Press, 1962–).

Jackson, Donald, and Dorothy Twohig, eds. *The Diaries of George Washington* (Charlottesville: University Press of Virginia, 1976).

Jefferson, Thomas. *The Jefferson-Dunglison Letters*. Edited by John M. Dorsey (Charlottesville: University of Virginia Press, 1960).

Jefferson, Thomas. *The Writings of Thomas Jefferson, Being His Autobiography, Correspondence, Reports, Messages, Addresses, and Other Writings, Official and Private* (Washington, DC, 1854).

Kaminski, John P., ed. *The Quotable Abigail Adams* (Cambridge, MA: Harvard University Press, 2009).

Koch, Adrienne, and William Peden, ed. *The Life and Selected Writings of Thomas Jefferson* (New York: Modern Library, 1944).

Larabee, Leonard W., ed., *The Papers of Benjamin Franklin* (New Haven, CT: Yale University Press, 1959-), vols. 1-14.

Lipscomb, Andrew, and Albert E. Bergh, eds. *The Writings of Thomas Jefferson* (Washington, DC: Thomas Jefferson Memorial Foundation, 1903).

Lopez, Claude A., ed., *The Papers of Benjamin Franklin* (New Haven, CT: Yale University Press, 1959-), vol. 27.

Madison, Dolley. *Memoirs and Letters of Dolly Madison* (Port Washington, NY: Kennikat Press, 1886; reprint 1971).

Madison, James. *Writings* (New York: Library of America, 1999).

Mather, Cotton. *A Letter about the Good Management under the Distemper of Measles, etc.* (Boston, 1979).

Mattern, David B., and Holly C. Shulman, eds. *The Selected Letters of Dolley Payne Madison* (Charlottesville: University of Virginia Press, 2003).

Miller, Lillian B. ed. *The Selected Papers of Charles Wilson Peale and His Family* (New Haven, CT: Yale University Press, 1988).

Mitchell, Stewart, ed. *New Letters of Abigail Adams, 1788-1801* (New York: Houghton Mifflin, 1947).

Oberg, Barbara B., ed. *The Papers of Benjamin Franklin* (New Haven, CT: Yale University Press, 1959-), vols. 28-35.

Peterson, Merrill D., ed. *Thomas Jefferson: Writings* (New York: Library of America, 1984).

Rives, William C., and Philip R. Fendall, eds. *Letters and Other Writings of James Madison* (Philadelphia, 1865).

Rush, Benjamin. *The Autobiography of Benjamin Rush: His "Travels through Life" Together with His Commonplace Book for 1789-1813.* Edited with introduction and notes by George W. Corner (Princeton, NJ: Princeton University Press, 1948).

Ryerson, Richard Alan, et al., eds. *Adams Family Correspondence*, vols. 5-6 (Cambridge, MA: Harvard University Press, 1963–).

Smith, James Morton. *The Republic of Letters: The Correspondence between Thomas Jefferson and James Madison, 1776-1826* (New York: Norton, 1995).

Sparks, Jared, ed. *The Writings of George Washington: Being His Correspondence, Addresses, and Messages, and Other Papers, Official and Private.* Vols. 1-9 (Boston: Little, Brown, 1885).

Tennent, John. *Every Man His Own Doctor* (Philadelphia: Printed and Sold by Benjamin Franklin, 1751).

Wilcox, William B., ed. *The Papers of Benjamin Franklin* (New Haven, CT: Yale University Press, 1959-), vols. 15-26.

Secondary Sources: Books

Arnett, Ethel Stephens. *Mrs. James Madison: The Incomparable Dolley* (Greensboro, NC: Piedmont Press, 1972).

Bayne-Jones, Stanhope. *The Evolution of Preventive Medicine in the United States Army, 1607-1939* (Washington, DC: Office of the Surgeon General, 1968).

Bedini, Silvio A. *Thomas Jefferson: Statesman of Science* (New York: Macmillan, 1990).

Bell, Whitfield J. Jr. *The Colonial Physician* (New York: Science History Publications, 1975).

Berkin, Carol. *Revolutionary Mothers: Women in the Struggle for America's Independence* (New York: Knopf, 2005).

Blanton, Wyndham Bolling. *Medicine in Virginia in the Eighteenth Century* (Richmond, VA: Garrett and Massey, 1931).

Bower, Catherine Drinker. *John Adams and the American Revolution* (New York: Grosset & Dunlap, 1950).

Brady, Patricia. *Martha Washington: An American Life* (New York: Viking, 2005).

Brands, H. W. *The First American* (New York: Doubleday, 2000).

Brant, Irving. *The Fourth President: The Life of James Madison* (New York: Bobbs Merrill, 1970).

Brieger, Gert H., ed. *Medical America in the Nineteenth Century: Reading from the Literature* (Baltimore, MD: Johns Hopkins University Press, 1972).

Brodie, Fawn. *Thomas Jefferson: An Intimate History* (New York: Norton, 1974).

Brookhiser, Richard. *James Madison* (New York: Basic Books, 1998).

Bumgarner, John R. *The Health of the Presidents: The 41 United States Presidents through 1993* (Jefferson, NC: MacFarland, 1994).

Burstein, Andrew. *Jefferson's Secrets: Death and Desire at Monticello* (New York: Basic Books, 2005).

Bynum, W. F., and Roy Porter, eds. *Medical Fringe and Medical Orthodoxy, 1750-1850* (London: Croom Helm, 1987).

Campbell, James. *Recovering Benjamin Franklin: An Exploration of a Life of Science and Service* (Chicago: Open Court, 1999).

Cassedy, James H. *Medicine in America: A Short History* (Baltimore, MD: Johns Hopkins University Press, 1991).

Chaplin, Joyce E. *The First Scientific American: Benjamin Franklin and the Pursuit of Genius* (New York: Basic Books, 2006).

Chernow, Ron. *Washington: A Life* (New York: Penguin, 2010).

Clagett, Martin. *Scientific Jefferson Revealed* (Charlottesville: University of Virginia Press, 2009).

Cohen, I. Bernard. *Science and the Founding Fathers* (New York: Norton, 1995.)

Crawford, Alan Pell. *Twilight at Monticello: The Final Years of Thomas Jefferson* (New York: Random House, 2008).

Decatur, Stephen. *Private Affairs of President Washington* (Boston: Houghton Mifflin, 1933).

Deppisch, Ludwig M. *The White House Physician: A History from Washington to George W. Bush* (Jefferson, NC: McFarland, 2007).

Duffy, John. *Epidemics in Colonial America* (Baton Rouge: Louisiana State University Press, 1953).

Duffy, John. *The Healers: A History of American Medicine* (Urbana: University of Illinois Press, 1976).

Duffy, John. *The Sanitarians: A History of American Public Health* (Urbana: University of Illinois Press, 1990).

Duran-Reynals, Mary Louise de Ayala. *The Fever Bark Tree: The Pageant of Quinine* (New York: Doubleday, 1946).

Ellis, Joseph J. *American Sphinx: The Character of Thomas Jefferson* (New York: Knopf, 1997).

Ellis, Joseph J. *First Family: Abigail and John* (New York: Knopf, 2010).

Ellis, Joseph J. *His Excellency George Washington* (New York: Knopf, 2004).

Estes, J. Worth, and Billy G. Smith, eds., *A Melancholy Scene of Devastation: The Public Response to the 1793 Philadelphia Yellow Fever Epidemic* (Canton, MA: Science History Publications, 1997).

Fenn, Elizabeth. *Pox Americana: The Great Smallpox Epidemic of 1775-82* (New York: Hill and Wang, 2001).

Ferling, John. *The Ascent of George Washington: The Hidden Political Genius of an American Icon* (New York: Bloomsbury, 2009).

Finger, Stanley. *Doctor Franklin's Medicine* (Philadelphia: University of Pennsylvania Press, 2006).

Flexner, James Thomas. *Washington: The Indispensable Man* (Boston: Little, Brown, 1974).

Gay, Peter. *The Enlightenment: An Interpretation.* Vol. 2, *The Science of Freedom* (New York: Knopf, 1969).

Gelles, Edith B. *Abigail and John: Portrait of a Marriage* (New York: Morrow, 2009).

Gevitz, Norman, ed. *Other Healers: Unorthodox Medicine in America* (Baltimore, MD: Johns Hopkins University Press, 1988).

Gillett, Mary G. *The Army Medical Department: 1775-1818* (Washington, DC: Center of Military History, 1981).

Gordon-Reed, Annette. *The Hemingses of Monticello: An American Family* (New York: Norton, 2008).

Gordon-Reed, Annette. *Thomas Jefferson and Sally Hemings: An American Controversy* (Charlottesville: University of Virginia Press, 1997).

Graff, Henry F. *The President: A Reference History* (New York: Scribners/Gale, 2002).

Gunderson, Joan. *To Be Useful to the World: Women in Revolutionary America, 1740-1790* (New York: Twayne, 1996).

Haines, Michael R., and Richard H. Steckel. *A Population History of North America* (New York: Cambridge University Press, 2000).

Halsey, Robert Hurtin. *How the President, Thomas Jefferson, and Doctor Benjamin Waterhouse Established Vaccination as a Public Health Procedure* (New York: privately printed, 1936).

Hawke, David Freeman. *Benjamin Rush: Revolutionary Gadfly* (Indianapolis: Bobbs-Merrill, 1971).

Holmes, John M. *Thomas Jefferson Treats Himself: Herbs, Physic, and Nutrition in Early America* (Fort Valley, VA: Loft Press, 1997).

Holton, Woody. *Abigail Adams* (New York: Free Press, 2009).

Hopkins, Donald R. *Princes and Peasants: Smallpox in Chicago* (Chicago: University of Chicago Press, 1983).

Horrocks, Thomas A. *Popular Print and Popular Medicine: Almanacs and Health Advice in Early America* (Amherst: University of Massachusetts Press, 2008).

Humphreys, Margaret. *Yellow Fever and the South* (New Brunswick, NJ: Rutgers University Press, 1992).

Isaacson, Walter. *Benjamin Franklin: An American Life* (New York: Simon & Schuster, 2003).

Ketcham, Ralph. *James Madison: A Biography* (Charlottesville: University Press of Virginia, 1990).

Ketcham, Ralph. *The Madisons of Montpelier* (Charlottesville: University of Virginia Press, 2009).

Klein, Herbert S. *A Population History of the United States* (New York: Cambridge University Press, 2004).

Langhorne, Elizabeth Coles. *Monticello: A Family Story* (Chapel Hill, NC: Algonquin Books, 1987).

Leavitt, Judith Walzer. *Brought to Bed: Childbearing in America, 1750 to 1950* (New York: Oxford University Press, 1986).

Leavitt, Judith Walzer, and Ronald L. Numbers. *Sickness and Health in America: Readings in the History of Medicine and Public Health* (Madison: University of Wisconsin Press, 1978).

Ledgin, Norm. *Diagnosing Jefferson: Evidence of a Condition That Guided His Beliefs, Behavior, and Personal Associations* (Arlington, TX: Future Horizons, 2000).

Lemay, J. A. Leo. *The Life of Benjamin Franklin: Soldier, Scientist, and Politician, 1748-1757* (Philadelphia: University of Pennsylvania Press, 2009).

Lopez, Claude-Anne. *Mon Cher Papa* (New Haven, CT: Yale University Press, 1990).

Lossing, Benson John. *Martha Washington* (New York: 1861).

Lynch, Jack, ed. *Critical Insights: Benjamin Franklin* (Pasadena, CA: Salem Press, 2010).

Maehle, Andreas-Holger. *Drugs on Trial: Experimental Pharmacology and Therapeutic Innovation in the Eighteenth Century* (Atlanta: Rodopi-B.V., 1999).

Makary, Marty. *Unaccountable: What Hospitals Won't Tell You and How Transparency Can Revolutionize Health Care* (New York: Bloomsbury Press, 2012).

Malone, Dumas. *Jefferson the President* (Boston: Little, Brown, 1970).

Martin, Edwin T. *Thomas Jefferson: Scientist* (New York: Henry Schuman, 1952).

Marx, Rudolph. *The Health of the Presidents* (New York: Putnam's, 1960).

Mayo, Bernard, ed. *Thomas Jefferson and His Unknown Brother* (Charlottesville: University of Virginia Press, 1981).

McCoy, Drew R. *The Last of the Fathers: James Madison and the Republican Legacy* (New York: Cambridge University Press, 1989).

McCullough, David G. *John Adams* (New York: Simon & Schuster, 2001).

McKeown, Thomas. *The Modern Rise of Population* (London: Edward Arnold, 1976).

McKeown, Thomas. *The Role of Medicine: Dream, Mirage, or Nemesis?* (Princeton, NJ: Princeton University Press, 1979).

Moss, Kay K. *Southern Folk Medicine, 1750-1820* (Columbia: University of South Carolina Press, 1999).

Mullan, Fitzhugh. *Plagues and Politics: The Story of the United States Public Health Service* (New York: Basic Books, 1989).

Murphy, Lamar Riley. *Enter the Physician: The Transformation of Domestic Medicine 1760-1860* (Tuscaloosa: University of Alabama Press, 1991).

Nagel, Paul C. *The Adams Women: Abigail and Louisa Adams, Their Sisters and Daughters* (New York: Oxford University Press, 1987).

Pepper, William. *The Medical Side of Benjamin Franklin* (New York: Argosy-Antiquarian, 1910; reprint 1970).

Porter, Dorothy, and Roy Porter. *Patient's Progress: Doctors and Doctoring in Eighteenth-Century England* (Stanford, CA: Stanford University Press, 1989).

Powell, John Harvey. *Bring Out Your Dead: The Great Plague of Yellow Fever in Philadelphia in 1793* (1949; reprint New York: Arno Press, 1970).

Randall, Henry S. *The Life of Thomas Jefferson* (New York: 1858).

Randolph, Sarah N. *The Domestic Life of Thomas Jefferson: Compiled from Family Letters and Reminiscences by His Great-Granddaughter* (New York: Ungar, 1878; reprint 1958).

Reiss, Oscar. *Medicine and the American Revolution: How Diseases and Their Treatments Affected the Colonial Army* (Jefferson, NC: MacFarland, 1998).

Reiss, Oscar. *Medicine in Colonial America* (Lanham, MD: University Press of America, 2000).

Riley, James C. *The Eighteenth-Century Campaign to Avoid Disease* (New York: St. Martin's Press, 1987).

Roberts, Cokie. *Founding Mothers: The Women Who Raised Our Nation* (New York: William Morrow, 2004).

Roberts, Cokie. *Ladies of Liberty* (New York: William Morrow, 2008).

Rocco, Fiammetta. *The Miraculous Fever-Tree: Malaria and the Quest for a Cure That Changed the World* (New York: HarperCollins, 2003).

Rorabaugh, W. J. *The Alcoholic Republic* (New York: Oxford University Press, 1979).

Rosen, George. *From Medical Police to Social Medicine: Essays on the History of Health Care* (New York: Science History Publications, 1974).

Rosenberg, Charles E. *Explaining Epidemics and Other Studies in the History of Medicine* (New York: Cambridge University Press, 1992).

Rosenberg, Charles E. *Our Present Complaint: American Medicine, Then and Now* (Baltimore, MD: Johns Hopkins University Press, 2007).

Rosenberg, Charles E. *The Cholera Years* (Chicago: University of Chicago Press, 1987).

Rothstein, William G. *American Physicians in the Nineteenth Century* (Baltimore, MD: Johns Hopkins University Press, 1972).

Savitt, Todd L. *Medicine and Slavery: The Diseases and Health Care of Blacks in Antebellum Virginia* (Urbana: University of Illinois Press, 1978).

Savitt, Todd L., and James Harvey Young, eds. *Disease and Distinctiveness in the American South* (Knoxville: University of Tennessee Press, 1988).

Shah, Sonia. *The Fever: How Malaria Has Ruled Humankind for 500,000 Years* (New York: Farrar, Straus, Giroux, 2010).

Shapiro, Arthur K., and Elaine Shapiro. *The Powerful Placebo: From Ancient Priest to Modern Physician* (Baltimore, MD: Johns Hopkins University Press, 1997).

Shorter, Edward. *Bedside Manners: The Troubled History of Doctors and Patients* (New York: Simon & Schuster, 1985).

Shryock, Richard H. *Medicine and Society in America, 1660-1860* (New York: New York University Press, 1960).

Smith, Page. *Jefferson: A Revealing Biography* (New York: McGraw-Hill, 1976).

Smith, Patricia Brady. *Nelly Custis Lewis's Housekeeping Book* (New Orleans: Historic New Orleans Collection, 1982).

Starr, Paul. *The Social Transformation of American Medicine* (New York: Basic Books, 1982).

Steele, Volney. *Bleed, Blister, and Purge* (Missoula, MT: Mountain Press, 2005).

Talbot, Page, ed. *Benjamin Franklin: In Search of a Better World* (New Haven, CT: Yale University Press, 2005).

Tannenbaum, Rebecca J. *The Healer's Calling: Women and Medicine in Early New England* (Ithaca, NY: Cornell University Press, 2002).

Tinterow, Maurice M. *Foundations of Hypnotism* (Springfield, IL: Charles C. Thomas, 1970).

Turner, Robert F., ed. *The Jefferson-Hemings Controversy: Report of the Scholars Commission* (Durham, NC: Carolina Academic Press, 2011).

Ulrich, Laurel Thatcher. *A Midwife's Tale: The Life of Martha Ballard; Based on Her Diary, 1785-1812* (New York: Knopf, 1990).

Ulrich, Laurel Thatcher. *Good Wives: Image and Reality in the Lives of Women in Northern New England, 1650-1970* (New York: Knopf, 1982).

Unger, Harlow Giles. *The Unexpected George Washington* (New York: Wiley, 2006).

Valencius, Conevery Bolton. *The Health of the Country: How American Settlers Understood Themselves and Their Land* (New York: Basic Books, 2002).

Vogel, Morris J., and Charles E. Rosenberg. *The Therapeutic Revolution: Essays in the Social History of American Medicine* (Philadelphia: University of Pennsylvania Press, 1979).

Whorton, James. C. *Nature Cures: The History of Alternative Medicine in America* (New York: Oxford University Press, 2002).

Wilbur, Keith C. *Revolutionary Medicine: 1700-1800* (Philadelphia: Chelsea House, 1980).

Willrich, Michael. *Pox: An American History* (New York: Penguin, 2011).

Wills, Garry. *James Madison* (New York: Henry Holt, 2002).

Winslow, Ola Elizabeth. *A Destroying Angel: The Conquest of Smallpox in Colonial Boston* (Boston: Houghton Mifflin, 1974).

Wood, Peter H. *Black Majority: Negroes in Colonial South Carolina* (New York: Knopf, 1974).

Woods, Gordon S. *The Americanization of Benjamin Franklin* (New York: Penguin, 2004).

Wooton, David. *Bad Medicine: Doctor Doing Harms since Hippocrates* (Oxford: Oxford University Press, 2006).

Secondary Sources: Articles

Abrams, Jeanne. "On the Road Again: Consumptives Traveling for Health in the American West, 1840-1925." *Great Plains Quarterly* 30 (Fall 2010): 271-85.

Adair, Douglass. "That Politics May Be Reduced to a Science." *Huntington Library Quarterly* 20 (August 1957): 343-60.

Barrett, John T. "The Inoculation Controversy in Puritan New England." *Bulletin of the History of Medicine* 12 (1942): 169-88.

Bell, Whitfield Jr. "Medicine in Boston and Philadelphia: Comparisons and Contrasts, 1750-1820," in *Medicine in Massachusetts, 1620 -1820* (Boston: Colonial Society of Massachusetts, 1980), 159-83.

Blanton, Wyndham B. "Washington's Medical Knowledge and Its Sources." *Annals of Medical History* 5 (1933): 52-61.

Caulfield, Ernest. "Early Measles Epidemics in America." *Yale Journal of Biology and Medicine* 15 (1942): 531-56.

Cheatham, Michael L. "The Death of George Washington: An End to the Controversy?" *American Surgeon* 74 (August 2008): 770-74.

Curfman, David R. "The Medical History of the Father of Our Country: General George Washington." The Order of Founders and Patriots of America. www.founderspatriots.org/articles/gw_medical_history.htm.

Estes, J. Worth. "George Washington and the Doctors." *Medical Heritage* 1 (January–February 1985): 44-57.

Ferling, John, and Lewis E. Braverman. "John Adams's Health Reconsidered." *William and Mary Quarterly* 55 (January 1998): 83-104.

Finger, Stanley, and Ian S. Hegeman. "Benjamin Franklin's Risk Factors for Gout and Stones: From Genes and Diet to Possible Lead Poisoning." *Proceedings of the American Philosophical Society* 152 (June 2008): 189-207.

Gensel, Lisa. "The Medical World of Benjamin Franklin." *Journal of the Royal Society of Medicine* 98 (December 2005): 534-38.

Hall, Courtney R. "Jefferson on the Medical Theory and Practice of the Day." *Bulletin of the History of Medicine* 31 (1957): 235-45.

Haller, John S. Jr. "Decline of Bloodletting: A Study in 19th-Century Ratiocinations." *Southern Medical Journal* 79 (April 1986): 469-75.

Hirschmann, J. V. "Benjamin Franklin and Medicine." *Annals of Internal Medicine,* December 6, 2005, 830-34.

Hunter, R. J. "Benjamin Franklin and the Rise of Free Treatment of the Poor by the Medical Profession of Philadelphia." *Bulletin of the History of Medicine* 30 (1957): 137-46.

Huth, Edward J. "Benjamin Franklin's Place in the History of Medicine." The James Lind Library. www.jameslindlibrary.org.

Jensen, John. "Before the Surgeon General: Marine Hospital in Mid-19th-Century America." *Public Health Reports* 112 (November/December 1997): 525-27.

Kopperman, Paul. E. "'Venerate the Lancet': Benjamin Rush's Yellow Fever Therapy in Context." *Bulletin of the History of Medicine* 78 (Fall 2004): 539-74.

Leavitt, Judith Walzer. "Science Enters the Birthing Room: Obstetrics in American since the Eighteenth Century." *Journal of American History* 70 (September 1983): 281-304.

Martin, Henry A. "Jefferson as a Vaccinator." *North Carolina Medical Journal,* January 1881, 32.

Mayo Clinic Staff. "The Medical History of George Washington (1732-1799)." *Proceedings of the Mayo Clinic,* February 11 and February 18, 1942, 92-96, 107-12, 116-21.

Merrens, H. Roy, and George D. Terry, "Dying in Paradise: Malaria, Mortality, and the Perceptual Environment in Colonial South Carolina." *Journal of Southern History* 50 (November 1984): 533-50.

Pernick, Martin S. "Politics, Parties, and Pestilence: Epidemic Yellow Fever in Philadelphia and the Rise of the First Party System." *William and Mary Quarterly* 29.4 (October 1972): 559-86.

Radbill, Samuel X. "Thomas Jefferson and the Doctors." *Transactions & Studies of the College of Physicians of Philadelphia* 37 (1969-1970): 106-14.

Ramsay, David. "A Review of the Improvement, Progress, and State of Medicine in the Eighteenth Century." Delivered January 1, 1800. *Transactions of the American Philosophical Society* 55 (1965): 96-217.

Ravenel, Mazyck. "Our Public Health Service." *American Journal of Public Health* 29 (September 1939): 1044-46.

Reed, Meribeth Meixner. "Describing the Life Cycle of U.S. Marine Hospital #17, Port Townsend, Washington, 1855-1933." *Military Medicine* 150 (April 2005): 259-66.

Riccards, Michael P. "The Presidency: In Sickness and in Health." *Presidential Studies Quarterly* 7 (December 1977): 215-31.

Rosen, George. "Political Order and Human Health in Jeffersonian Thought." *Bulletin of the History of Medicine* 26 (1952): 32-44.

Rusnock, Andrea. "Catching Cowpox: The Early Spread of Smallpox Vaccination." *Bulletin of the History of Medicine* 83 (2009): 17-36.

Ruttman, Darrett B., and Anita H. Ruttman. "Of Agues and Fevers: Malaria in the Early Chesapeake." *William and Mary Quarterly* 33 (January 1976): 31-60.

Schneeberg, Norman G. "The Medical History of Thomas Jefferson." *Journal of Medical Biography* 16 (2008): 118-25.

Steckel, Richard. "Nutritional Status in the Colonial American Economy." *William and Mary Quarterly* 56 (January 1999): 31-52.

Sullivan, Robert B. "Sanguine Practices: A Historical and Historiographic Reconsideration of Heroic Therapy in the Age of Rush." *Bulletin of the History of Medicine* 68 (Summer 1994): 211-34.

Tannenbaum, Rebecca J. "Mary Hale and Ann Edmonds: Gender, Women's Work, and Health in Colonial Massachusetts," in Eric Arnesen, ed., *The Human Tradition in American Labor History* (Wilmington, DE: Scholarly Resources, 2004), 1-14.

Tannenbaum, Rebecca J. "'What Is Best to Be Done for These Fevers': Elizabeth Davenport's Medical Practice in New Haven Colony." *New England Quarterly* 70 (June 1997): 265-84.

Thorup, Oscar A. "Jefferson's Admonition." *Mayo Clinic Proceedings* 47 (May 1971): 199-201.

Wang, Shirley S. "Why Placebos Work Wonders." *Wall Street Journal,* January 3, 2012, D1-D2.

Watson, Patricia A. "The 'Hidden Ones': Women and Healing in Colonial New England," in *Medicine and Healing,* Dublin Seminar for New England Folklore (Boston: Boston University, 1992).

Will, Drake W. "The Medical and Surgical Practice of the Lewis and Clark Expedition." *Journal of the History of Medicine and Applied Sciences* 14 (July 1959): 273-97.

Wood, Gordon S. "The Pursuit of Happiness." *New Republic Online,* April 8, 2004.

INDEX

Academy of Natural Sciences (Philadelphia), 98

Act for the Relief of Sick and Disabled Seamen (1798), 155–156

acupuncture, 234

Adams, Abigail, 119–168; Alien and Sedition Acts, 159; Bark (quinine from cinchona tree bark), 139; Battle of Bunker Hill (1775), 127; birth, 119; bloodletting, 16, 147–148, 152; childbirths, 130; common good, devotion to, 128; death, 167; Declaration of Independence, 137; *Domestic Medicine* (Buchan), 20, 148; in England, 145; exercise, 145–147; as family healer, 132–141; as first lady, 159–160; in France, 145, 146; general welfare, government's role in promoting, 137; on health, 1, 157–158, 160; health, concerns with, 1, 3–4, 119, 122, 127, 134–135, 144, 162–163; herbal remedies, 18, 133; homeschooling, 120; intellectual capabilities, 129; landownings, 160–161; laudanum (an opiate), 19; letters/correspondence, 128; in London, 146; marriage, 120, 122; medical guides, access to, 19; medical treatment, approach to, 7, 135; ocean voyages, 141, 144–145, 149; personality, 162; in Philadelphia, 151–152, 154–155; political interests, 126; portrait of, *160*; post-presidential years, 160–166; predeceased children, 4, 126, 129, 139–141, 158, 165; preventative health, notion of, 153; purging (laxatives), 148; religious faith, 140–141, 149, 165; Richmond Hill house, 150; smallpox immunization, 1–2, 31, 136, 137, 138–139; stoicism, 140; Stonyfield (or Peacefield), 149, 161; tuberculosis, understanding of, 150–151; in Washington, D.C., 159
—illnesses/conditions: ague, 152, 161; arthritis, 151, 152, 166; bacterial ailment, 133; colds, 134; diabetes, 156; dysentery, 156; eye problems, 162; headaches, 119; insomnia, 119, 156, 162; jaundice, 134; malaria, 156; obesity, 146; rheumatic fever, 119; rheumatism, 18, 134, 145, 151, 152–153, 162, 166; St.

Anthony's erysipelas (skin condition), 162; seasickness, 145; skin rashes, 162; stomach ailments, 146, 155; stroke, 166–167; toothaches, 152; whooping cough, 129
—personal relations: Adams, Abigail (Nabby) (daughter), 145, 152, 153, 156–157, 167, 187; Adams, John (husband), 44, 56, 107–108, 119–122, 126 –128, 132, 135–140, 144, 158, 159, 166; Adams, John Quincy (son), 146, 147; Adams, Louisa Catherine Johnson (daughter-in-law), 163; Adams, Susanna (mother-in-law), 125, 154; Adams, Thomas Boylston (son), 1, 149, 153, 160; Brisler, Mrs. (housekeeper), 152; Cranch, Mary (sister), 108, 130, 145, 146, 150, 151, 164, 167, 186; Cranch, Richard (brother-in-law), 164, 167; Franklin, Benjamin, 99, 108; George (footman), 150; Jefferson, Maria (Polly) (Jefferson's daughter), 187, 188; Jefferson, Thomas, 140, 145, 146–147, 165, 186, 188, 189, 190, 209, 215, 216; Johnson, Catherine, 160; Patsy (maidservant), 133; Peabody, Elizabeth Smith Shaw (sister), 133, 150; Rush, Dr. Benjamin, 128, 152; Shaw, Elizabeth (later Elizabeth Shaw Peabody), 145–146; Shaw, William (nephew), 157–158; Smith, Caroline (granddaughter), 166; Smith, Elizabeth Quincy (mother), 130, 133–134; Smith, Elizabeth (Betsy) (sister), 162; Smith, Isaac (uncle), 136; Tufts, Dr. Cotton, 119–120, 148; Warren, Mercy Otis, 162, 166; Washington, George, 66–67, 77, 151; Waterhouse, Dr. Benjamin, 148, 166

Adams, Abigail (Nabby) (John & Abigail's daughter): birth, 129; children, 149; death, 164–166; financial straits, 154–155, 158; in London, 146; marriage, 146; ocean voyage, 145; predeceased children, 149; smallpox immunization, 137; swimming, 146
—illnesses/conditions: breast cancer, 25, 163–164; mumps, 135; smallpox, 137; whooping cough, 129
—personal relations: Adams, Abigail, 145, 152, 153, 156–157, 167, 187; Adams, John, 165; Rush, Dr. Benjamin, 25, 164

ideas, 89–90; medicine, interest in/knowledge of, 7, 27, 81–82, 83, 88–89, 90, 100–101, 106, 111; medicine, scientific approach to, 81; medicine, skepticism about contemporary, 101, 109; microscopes, 91; moderation, commitment to, 109; *New England Courant* (newspaper), 83, 85; Pennsylvania Assembly, 81, 102–103; *Pennsylvania Gazette* (newspaper), 84, 85, 91, 116; Pennsylvania Hospital, 80–81; personality, 100, 107; Philadelphia Hospital, 87–88; physician friends, 50; "placebo effect," notion of, 95–96; *Poor Richard's Almanac*, 27, 84, 91, 93–94; portrait, *80*; postal system, 98; predeceased children, 85; preventative health, notion of, 93, 94–98, 111, 115; printing industry, 82–84, 86, 92, 112; public health care, 5–6, 7, 231; religiosity, good works in, 79–80; sanitation reform, interest in, 100; scientific interests, 81–82; smallpox immunization, 2, 28, 31, 84–86, 91, 93, 136, 232; *Some Account of the Pennsylvania Hospital*, 87–88; sponge bathing, 89; Stamp Act (1765), 89, 98; swimming, 83–84, 93, 95, 98; tracheotomy, 76; *Tract on Yellow Fever* (Mitchel), 90–91; Treaty of Paris (1783), 99, 109; University of Pennsylvania, 81; urbanization, 195; utopianism, 235; vegetarianism, 95; war updates sent to, 57; wine, 111
—illnesses/conditions: ague, 93; bladder stones, 106, 107–108, 108–109, 184; on cancer, 90; colds, 89, 93, 103; depression, 95, 96; dizziness, 104–105; epilepsy, 95; gout, 93, 95, 100, 103, 104–105, 106–108, 113–114, 115, 184; influenza, 89, 94; insomnia, 104; kidney stones, 88, 93, 109, 113; lead poisoning, 112, 118; on malaria, 93; melancholy, 96; mental health, 92; palsy/tremors, 95; pleurisy, 15, 84, 92, 116; pneumonia, 84; psoriasis, 99–100, 103, 106, 113; rheumatism, 94; scurvy, 89; skin rashes, 99; smallpox, 94; stomach ailments, 93, 112; throat infection, 105; tobacco use, disapproval of, 112; on typhus (Goal Fever), 91–92
—personal relations: Adams, Abigail, 99, 108; Adams, John, 94, 99, 107–108, 116, 141, 143, 236; Barbeu-Dubourg, Dr., 94–95; Bard, Dr. John, 64; Belcher, Jonathan, 95; Bond, Dr. Thomas, 87, 101; Brillion, Madame, 106; Cabanis,

Pierre-Jean-Georges, 101, 109; Colden, Dr. Cadwallader, 82, 90–91; Denham (Philadelphia merchant), 83–84; Diderot, Denis, 101; Evans, Dr. Cadwallader, 87; Fothergill, Dr. John, 100, 103; Franklin, Abiah Folger (mother), 81, 88; Franklin, Deborah (Debby) Read (wife), 85, 88, 99, 104–106; Franklin, James (brother), 82–83; Franklin, John (brother), 96–97; Franklin, Josiah (father), 82; Franklin, Sally (Sarah) (daughter), 86; Franklin, William (son), 79, 98; Franklin, William Temple (grandson), 109; Heberden, Dr. William, 86; Hewson, Mary Stevenson, 108; Hume, David, 101; Ingenhousz, Dr. Jan, 96; Jackson, Richard, 89; Jay, John, 108; Jefferson, Thomas, 109, 115, 170, 173, 184–185, 190; Johnson, Samuel, 93, 94; Jones, Dr. John, 66; Keimer, Samuel, 83, 84; Keith, William, 83; Louis XVI, King of France, 186; Mecom, Jane Franklin (Benjamin Franklin's sister), 97, 100; Mesmer, Dr. Franz Anton, 101–102, 104, 185; Morgan, Dr. John, 58, 101; Pringle, Dr. John, 91, 100, 112; Rush, Dr. Benjamin, 15, 22, 25, 86, 89, 91, 94, 101, 111–112, 116; Shipley, Jonathan, 112–113; Shippen, Dr. William, 101; Small, Dr. Alexander, 106–107; Temple, John, 107; Vergennes, Comte de, 108; Vicq d'Azyr, Dr. Félix, 100–101; Voltaire, 117; Washington, George, 34, 65, 93, 113, 114; Wistar, Dr. Caspar, 101
Franklin, Deborah (Debby) Read (Benjamin's wife), 85, 88, 99, 104–106
Franklin, Frances (Franky) Folger (Benjamin's son), 85–86
Franklin, James (Benjamin's brother), 82–83
Franklin, Jane (Benjamin's sister), 97
Franklin, John (Benjamin's brother), 96–97
Franklin, Josiah (Benjamin's father), 82, 88
Franklin, Mary (Benjamin's sister), 90, 97
Franklin, Sally (Sarah) (Benjamin's daughter), 85, 86
Franklin, William (Benjamin's son), 79, 85, 98, 109
Franklin, William Temple (William's son), 109
Franklin stove, 110
fresh air: Adams, John, 94, 137, 236; Franklin, Benjamin, 94–95, 116, 236; Jefferson, Thomas, 185; Rush, Dr. Benjamin, 116

ABOUT THE AUTHOR

Jeanne E. Abrams is Professor at Penrose Library and the Center for Judaic Studies at the University of Denver. She received her Ph.D. in American history from the University of Colorado at Boulder with a specialization in archival management. She is the author of *Jewish Women Pioneering the Frontier Trail: A History in the American West* (New York University Press) and *Dr. Charles David Spivak: A Jewish Immigrant and the American Tuberculosis Movement* (University Press of Colorado), as well as numerous articles in the fields of American, Jewish, and medical history that have appeared in scholarly journals and popular magazines.